CLINICS IN DEVELOPMENTAL MEDICINE NO. 120

THE NEUROPHYSIOLOGICAL EXAMINATION OF THE NEWBORN INFANT

Clinics in Developmental Medicine No. 120

THE NEUROPHYSIOLOGICAL EXAMINATION OF THE NEWBORN INFANT

Edited by
J.A. EYRE

1992
Mac Keith Press

Distributed by:
OXFORD: Blackwell Scientific Publications Ltd
NEW YORK: Cambridge University Press

5a Netherhall Gardens, London NW3 5RN

First published 1992

British Library Cataloguing in Publication Data

The neurophysiological examination of the newborn infant.—
(Clinics in developmental medicine; 120)
I. Eyre, J. A. II. Series
618.928

ISBN (UK) 0 901260 89 4
(USA) 0 521 41276 5

Printed in Great Britain at The Lavenham Press Ltd, Lavenham, Suffolk
Mac Keith Press is supported by **The Spastics Society, London, England**

CONTENTS

CONTRIBUTORS

J. CONNELL	Consultant Paediatrician, Wexham Park Hospital, Slough, Berkshire.
R.W.I. COOKE	Professor of Paediatric Medicine, Institute of Child Health, Royal Liverpool Children's Hospital, Alder Hey, Liverpool.
L. DUBOWITZ	Research Lecturer, Department of Paediatrics and Neonatal Medicine, Hammersmith Hospital, London.
V. DUBOWITZ	Professor of Paediatrics, Department of Paediatrics and Neonatal Medicine, Hammersmith Hospital, London.
BERNARD DURON	Professor, Laboratoire de Neurophysiologie, Faculté de Médicine, Université de Picardie à Amiens, France.
J.A. EYRE	Professor of Paediatric Neuroscience, Department of Paediatrics, University of Newcastle upon Tyne.
PHYLLIS M. GOOTMAN	Professor of Physiology and Neural and Behavioral Science, State University of New York Health Center at Brooklyn, New York.
NORMAN GOOTMAN	Professor of Pediatrics, State University of New York Health Center at Brooklyn, New York.
G.F.A. HARDING	Professor of Clinical Neurophysiology, Aston University, Birmingham.
JOSETTE KHATER-BOIDIN	Laboratoire de Neurophysiologie, Faculté de Médicine, Université de Picardie à Amiens, France.
C.R. KENNEDY	Consultant Paediatric Neurologist, Child Health Department, Southampton General Hospital.
S. MILLER	Professor of Anatomy, Division of Clinical Neurosciences, University of Newcastle upon Tyne.

D. MURDOCH EATON	Research Fellow, Department of Paediatrics and Neonatal Medicine, Hammersmith Hospital, London.
OSMUND REYNOLDS	Professor of Neonatal Paediatrics, University College and Middlesex School of Medicine, London.
MARGOT J. TAYLOR	Department of Paediatrics, Division of Neurology, The Hospital for Sick Children, Toronto.
KAZUYOSHI WATANABE	Professor of Pediatrics, Department of Pediatrics, Nagoya University School of Medicine, Japan.
ANDREW R. WILKINSON	Reader and Honorary Consultant, Department of Paediatrics, University of Oxford.

FOREWORD

Investigating the nervous system of the newborn infant, especially if very small and ill, is a formidable problem. Yet it is one that is attracting a large and increasing amount of attention. This is partly because learning how the nervous system develops is exciting in its own right. Those who care for ill babies also need information, preferably obtained by noninvasive techniques, about the structure and function of the brains of the babies they treat. The availability of these techniques enables questions to be addressed about the prevalence and mechanisms of brain injury, the effects of preventive strategies and treatment, and about the prognostic significance of abnormalities.

For this book Professor Janet Eyre has brought together an international group of distinguished contributors, all of whom have advanced our understanding of the neurophysiology of the newborn infant. She sets the scene with an account of the development of the nervous system, and the chapters that follow provide an up-to-date account of the relevant electrophysiological disciplines, ranging from established ones such as electroencephalography to those that are new and promising (for example the assessment of motor pathways by electromagnetic stimulation of the motor cortex). Normal aspects of development are emphasised, so that clear definitions of abnormality—difficult to find in this field—can be established. One chapter deals with the assessment of the autonomic nervous system, and another with the difficult issue of brain death.

The contribution in recent years of noninvasive techniques (including electrophysiological ones) to our understanding of the brain in newborn infants has been very great. The new developments in the field are exciting. The following chapters give a comprehensive account of what has so far been achieved.

OSMUND REYNOLDS
November 1991

1
THE DEVELOPMENT OF THE NERVOUS SYSTEM

J.A. Eyre

Central to the interpretation of neonatal neurophysiological assessments is an understanding of the processes underlying neuronal development and the ontogenesis of the nervous system. The purpose of this review, therefore, is to provide a foundation for the chapters that follow by reviewing the development of the human brain. First, it deals with the most important concepts and themes in the ontogenesis of the brain which are relevant to an interpretation of the neurophysiological investigations in the newborn infant. A more detailed review of human cortical development is then given to illustrate the processes occurring in all areas of the developing nervous system, which may differ only in magnitude or timing.

Development of the nervous system

This involves a number of fundamental processes which can vary in prominence in different areas: cell proliferation, cell migration, progressive cell growth and differentiation, and cell degeneration and death. These processes are not necessarily sequential but occur at the same time within and between different regions (Altman and Bayer 1988).

The cells of the nervous system arise from the neural plate, a thickening of embryonic ectodermal tissue. As the neural plate grows, its margins become raised to form the neural folds and a longitudinal neural groove develops between them. As the neural groove deepens, the neural folds come into contact and fuse to convert the groove into a slit-like canal and the neural plate into the neural tube.

Fusion of the neural folds occurs first in the hindbrain or upper cervical region, towards the end of the third week of gestation, and extends both rostrally and caudally until the process of fusion is completed at the end of the fourth week.*

The neural plate and early neural tube initially comprise a single layer of epithelial stem cells, the neuroepithelium. The cells which lie in the line of fusion of the dorsal edges of the neural plate constitute the neural crest. The primary neuroepithelium gives rise to all cell types in the central nervous system (CNS) except the microglia. This includes neurons which are wholly confined to the CNS

* In this chapter, and in the rest of the book, *gestational age* refers to the length of time from the mother's last menstrual period and before birth; while *post-conceptional age* refers to the gestational age plus postnatal age.

and also those somatic motor and preganglionic efferent neurons with somata within the CNS and axons which pass into the peripheral nervous system. The neural crest cells first form a strip of tissue flanking the neural tube and subsequently migrate widely to form (amongst other structures) the sensory neurons of the dorsal root ganglia of the spinal nerves, the principal postganglionic neurons of the sympathetic and parasympathetic nervous system, the Schwann cells, and the glial elements of the autonomic ganglia and peripheral receptors (Williams *et al.* 1989).

Within the primary neuroepithelium there are time-dependent differences from one region to the next in the dynamics of cell proliferation. Initially the overall trend for neuronal development is in a caudal-to-rostral sequence. For example the brainstem neurons, which send projections to the forebrain, cease division and begin differentiation before local circuit neurons within the neocortex. The early differentiation of brainstem neurons ensures that the vital circuitry in the pons medulla and diencephalon is assembled and functioning in the prenatal period. In contrast the more rostral systems, which subserve more complex functions, differentiate primarily in the latter stages of gestation and during the postnatal period.

There is also a timed sequence of development within any one region; in the neural tube forming the spinal cord, for example, there is a ventral-to-dorsal chronological gradient in proliferative activity. The ventral zone produces the motor neurons of the ventral horn before the intermediate zone produces interneurons; the last to be generated are the receiving neurons of the dorsal horn (Altman and Bayer 1988).

During genesis of the various cell types within the CNS, neuroblasts are the first to be formed, followed by glioblasts (Sidman and Rakic 1973). Most neuroblasts are formed prenatally within the first 24 weeks of gestation, but significant postnatal neurogenesis does occur. Indeed in the cerebellum most of the nerve cells are formed after birth. Only the Purkinje cells and the neurons in the deep cerebellar nuclei are formed prenatally, while Golgi cells are generated perinatally. Cerebellar interneurons (apart from the Golgi cells) are produced for several months after birth and granule cells, the most abundant interneurons in the cerebellum, increase substantially in number for the first two years after birth (Larroche 1966, Gadsdon and Emery 1976). Furthermore, neurogenesis in the dentate gyrus of the hippocampus may continue not only in childhood but also into adult life (Kaplan and Hinds 1977, Kaplan and Bell 1983).

Gliogenesis in the periventricular area of the cerebral cortex and in other sites in the nervous system occurs predominantly in the postnatal period and continues during the first two years after birth (Dobbing 1970, Brasel and Gruen 1986).

The primary neuroepithelium constitutes the wall of the embryonic cerebrospinal ventricular system and within it cell mitosis typically takes place near the lumen. The progeny of the divisions largely move away from the ventricular zone to form an intermediate zone where they lose their proliferative capacity and differentiate into neuroblasts (Sidman and Rakic 1973, Altman and Bayer 1988).

Some cells, however, leave the primary ventricular germinal matrix but do not lose their proliferative capacity and form a subventricular secondary germinal matrix between the ventricular and intermediate layers, there continuing to multiply to provide further generations of neuroblasts and later in development to form glioblasts. In some regions of the nervous system, for example the cerebellum, some mitotic subventricular stem cells migrate across the entire neural wall to form a subpial secondary germinal matrix. These secondary germinal matrices tend to be formed relatively late during development (Rakic 1975, Altman and Bayer 1988).

Cells that leave the primary or secondary germinal matrices lose their proliferative capacity and begin the process of migration and differentiation. In some areas of the CNS there is simple passive translocation, where neuroblasts which are beginning differentiation accumulate outside the neuroepithelium. More commonly neuroblasts settle some distance from their germinal matrix and get there by a process of active migration. Such migration may be accretionary, convergent or divergent in pattern. Accretionary migration occurs when neurons from a single germinal source migrate by a common route to constitute the entire population of a specific region. This pattern is seen in the formation of layers II to VI of the cerebral cortex (Berry and Rogers 1965, Rakic 1972). Convergent migration refers to the assembly of a specific structure from neurons derived from many different sources and which all followed a different migratory path. The formation of the cerebellum occurs from such convergent migration of neuroblasts (Altman 1982). In contrast the formation of the suprasegmental precerebellar nuclei of the pons and medulla arise from divergent migration, where the neurons forming each of these nuclei arise in sequence from a common source but migrate to a different site (Altman and Bayer 1978).

Following the period of migration the neuron undergoes differentiation and maturation. There may be a period of rapid somatic growth, when the cell body volume can increase fivefold (Miller 1988). Despite the increase in size of cell bodies, the cell body : neuropil ratio decreases because of an even more dramatic increase in the volume of the neuropil (Conel 1939–1960). The increase in neuropil primarily involves the extension of dendrites, an increase in the complexity of dendritic trees and the production of dendritic spines (Marin-Padilla 1970). The arborisation of dendrites with the formation of dendritic spines is a critical event in the development of the CNS, since dendrites provide the major proportion of membrane surface area for synapse formation and for the integration of both excitatory and inhibitory synapse activity (Purpura 1975). Dendritic differentiation begins as soon as neurons complete their migration, and continues well into the postnatal period in relation to ongoing elaboration of axons and synapses within the neuropil (Molliver *et al.* 1973). The final growth of the dendritic tree is influenced by patterns of afferent connections and their activity (Greenough and Chang 1988). If deprived of afferents experimentally, dendrites fail to develop fully and after a critical period may become permanently affected, even if functional inputs are restored: as in the visual systems of young animals, for instance (Blakemore 1974).

Metabolic factors also affect the final branching patterns of dendrites; thus gross nutritional deficiency, endocrine abnormalities and anoxia may all disturb the normal pattern (Horn 1955, Bedi and Warren 1988).

At this stage of development, neurons also begin to elaborate axonal projections. These axonal projections are thought initially to be numerous and diffuse (Innocenti 1981, Ivy *et al.* 1984) with a subsequent decrease in the number of projections by elimination of axon collaterals. Thus it appears likely that neurons initially elaborate more axonal processes than will eventually be maintained, and that there is selective elimination of many of these.

More than 60 years ago, Ramon y Cajal (1929) suggested that developing nerves establish more than the required number of connections when they initially invade their targets, with the selection of which axons are to be maintained taking place on the basis of appropriate neural activity. Cajal's original hypothesis is receiving increasing support, with accumulating evidence not only of axon collateral withdrawal but also of the formation initially of an excess of synapses. The peak density of synapses occurs in the immediate postnatal period in primates and is followed by a significant reduction in synapse numbers (Rakic *et al.* 1986). Synapse elimination may be a general feature of neural ontogeny with synapse elimination occurring in skeletal muscle, autonomic ganglia and the CNS (Greenough and Chang 1988). There is also excess production of neurons during development; subsequent phases of cell death may claim between 15 and 85 per cent of the initially formed neurons within different regions of the CNS (Adler 1988).

During this period the retained axons increase in diameter. In corticospinal tract fibres, for example, there is a threefold increase in diameter in the first three postnatal months, and a sevenfold increase in the first six postnatal months (Nathan and Smith 1955). Experimental evidence suggests that myelination of axons occurs in proportion to the growth in diameter of the axon, and that axonal growth in turn occurs in proportion to growth of neural perikayon. In development of cortical areas, the order of cytoarchitectural maturation correlates well with myelogenesis in the axons of the same cells (Yakovlev 1962). The appearance of myelin on a given axon is thus closely correlated with maturation of synaptic connections and the dendritic tree of the neuron, and neuronal maturation is likely to be a prerequisite for the onset of myelination. It is possible that the chronological and topographical sequences of CNS myelination are ultimately determined by and follow neuronal maturation.

Yakovlev and Lecours (1967) were the first to describe the temporal sequence of myelination in man. Myelination proceeds proximal to distal along an axon from the neuron of origin. In the peripheral nervous system the ventral roots of the cerebrospinal nerves to somatic musculature myelinate earliest and rapidly before those of the dorsal root fibres. Myelination of the dorsal and ventral roots begins at 20 weeks gestational age (GA). Axon diameter growth and myelination in the peripheral nerves are essentially completed in the first five postnatal years. In contrast, in the CNS the myelination of fibre systems mediating sensory input to the thalamus and the cerebral cortex precedes myelination of the fibre systems of the motor pathways. Myelination in the CNS begins at 18 weeks gestational age but the period of most rapid myelination is in the first eight postnatal months. Unlike the peripheral nervous system, however, myelination continues in many pathways until adulthood, probably reflecting a progressive increase in axon fibre diameter throughout this period.

These morphological changes (in neuronal size, dendritic tree, synapse distribution and density, and axon diameter) are also associated with changes in the neurophysiological functioning of the neurons. The threshold for excitation of a neuron will change with the increasing soma volume (Kernell 1966) and the decreasing soma to dendritic ratios (Rall *et al.* 1967). Excitatory and inhibitory postsynaptic potentials in immature neurons characteristically have a slow rise time, a long duration and a low peak amplitude compared with mature neurons (Purpura and Shofer 1972). Temporal dispersion of impulses in immature axons may contribute to the slow rise time and long duration of the postsynaptic potentials; so too will the predominance of axodendritic synapses and the lack of axosomatic synapses in immature neurons (Rall *et al.* 1967). Spike potentials, however, are longer in duration in immature neurons, suggesting that there are also fundamental differences in the kinetics of ionic processes in the cell membrane of immature neurons (Purpura and Shofer 1972, Vernadakis 1988). In the peripheral nerves the increasing fibre diameters and progressive myelination are reflected in increasing conduction velocities and decreased thresholds for activation (Hursh 1939).

Development of the cerebral cortex

In mammalian embryos, the evagination of the dorsolateral walls of the prosencephalon marks the beginning of the development of the cerebral vesicles. The progressive transformation of the undifferentiated neuroepithelium of the prosencephalon into mammalian neocortical organisation begins from 33 days GA (see Table 1.I). It is characterised by at least three fundamental events:

(1) the arrival of afferent fibres at the cerebral vesicle (day 35). The origin of these fibres remains unknown; some are thought to arise from the developing thalamus and some from the mesencephalic tegmentum
(2) establishment of a primitive cortical organisation, and
(3) the appearance of the cortical plate within the pre-existing cortical organisation (Marin-Padilla 1988).

Following the formation of the cerebral vesicles (day 35), primitive corticopetal fibres start to pass into them. At the time of their arrival cortical ontogenesis begins. The primitive neurons of the subpial marginal zone start to differentiate and to establish a primitive cortical organisation comprising a population of well differentiated neurons (Cajal-Retzius cells) with synapses, neuropeptides and receptors (Marin-Padilla 1988). The function of this primitive neural network is still

TABLE 1.I
Thickness and differentiation of various layers of the human cerebral (motor) cortex during the fetal period

Gestation (wks)	*Cortical plate (μm)*	*Development of cortical plate*
7–11	100–120	Undifferentiated
15–16	300–500	VI and V differentiated
18–20	700–800	IV differentiated
24–26	900–1000	IIIc differentiated
28–30	1300–1500	IIIb
38–40	1800–2100	IIIa and IIb

Adapted from Marin-Padilla (1988)

the subject of debate: whether it acts transiently in a primitive neural network, as a temporary target for waiting afferent systems, or as a scaffold for the ensuing development of the cortical layers.

The cortical plate, from which the cortical layers II to VI are derived, grows within the primitive neural network and splits it into a superficial lamina (from which ultimately layer I of the cerebral cortex is derived) and a deep lamina (which will ultimately form part of the subcortical white matter). The mammalian cortical plate starts to form by day 54. All cortical neurons originate from a proliferative zone in the periventricular area (Sidman and Rakic 1973, Marin-Padilla 1988). Cortical neuroblasts initially migrate from the proliferative zone to form the lower border of the cortical plate. Subsequent neuroblasts migrate past previously formed neurons to reach more superficial layers of the cortical plate. Thus the neurons located closest to the ventricular border of the cortical plate are the oldest and those at its pial surface the youngest. Differentiation of the cortical plate also follows an 'inside out' progression which starts with layer VI and proceeds to layer I (Table 1.I).

Early in cortical ontogenesis the cortical plate grows rapidly but is undifferentiated. The arrival of new afferent fibres, at approximately 15 weeks GA, appears to induce differentiation of layers VI, V and IV. The subsequent arrival of other afferent fibres results in the progressive maturation of other layers; layer III differentiates with the arrival of interhemispheric callosal fibres and that of layer II with the arrival of cortico-cortical fibres (see table).

The arrival of afferent input is associated with the rapid development of the dendritic trees of cortical neurons and the formation of synapses within the cortical plate. The earliest synapses reported within the cortical plate in the developing human fetus were observed at 23 weeks of gestation (Molliver *et al.* 1973). The process of dendritic tree development and synapse formation continues throughout the later part of gestation and in the postnatal period.

It is likely that excitatory postsynaptic potentials of pyramidal cells are the most significant events in generating the membrane currents contributing to cortical evoked potentials (Mitzdorf 1985). The changing pattern of cortical evoked potentials, therefore, is likely to reflect progressive development of the dendritic tree and synapse formation in succeeding layers of the cerebral cortex.

At birth there is little differentiation of the basal ramifications of the pyramidal cells of the cortex (Schade and Van Groenigen 1961). In the postnatal period there follows a rapid increase in the length, diameter and branching pattern of dendritic trees. There may be a tenfold increase in length of the dendritic trees in first three months after birth.

In studies of fetal sheep, Bernhard and Meyersson (1972) and Persson (1973) correlated changes in cortical evoked potentials with the progressive development of the cortical neurons. These authors demonstrated that the first somatosensory evoked potentials occurred in the fetal sheep on 42 to 60 days GA (roughly equivalent to 18 to 20 weeks GA in the human fetus). These were entirely positive in sign and were probably due to 'blind end' recordings from unterminated afferent fibres. At 68 to 80 days GA cortical evoked potentials became positive and negative in sign and this correlated with the differentiation of layers IV, V and VI of the cortex. Subsequent changes in the shape of the evoked potential correlated well with the predicted current changes consequent upon the progressive development of the dendritic tree of more superficial layers of the cortical plate.

The changes in cortical evoked potentials may also reflect the developing physiological function of the cortical neurons. For example, there is a slower rise time and longer duration for excitatory postsynaptic potentials in immature cortical cells, often lasting about 100 milliseconds (ms) compared with 5 to 20ms in the adult cortex (Purpura and Shofer 1972). These long durations are likely to arise from temporal dispersion of the afferent volley in the immature afferent fibres and from the relative density and position of synapses on the dendritic tree and soma of the neuron (see p. 3). Such long durations complement the slower rise time and longer time course of cortical evoked potentials in the immature cortex, which can be up to five to 10 times as long as in the adult.

Cortical projection neurons begin to elaborate their axons while they are still migrating (Miller 1988). The axons of the corticospinal tracts, for example, begin to develop in the ninth week of fetal life and have reached their caudal limits by the 29th week. The commissural links between the hemispheres begin before 10 weeks of gestation. The first to appear is the anterior commissure between pyriform cortices and olfactory bulbs. Soon afterwards the relatively small hippocampal commissure joins the hippocampal areas. The corpus callosum first appears as a few axons passing over the hippocampal commissure at 10 weeks GA. It continues to grow long after birth but the increase in size is a consequence of axon diameter increase and myelination, and masks a substantial loss of axon number accompanying cortical differentiation (Williams *et al.* 1989).

Myelination of the axons of cortical neurons follows the temporal order of cytoarchitectural maturation (Yakovlev 1964). Thus the degree of myelination of a fibre tract is likely to be a marker for the level of maturation of its neurons. This observation may explain why the progressive decrease in latency of cortical evoked potentials is also associated with a progressive maturation in the waveform of the potential.

Conclusion

During the perinatal period there is very rapid growth and maturation of the neurons within the central and peripheral nervous systems, the complexity of which has been illustrated by this review. The neurobiological process, however, will be reflected in neurophysiological function and thus in the patterns of evoked motor and sensory potential activity. Increasing our knowledge of human nervous system development, and correlating this with a detailed study of the normal postnatal changes in both sensory and motor evoked potentials, is likely to allow the identification of children who are following a normal pattern of development and those in whom abnormal development is occurring. A more detailed understanding of the origin and development of evoked potentials is also likely to allow the assessment of the efficacy of interventions designed to promote more normal patterns of neural development in those with perinatal or congenital brain damage.

REFERENCES

Adler, R. (1988) 'Trophic factors in neural development.' *In* Meisami, E., Timiras, P.S. (Eds) *Handbook of Human Growth and Developmental Biology, Vol. 1: Part A*. Florida: CRC Press. pp. 67–74.

Altman, J. (1982) 'Morphological development of rat cerebellum and some of its mechanisms.' *In* Paray, S.L., Chan Palay, V. (Eds) *The Cerebellum: New Vistas*. Berlin: Springer. pp. 63–78.

—— Bayers, S.A. (1978) 'Perinatal development of the cerebellar system in the rat. II: Cytogenetics and histogenesis of the inferior olive, pontine grey and pre cerebellar reticular nuclei.' *Journal of Comparative Neurology,* **179**, 49–69.

—— —— (1988) 'The development of neurons.' *In* Meisami E., Timiras P.S. (Eds) *Handbook of Human Growth and Developmental Biology, Vol. 1: Part A*. Florida: CRC Press. pp. 1–26.

Bedi, K.S., Warren, M.A. (1988) 'Effects of nutrition on cortical development.' *In* Peters, A., Jones, E.G. (Eds) *Cerebral Cortex, Vol. 7: Development and Maturation of Cerebral Cortex*. New York: Plenum Press. pp. 441–473.

Berry, M., Rogers, A.A. (1965) 'The migration of neuroblasts in the developing cerebral cortex.' *Journal of Anatomy*, **99**, 691–709.

Bernhard, C.G., Meyersson, B.A. (1973) 'Morphological and physiological aspects of recipient functions in the cerebral cortex.' *In* Cromline, S., Cross, K., Dawes, G.S., Nathanielz, P.W. (Eds) *Foetal and Neonatal Physiology*. London: Cambridge University Press. pp. 1–19.

Blakemore, C. (1974) 'Development of functional connections in the mammalian visual system.' *British Medical Bulletin*, **30**, 152–157.

Brasel, J.A., Gruen, R.K. (1986) 'Cellular growth.' *In* Falkner, K., Tanner, J.M. (Eds) *Human Growth, Vol. 1: Developmental Biology, Prenatal Growth*. New York: Plenum Press. pp. 54–57.

Cajal, S.R. (1959) *Studies on Vertebrate Neurogenesis*. (Originally published 1929.) Translated by Goth, L. Springfield, IL: Charles C. Thomas.

Conel, J. (1939–1960) *The Postnatal Development of the Human Cerebral Cortex, Vols I–VI*. Cambridge, MA: Harvard University Press.

Dobbing, J. (1970) 'Undernutrition and the developing brain: the relevance of animal models to the human problem.' *American Journal of Diseases of Children*, **120**, 411–419.

Gadsdon, D.R., Emery, J.L. (1976) 'Some quantitative morphological aspects of human post-natal cerebellar growth.' *Journal of Neurological Science*, **29**, 137–146.

Greenough, W.T., Chang, F.F. (1988) 'Plasticity of synapse structure and pattern in the cerebral cortex.' *In* Peters, A., Jones, E.G. (Eds) *Cerebral Cortex, Vol. 7: Development and Maturation of Cerebral Cortex*. New York: Plenum Press. pp. 391–429.

Horn, G. (1955) 'Thyroid deficiency and inanition. Effects of replacement therapy on the development of the cerebral cortex in young albino rats.' *Anatomical Record*, **121**, 63–71.

Hursh, J.B. (1939) 'Conduction velocity and diameter of nerve fibres.' *American Journal of Physiology*, **127**, 131–139.

Innocenti, G.M. (1981) 'Growth and reshaping of axons in establishment of visual callosal connections.' *Science*, **212**, 824–831.

Ivy, G.O., Yould, H.J., Killackery, H.P. (1984) 'Variability in the distribution of callosal projections in adult parietal cortex.' *Brain Research*, **306**, 53–61.

Kaplan, M.S., Hinds, J.W. (1977) 'Neurogenesis in the adult rat: electron microscope analysis of light autoradiographs.' *Science*, **197**, 1092–1101.

—— Bell, D.H. (1983) 'Neuronal proliferation in the 9 month old rodent—autoradiographic study of granule cells in the hippocampus.' *Experimental Brain Research*, **52**, 1–5.

Kernell, D. (1966) 'Input resistance, electrical excitability and size of ventral horn cells in cat spinal cord.' *Science*, **152**, 1637–1640.

Larroche, J.C. (1966) 'The development of the central nervous system during intrauterine life.' *In* Falkner, F. (Ed.) *Human Development*. Philadelphia: W.B. Saunders. p. 257.

Marin-Padilla, M. (1970) 'Prenatal and postnatal ontogenesis of the human motor cortex: a Golgi study. 1: The sequential development of the cortical layers.' *Brain Research*, **23**, 167–183.

—— (1988) 'Early ontogenesis of the human cerebral cortex.' *In* Peters, A., Jones, E.G. (Eds) *Cerebral Cortex, Vol. 7: Development and Maturation of Cerebral Cortex*. New York: Plenum Press. pp. 1–30.

Miller, M.W. (1988) 'Development of projection and local circuit neurons in neocortex.' *In* Peters, A., Jones, E.G. (Eds) *Cerebral Cortex, Vol. 7: Development and Maturation of Cerebral Cortex*. New York: Plenum Press. pp. 133–166.

Mitzdorf, U. (1985) 'Current source density method and application in cat cerebral cortex: investigation of evoked potentials and EEG phenomena.' *Physiological Review*, **65**, 37–99.

Molliver, M.E., Kostovic, I., Van der Loos, H. (1973) 'The development of synapses in cerebral cortex of the human fetus.' *Brain Research*, **50**, 403–407.

Nathan, P.W., Smith, M.C. (1955) 'Long descending tracts in man. I. Review of present knowledge.' *Brain*, **78**, 249–303.

Persson, H.E. (1973) 'Development of somatosensory cortical functions: an electrophysiological study in prenatal sheep.' *Acta Physiologica Scandinavica* (Suppl.), **394**, 1–64.

Purpura, D.P. (1975) 'Normal and aberrant neuronal development in the cerebral cortex of the human fetus and young infant.' *In* Buchwald, N.A., Brazier, M.A.B. (Eds) *Brain Mechanisms in Mental Retardation*. New York: Academic Press. pp. 141–170.

—— Shofer, R.J. (1972) 'Principles of synaptogenesis and their application to ontogenetic studies of mammalian cerebral cortex.' *In* Clemente, C.D., Purpura, D.P., Mayer, F.E. (Eds) *Sleep and the Maturing Nervous System*. New York: Academic Press. pp. 3–31.

Rakic, P. (1972) 'Mode of cell migration of the superficial layers of fetal monkey neocortex.' *Journal of Comparative Neurology*, **146**, 61–84.

—— (1975) 'Timing of major ontogenetic events in the visual cortex of the rhesus monkey.' *In* Buchwald, N.A., Brazier, M.A.B. (Eds) *Brain Mechanisms in Mental Retardation*. New York: Academic Press. pp. 3–40.

—— Bourgeois, J.P., Eckenhoff, M.F., Zecevic, N., Goldman Rakic, P. (1986) 'Concurrent over production of synapses in diverse regions of the primate cerebral cortex.' *Science*, **232**, 232–235.

Rall, W., Burke, R.E., Smith, T.G., Nelson, P.G., Frank, K. (1967) 'Dendritic location of synapses and possible mechanisms for the monosynaptic EPSP in motoneurons.' *Journal of Neurophysiology*, **30**, 1169–1193.

Schade, J.P., Van Groenigen, W.B. (1961) 'Structural organisation of the human cerebral cortex.' *Acta Anatomica*, **47**, 74–111.

Sidman, R.L., Rakic, P. (1973) 'Neuronal migration with special reference to the developing human brain: a review.' *Brain Research*, **62**, 1–35.

Vernadakis, A. (1988) 'Synaptogenesis: morphological, biochemical, and electrophysiological correlates.' *In* Meisami, E., Timiras, P.S. (Eds) *Handbook of Human Growth and Developmental*

Biology, Vol. 1: Part A. Florida: CRC Press. pp. 75–94.
Williams, P.I., Warwick, R., Dyson, M., Bannister, L.H. (1989) *Gray's Anatomy*. London: Churchill Livingstone. pp. 133–135.
Yakovlev, P.I. (1962) 'Morphological criteria of growth and maturation in man.' *Mental Retardation, Research Publication of the Association for Nervous and Mental Disease, Vol. 39*. New York: Association for Nervous and Mental Disease. pp. 3–46.
—— Lecours, A. (1967) 'The myelogenetic cycles of regional maturation of the brain.' *Regional Development of the Brain in Early Life*. Oxford: Blackwell Scientific. pp. 3–70.

2
THE NEONATAL ELECTROENCEPHALOGRAM AND SLEEP-CYCLE PATTERNS

Kazuyoshi Watanabe

In the newborn infant, the electroencephalogram (EEG) provides an extremely useful noninvasive test for evaluating brain function at the bedside. It has been used to diagnose neonatal seizures, to evaluate the degree of perinatal brain damage and its prognosis, to assess maturity, for continuous monitoring of brain function and as an ancillary diagnosis of neurological disorders.

In addition to the conventional multichannel recording, continuous monitoring systems using the continuous ambulatory EEG monitor (Medilog) (Eyre *et al.* 1983, 1988; Bridges *et al.* 1986; Connell and Oozeer 1988; Connell *et al.* 1987*a*,*b*, 1988, 1989*a*,*b*) and the cerebral function monitor (CFM) (Bjerre *et al.* 1983, Archbald *et al.* 1984, Verma *et al.* 1984, Viniker *et al.* 1984, Greisen *et al.* 1987, 1989) have recently proved to be useful diagnostic and prognostic tools in perinatal encephalopathy. But this chapter deals mainly with findings obtained with conventional EEG recordings, because they should be the basis for the interpretation of those obtained with other methods.

The development of the brain in the last trimester of pregnancy is reflected in the rapid evolutionary changes of EEG patterns in this period. This development is dependent on post-conceptional age (PCA) rather than postnatal age or birth-weight.* The EEG changes with behavioural state cycles, which also show an increasing organisation with advancing PCA age. Recording in all states is essential for the proper assessment of the neonatal EEG.

Behavioural states of the newborn infant

Sleep states of the newborn infant are usually defined by EEG pattern, eye movements, body movements, respiration and chin electromyogram (EMG), but non-sleep states cannot be determined by polygraphic criteria alone (Anders *et al.* 1971). The usefulness of the above parameters in the definition of states changes with maturation (Parmelee and Stern 1972). The submental EMG is least useful in the neonatal period and becomes useful only around or after term. The EEG shows a dramatic change with increasing PCA and undergoes various alterations under pathological conditions. Therefore we have defined sleep states using three

* For definition of gestational age and post-conceptional age, see footnote on page 1.

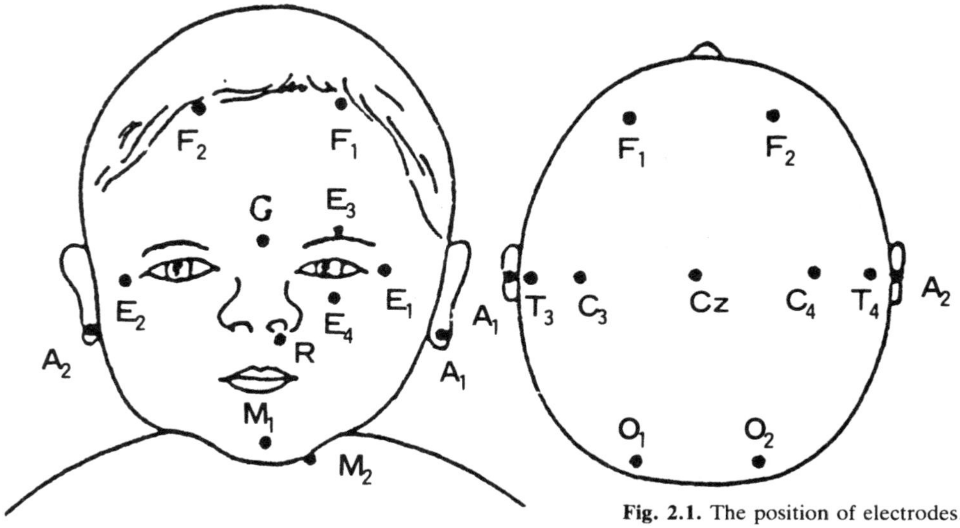

Fig. 2.1. The position of electrodes.

parameters: body movements, eye movements and respiration.

Awake (AW): eyes open or crying.

Drowsiness (DR): eyes slightly open, or eyes opening and closing.

Active sleep (AS): eyes closed, eye movements positive, body movements positive or negative, respiration irregular.

Quiet sleep (QS): eyes closed, eye movements negative, body movements negative, respiration regular.

Indeterminate sleep (IS): sleep states which could not be classified as either AS or QS.

Method of recording neonatal EEG

The method of neonatal EEG recording has been described in detail elsewhere (Werner *et al.* 1977) and minimal technical standards of neonatal EEG have been published (American Electroencephalographic Society 1986). Sixteen-channel recordings including two or more non-EEG polygraphic variables are recommended, but usually 13 or 14 channels including 10 to 12 EEG channels and other parameters are sufficient (Fig. 2.1). The other parameters most frequently monitored are respiration, electro-oculogram, electrocardiogram and chin EMG. The minimum scalp electrode positions are F_1, F_2, C_3, C_4, C_z, T_3, T_4, O_1 and O_2 and the various montages are used by different laboratories. The montages often used are F_1–C_3, C_3–O_1, F_2–C_4, C_4–O_2, F_1–T_3, T_3–O_1, F_2–T_4, T_4–O_2, T_3–C_3, C_3–C_z, C_z–C_4, C_4–T_4 (or T_3–C_z, C_z–T_4 in place of the last four). F_1 and F_2 are halfway between Fp_1 and F_3, and Fp_2 and F_4, respectively. C_z should always be included because positive Rolandic sharp waves may occur only at C_z. The time constant should not be less than 0.3 seconds, because very slow waves are predominant in newborn infants. It is advantageous to schedule the EEG at feeding time and arrange to feed the infant after electrodes have been applied but before beginning the recording as babies tend to sleep after feedings. It is necessary to obtain at least 60 minutes of recording to sample all states. At least AS, before and after QS, and a full episode of QS should be recorded. Sedatives should not be used to obtain a sleep recording.

Normal development of EEG and sleep cycle pattern

Developmental changes of EEG and cyclic organisation of states have been described in detail by various authors (Parmelee *et al.* 1968; Dreyfus-Brisac 1979; Karch *et al.* 1982; Anderson *et al.* 1985; Lombroso 1985, 1987; Torres and Anderson 1985; Mizrahi 1986; Nolte and Haas 1987; Curzi-Dascalova *et al.* 1988) and will be described briefly (Figs 2.2 to 2.7). Three-digit codes are used to classify various EEG patterns according to Parmelee *et al.* (1968) with some modifications. The first two digits represent PCA and the last one an EEG pattern. For example, the code 287 refers to an EEG pattern with maturity corresponding to 28 weeks PCA and an intermittent pattern. The code 200 refers to an EEG pattern with maturity less than 30 weeks and nonspecific pattern.

24 to 25 weeks PCA (Fig. 2.2)

Infants spend most of their time in IS. The EEG is almost always discontinuous, displaying intermittent bursts of high-voltage activity on a flat background (247). The burst consists of very high-voltage ultraslow waves usually accompanied by rhythmic theta, alpha and beta activities. These complexes are called delta brushes, spindle delta or beta-delta complexes. The flat period tends to be shorter in AS or IS with body movements than in QS or IS without body movements. Occasionally only high-voltage slow waves of smaller amplitude occur without superimposed rhythmic faster activities. This nonspecific pattern (200) is seen in infants under 30 weeks PCA.

26 to 28 weeks PCA (Fig. 2.3)

IS still occupies most of the infant's sleeping time. The EEG is still mostly discontinuous (287), but becomes more continuous in AS or IS with body movements (282). The EEG of QS is similar to that of the previous period (287).

29 to 31 weeks PCA (Fig. 2.3)

IS is still the predominant sleep state, but behavioural state cycles begin to emerge towards the end of this period. The EEG tends to be less discontinuous in AS or IS with body movements, showing two types of EEG patterns: medium-voltage semicontinuous (similar to 282) and high-voltage semicontinuous or continuous slow-wave patterns with theta bursts (similar to 283). The EEG of QS is still mostly discontinuous. The high-voltage slow waves of the burst show a gradual decrease in amplitude and a gradual increase in frequency. Until this age, theta delta complexes and high-voltage theta bursts are the characteristic EEG pattern, in addition to delta brushes.

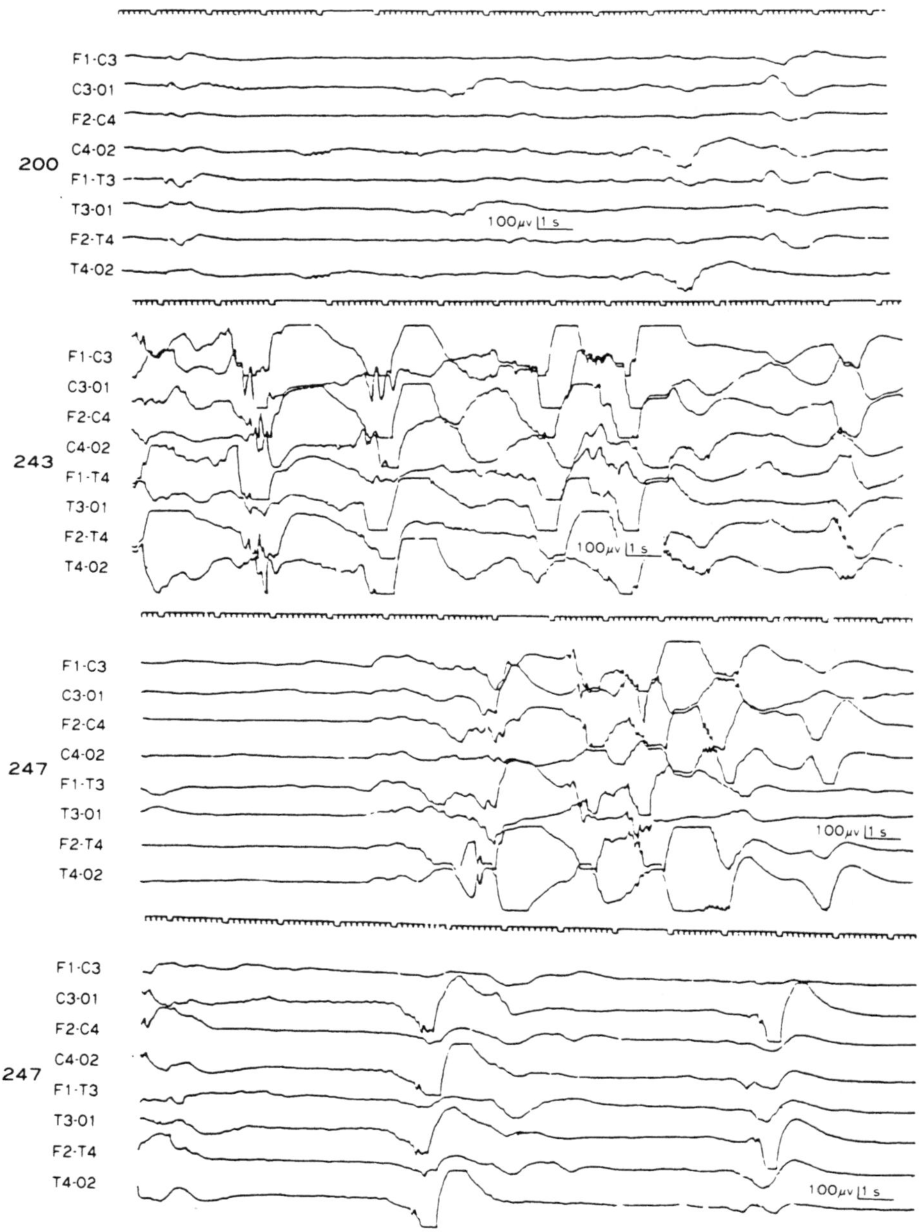

Fig. 2.2. EEGs at 24 weeks PCA. The figures on the left side in this figure and in subsequent figures indicate the EEG code according to Parmelee *et al.* (1968), with modifications.

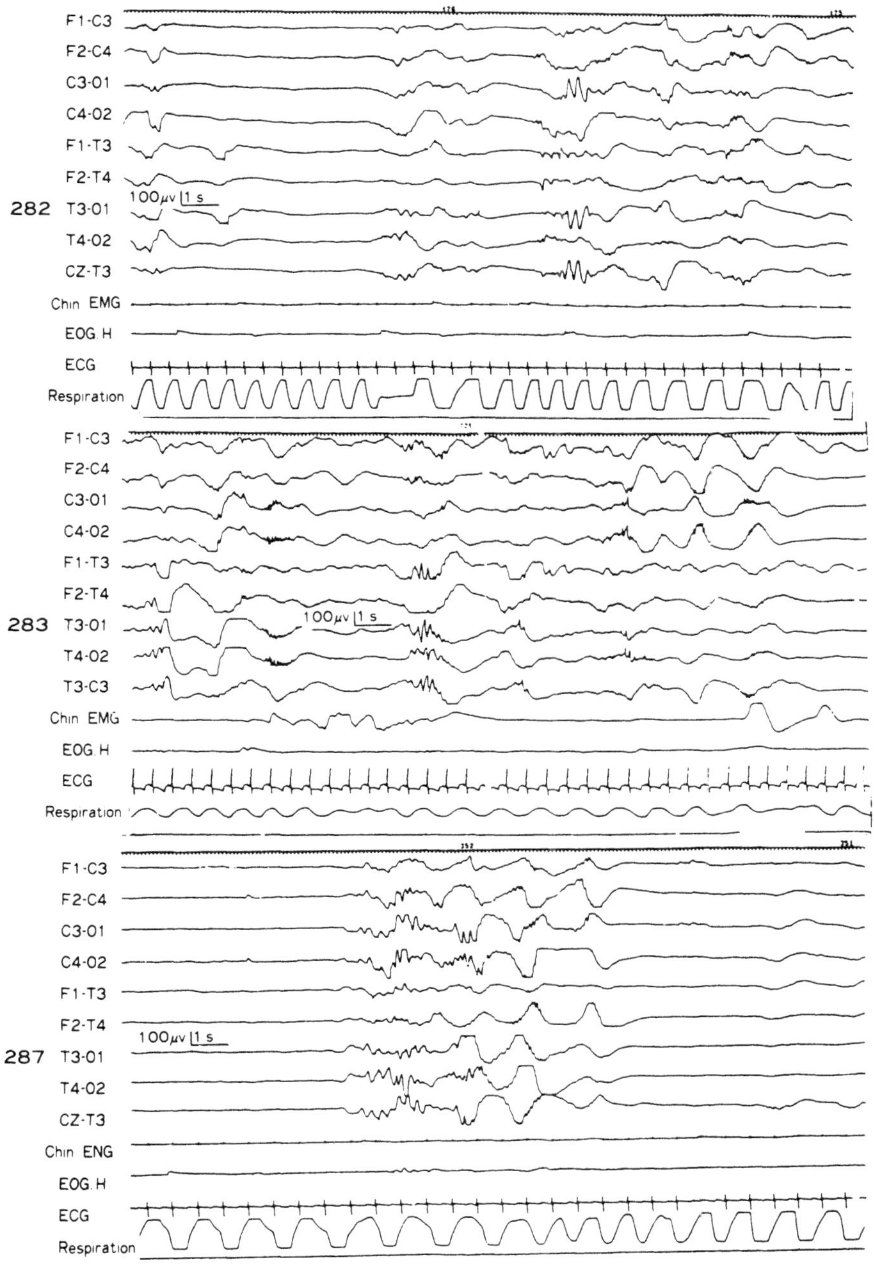

Fig. 2.3. EEGs at 28 weeks PCA.

32 to 33 weeks PCA (Fig. 2.4)
This period is characterised by an emergence of behavioural state cycles with concomitant changes of EEG patterns, although the continuity of each sleep state is still incomplete and IS is still abundant.

The EEG is mostly continuous in AS and discontinuous (327) in QS. Theta-delta complexes or high-amplitude theta bursts are no longer the prevailing pattern at this age; delta brushes become the predominant pattern. The EEG of AS displays two patterns, *i.e.* continuous low- to medium-voltage activity with occasional delta brushes (322) and high-voltage slow pattern consisting mainly of delta brushes (323). These slow waves show a further decrease in amplitude and increase in frequency. They are occipital dominant at early PCA (Inokuma *et al.* 1984).

34 to 35 weeks PCA
This period is characterised by a decrease in the occurrence of delta brushes and the overall amplitude of the background in AS. On the other hand, the EEG of QS still shows a discontinuous pattern with a further decrease in the amplitude and a further increase in frequency of delta waves. The burst-to-burst interval shows a further decrease, with most intervals below 20s.

36 to 37 weeks PCA (Fig. 2.5)
There is now a clearly defined sleep cycle consisting of relatively well sustained AS and QS. The EEG of AS is characterised by relatively low-voltage irregular activity with some medium-voltage slow waves superimposed with a few low-voltage fast waves (362). The EEG of QS still shows a discontinuous tracing (367), but with some low-voltage irregular activity appearing in the interburst phase in the occipital regions. A considerable amount of delta brushes still occur in the high-voltage burst phase. A continuous high-voltage slow pattern seen in the term infant begins to emerge at this age, but the frequency is slower with some superimposed low-voltage fast waves (363).

38 to 39 weeks PCA
Four EEG patterns are established: *i.e.* low-voltage irregular (LVI, 402), mixed (M, 403), high-voltage slow (HVS, 405), and trace alternant (TA, 407) pattern. A few delta brushes still occur in QS.

40 to 41 weeks PCA (Fig. 2.6)
The cyclic organisation of sleep is fully established with concomitant EEG changes. LVI and M patterns are mainly observed in AS, and HVS and TA in QS. M patterns usually occur in AS immediately before QS, and HVS patterns in the initial phase of QS before TA patterns appear.

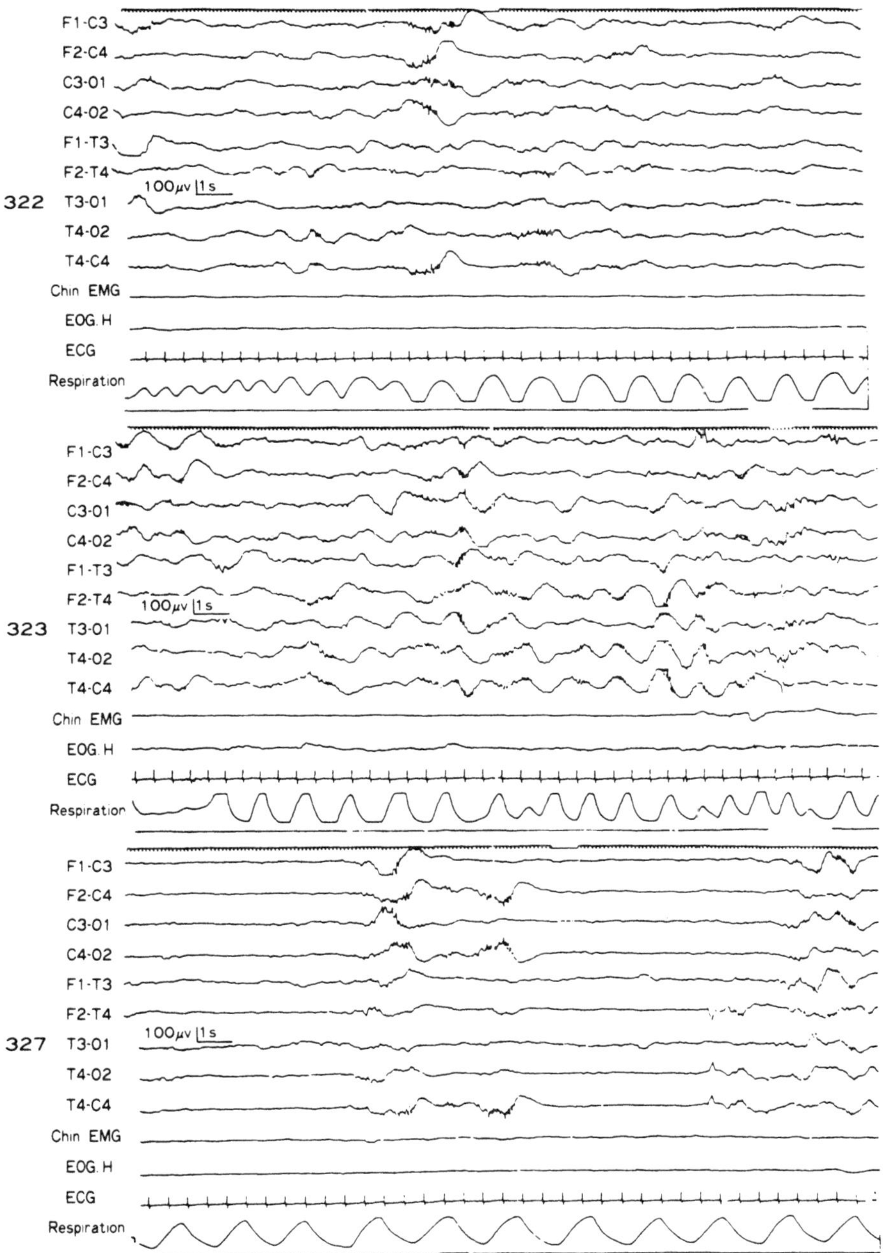

Fig. 2.4. EEGs at 32 weeks PCA.

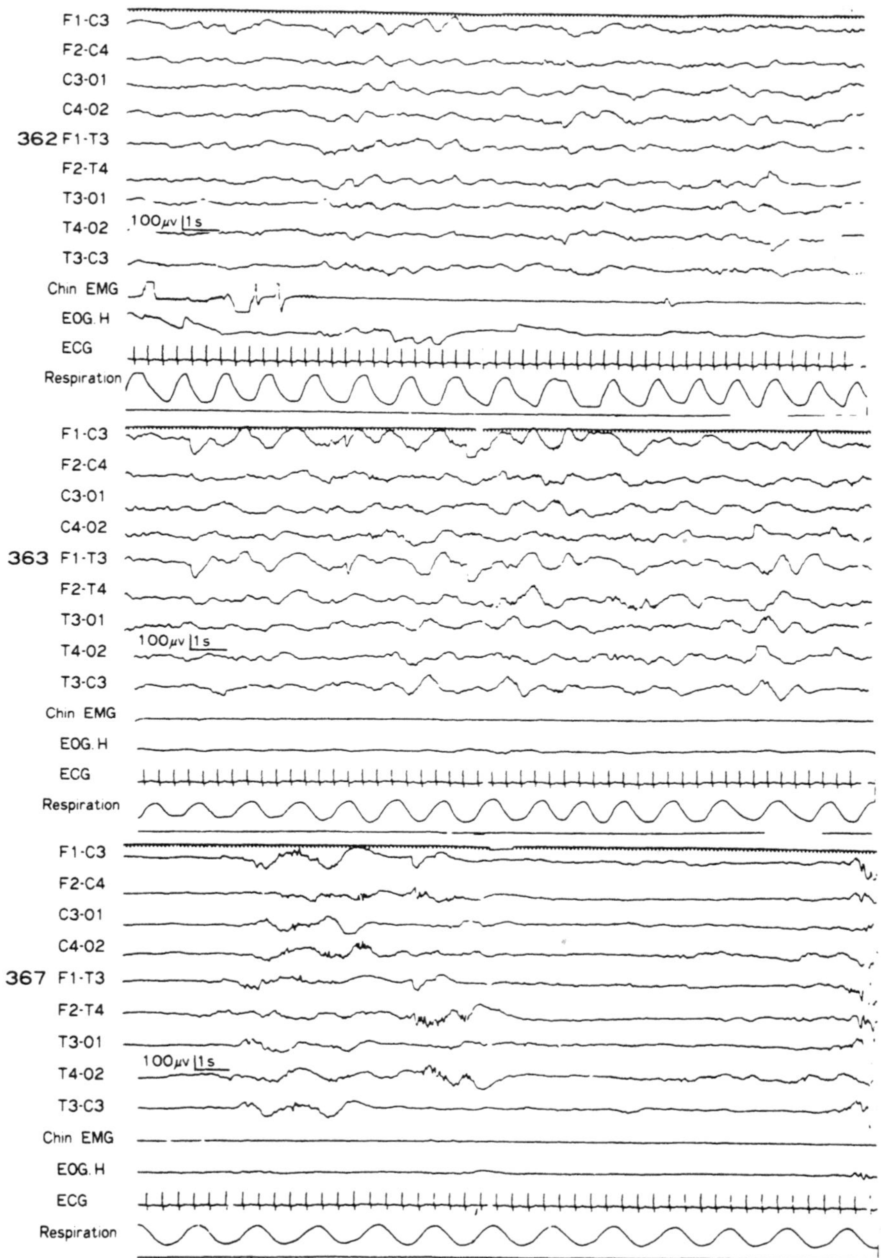

Fig. 2.5. EEGs at 36 weeks PCA.

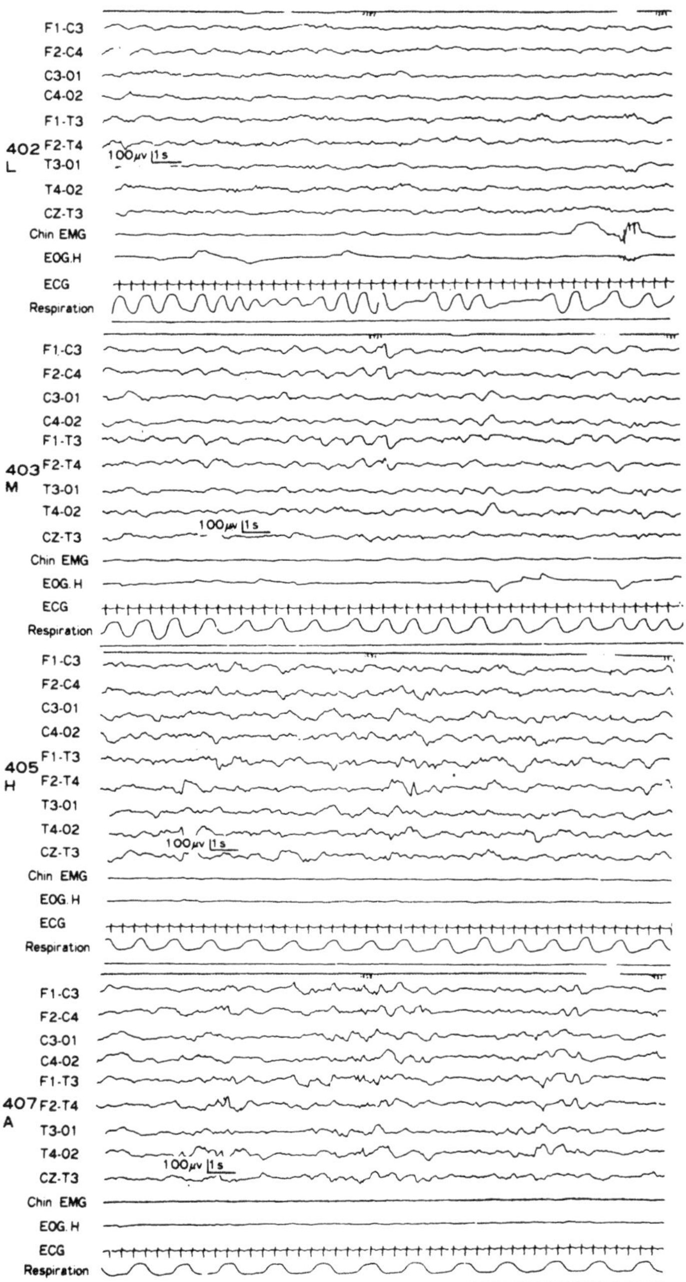

Fig. 2.6. EEGs at 40 weeks PCA.

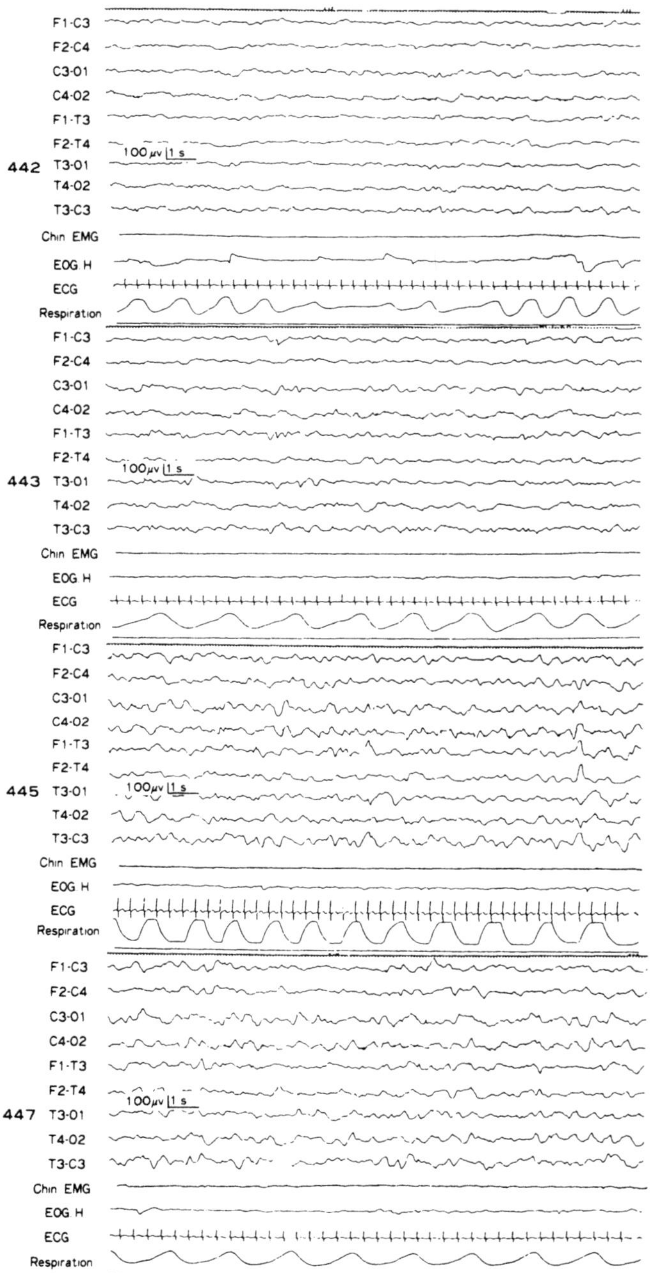

Fig. 2.7. EEGs at 44 weeks PCA.

42 to 46 weeks PCA (Fig. 2.7)
HVS patterns gradually replace TA patterns in quiet sleep, becoming the main EEG pattern of QS after 46 weeks PCA (Watanabe *et al.* 1974, Ellingson and Peters 1980). TA patterns disappear in the occipital region earlier than in the frontal.

Characteristic EEG waveforms in the normal newborn infant
Delta brushes, spindle-delta, beta-delta complexes
This pattern occurs most frequently at 31 or 32 weeks PCA and decreases gradually to disappear first in AS at around 37 weeks and then in QS around 40 weeks PCA (Watanabe and Iwase 1972). The frequency of brushes is often slower under 32 weeks PCA.

High-voltage rhythmic theta bursts
This pattern occurs most frequently at 27 or 28 weeks PCA, and is seldom seen at or after 34 weeks PCA. The bursts occur most frequently in temporal regions. Hughes *et al.* (1987) called the pattern 'premature temporal theta', including low-amplitude patterns, and reported that it maximised at 29 to 31 weeks and then diminished and disappeared near term.

Intermittent pattern ('tracé disontinu', 'trace alternant')
The low-amplitude phase of this intermittent pattern decreases in duration with increasing PCA. The maximum burst-to-burst interval decreases with increasing PCA but the modal value remains about 7 to 10s. The burst phase shows a gradual decrease in amplitude and a gradual increase in frequency with increasing age. There have been several quantitative studies on this pattern (Parmelee *et al.* 1969, Miyazaki *et al.* 1978, Hughes *et al.* 1983*a*, Connell *et al.* 1987*a*, Eyre *et al.* 1988, Hahn *et al.* 1989). The degree of discontinuity has been used to assess the normal development and the extent of acute brain damage in abnormal infants (Connell *et al.* 1987*b*, 1988, 1989*a*,*b*).

Bifrontal sharp transients, bifrontal slow-wave bursts, bifrontal sharp and slow waves
Biphasic hump-like sharp waves and slow-wave bursts begin to appear and become well defined at 35 weeks and disappear by 46 weeks PCA (Ellingson and Peters 1980). They may be absent in 20 or 30 per cent of normal infants. These waves are often combined to form waveforms resembling sharp and slow-wave complexes (Watanabe 1978). They usually occur in AS immediately before QS (Statz *et al.* 1982) and are associated with M pattern.

FZ theta/alpha bursts
These bursts are recorded mainly in the midline frontal area, consisting of 5 to 9HZ, 50 to 200μv, multiple, often sharp theta or alpha waves lasting between 0.3 and 1.5s (Hayakawa *et al.* 1987). They are observed mainly in infants at 38 to 43 weeks PCA.

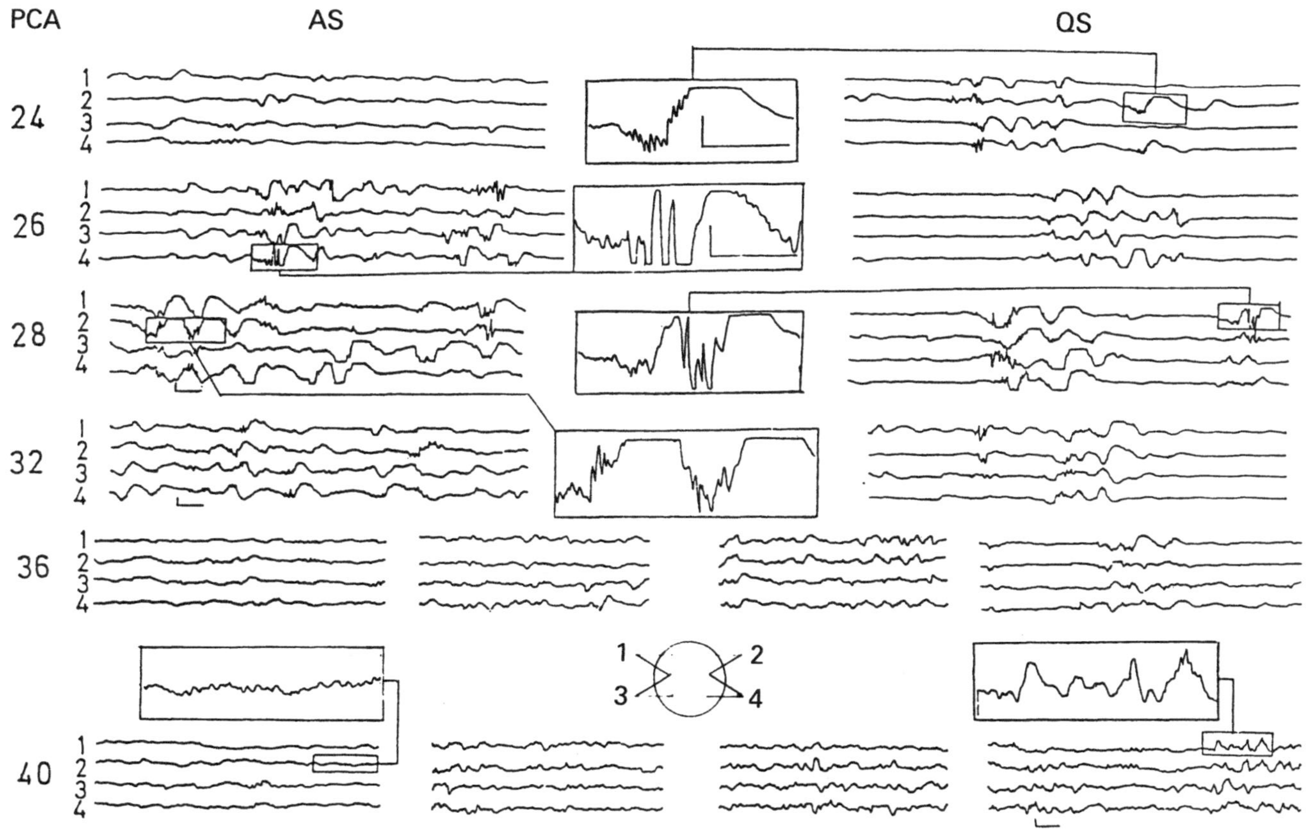

Fig. 2.8. Developmental changes in EEG from 24 to 40 weeks PCA in relation to sleep state. AS, active sleep; QS, quiet sleep. Calibration: 100μv, 1s.

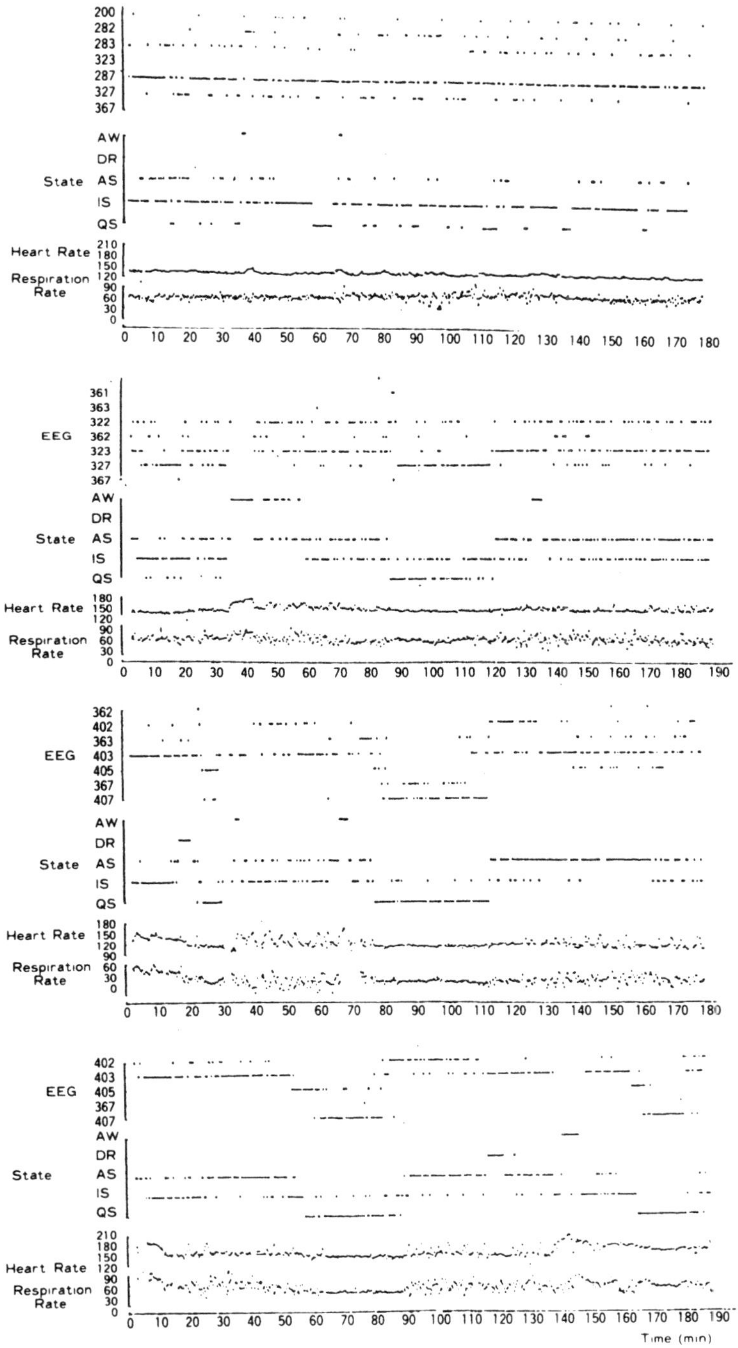

Fig. 2.9. Developmental changes in sleep-cycle patterns at (*top to bottom*): 29 weeks, 32 weeks, 37 weeks and 40 weeks PCA; AW, awake; DR, drowsiness; AS, active sleep; QS, quiet sleep; IS, indeterminate sleep.

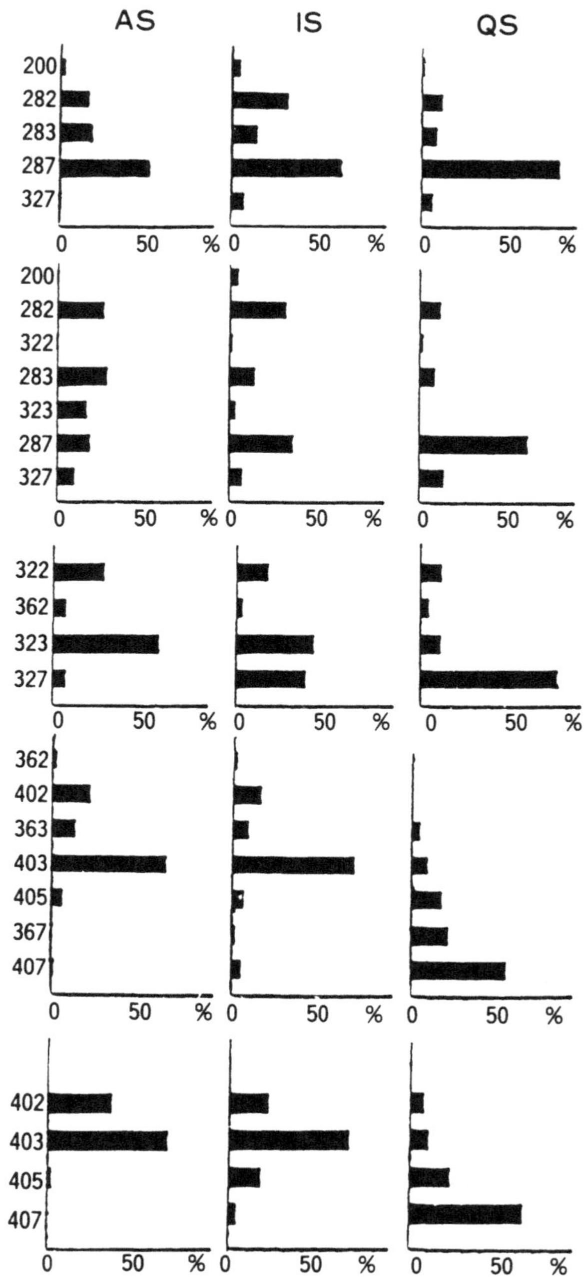

Fig. 2.10. Developmental changes in the relationship between sleep states and EEG patterns, at (*top to bottom*) 25 weeks, 29 weeks, 32 weeks, 37 weeks and 40 weeks PCA. AS, active sleep; IS, indeterminate sleep; QS, quiet sleep.

Temporal sharp transients
These bi- or triphasic sharp transients are seen mainly during transition from AS to QS, and occur most frequently in the right mid-temporal area (Karbowski and Nencka 1980).

Transient flattenings
Background activity often shows attenuation lasting up to 10s following acoustic or tactile stimuli, or startles. It usually occurs in QS.

Transient flattenings of background activity are observed in 24 per cent of term infants at or near the onset of the first QS in a sleep episode, and last for about a minute, followed by a variable period of discontinuous activity (O'Brien *et al.* 1987).

Relation between sleep states and EEG patterns
EEG patterns are classified using a three-digit code invented by Parmelee *et al.* (1968), and supplemented by Nolte and Haas (1987) and ourselves. An improving correlation between sleep states and EEG patterns is observed with increasing PCA (Figs 2.8 to 2.10).

Abnormal EEGs in the term newborn infant
There have been many classification systems for abnormal neonatal EEGs (Engel 1975, Dreyfus-Brisac 1979, Holmes *et al.* 1982, Coen and Tharp 1985, Lombroso 1985, Pezzani *et al.* 1986) and it is difficult to review them all and integrate them. Table 2.I shows our own classification. EEG abnormalities are usually described in terms of background and paroxysmal activity. Background activity refers to any EEG activity representing the setting in which a given normal or abnormal pattern appears and from which such pattern is distinguished. Paroxysmal activity denotes electrical phenomena with abrupt onset and termination and showing higher amplitude than the background.

Background EEG and sleep cycle abnormalities
In the acute stage of perinatal encephalopathy, the EEG usually shows varying degrees of depression. In order to analyse quantitative pattern changes in relation to sleep states and to confirm the validity of the classification, each 20s epoch of EEG was coded as follows (Watanabe *et al.* 1980): F, flat pattern or almost isoelectric activity of 0 to 5μv; P, poor activity or very low-voltage activity of 5 to 20μv; L, low voltage irregular activity of 20 to 50μv; M, medium-voltage slow activity of 30 to 100μv; H, continuous high-voltage slow activity of 50 to 150μv; A, alternating or trace alternant pattern; and D, discontinuous pattern.

MINIMAL DEPRESSION (Figs 2.11 to 2.13)
The low-voltage phase of pattern A is often abnormally attenuated, constituting pattern D. In infants whose EEG is minimally depressed in the first weeks, the sleep

TABLE 2.I
Classification of abnormal EEGs

I. Background EEG

A. Depression
1. minimal depression
2. mild depression
3. moderate depression
4. marked depression
5. maximal depression
6. low voltage

B. Hyperexcitability
1. increased theta/alpha waves
2. high-voltage rhythmic alpha-beta waves

C. Continuous pattern without sleep cycles
1. intermittent asynchronous delta activity
2. low- to medium-voltage continuous activity with semirhythmic theta waves

D. Topographic abnormality
1. asymmetry
2. asynchrony
3. localised low voltage
4. localised activity on a flat background
5. fronto-occipital voltage gradient

E. Transient patterns
1. semirhythmic theta or delta bursts
2. excessive, very high-voltage or very slow bifrontal humps

F. Dysmature pattern

II. Paroxysmal abnormalities

A. Interictal
1. focal spikes, sharp waves
   (1) negative spikes
   (2) positive spikes
2. multifocal spikes
3. periodic paroxysm
4. subclinical discharges or ictal abnormalities

B. Ictal
1. repeated spikes or sharp waves
2. paroxysmal delta
3. paroxysmal theta
4. paroxysmal alpha (rhythmic alpha discharge)
5. repeated stereotyped wave complexes
6. paroxysmal irregular slow waves
7. desynchronisation, flattening
8. recruiting rhythm
9. fast-wave bursts
10. no change

C. Status
1. subclinical or clinical status epilepticus with various electrical discharges
2. subclinical delta status epilepticus

cycle is often slightly disturbed although gross cyclic organisation is usually maintained. Patterns L and M are usually associated with AS, and intermittent patterns A and D with QS, although pattern A is mostly replaced by pattern D.

MILD DEPRESSION (Figs 2.11, 2.12, 2.14)

The H pattern is decreased and hardly seen, and the low-voltage phase of pattern A is abnormally attenuated. L, M and D are the main EEG patterns. In infants with mildly depressed EEGs in the first week, the sleep cycle is more often disturbed, although the cyclic organisation is still maintained. Patterns L and M are mainly seen in AS, although the former occurs more frequently and the latter less frequently than in normal infants. Pattern D is mainly associated with QS but pattern H is no longer observed. Pattern L is seen more frequently and pattern A less often in QS, compared with normal infants. Infants with mildly depressed EEGs in the first week will usually show normal or minimally depressed EEGs with normalisation of the sleep cycle in the second week (Fig. 2.15).

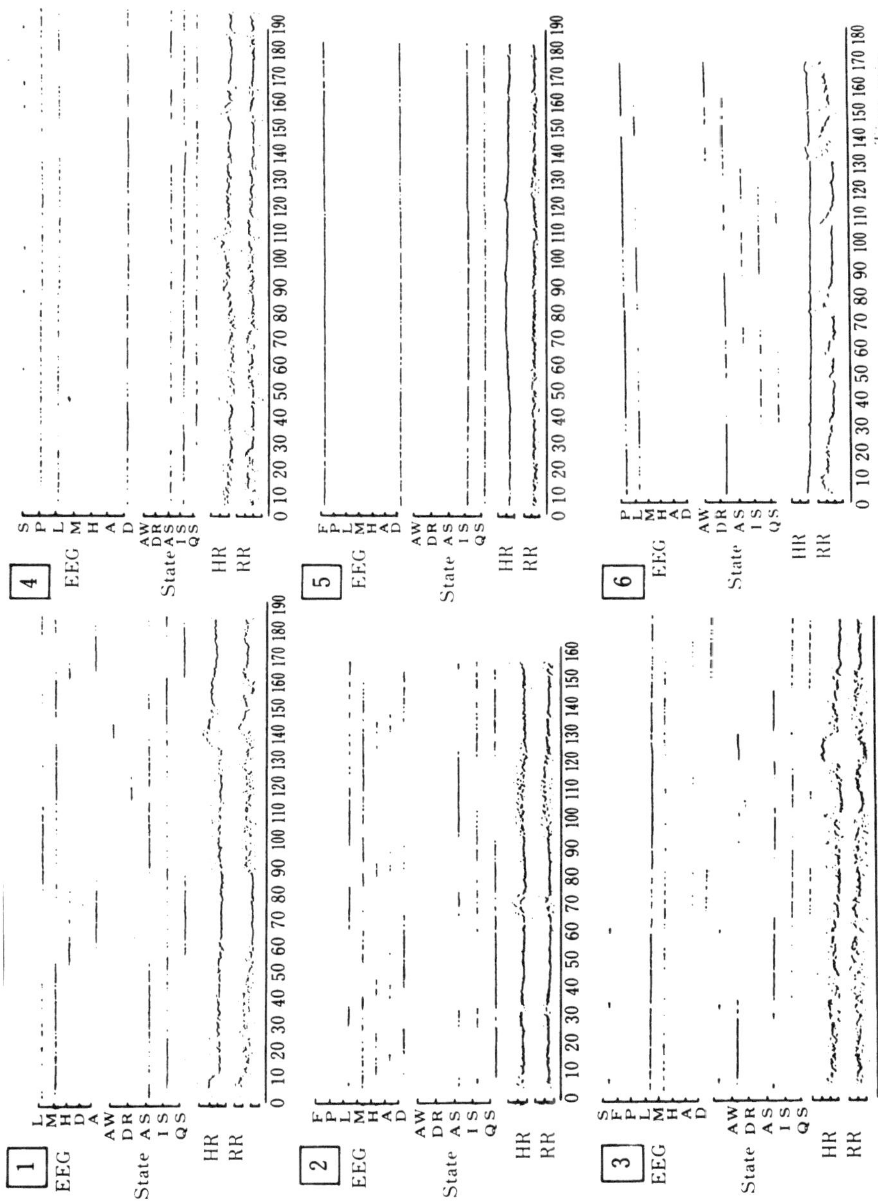

Fig. 2.11. Sleep cycle patterns in normal and abnormal term newborn infants. 1, normal; 2, minimal depression; 3, mild depression; 4, moderate depression; 5, marked depression (1–5 in the first week); 6, low voltage. The EEG is coded using the classification of Watanabe *et al.* (1980): S, seizure; F, flat pattern; P, very low-voltage activity, L, low-voltage irregular activity; M, medium-voltage slow activity; H, continuous high-voltage slow activity; A, trace alternant pattern; D, discontinuous pattern. The sleep states are classified: AS, active sleep; IS, indeterminate sleep; QS, quiet sleep. HR, heart rate; RR, respiration rate.

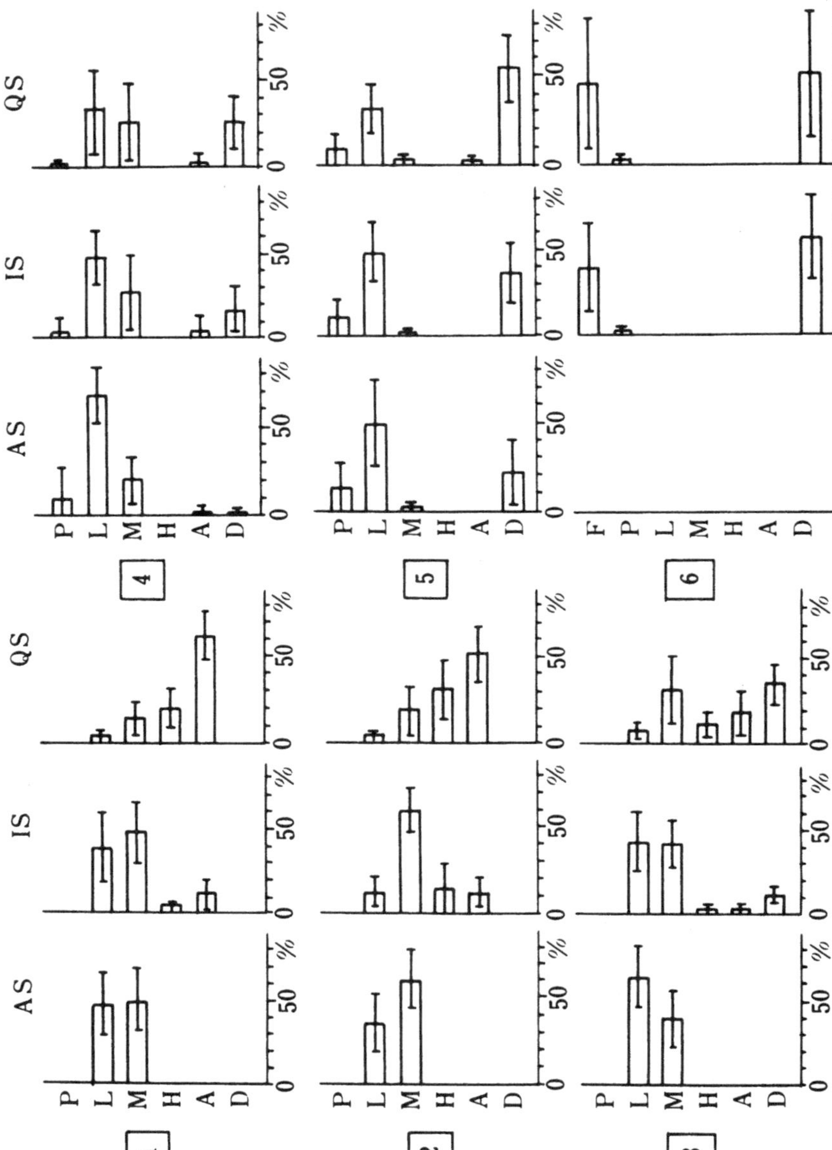

Fig. 2.12. Relationship between sleep states and EEG patterns in normal and abnormal term newborn infants; 1, normal; 2, abnormal infant with normal background EEG; 3, minimal depression; 4, mild depression; 5, moderate depression; 6, marked depression. The EEG is coded using the classification of Watanabe *et al.* (1980): S, seizure; F, flat pattern; P, very low-voltage activity; L, low-voltage irregular activity; M, medium-voltage slow activity; H, continuous high-voltage slow activity; A, trace alternant pattern; D, discontinuous pattern. The sleep states are classified: AS, active sleep; IS, indeterminate sleep; QS, quiet sleep.

MODERATE DEPRESSION (Figs 2.11, 2.12, 2.16)
Only three EEG patterns—low-voltage continuous patterns of P and L, and discontinuous pattern D—can be recognised without patterns M and H. In infants with this finding in the first week, the sleep cycle is usually moderately disrupted with loss of regular alternation of the two sleep states, although both can be identified. Pattern L is seen more frequently in QS, compared with normal infants. Pattern D (which, in infants with minimally and mildly depressed EEG, is almost exclusively seen in QS) occurs frequently in AS. Although patterns L and D are observed in both sleep states, the former still occurs more frequently in AS and the latter in QS. Infants initially showing moderately depressed EEGs will have mildly or minimally depressed or normal EEGs in the second week with progressive improvement in the cyclic organisation of sleep (Fig. 2.17). Reactive burst-suppression may be classified here (Holmes *et al.* 1983).

MARKED DEPRESSION (Figs 2.11, 2.12, 2.18)
The EEG consists of patterns D and F, corresponding to a burst-suppression pattern with long flat periods. Infants displaying this finding in the first week demonstrate no sleep cycle at all, with loss of variability of heart and respiratory rates. They are in apparent IS or QS, which is not sleep. Most of them will show moderately or mildly depressed EEGs in the second week (Fig. 2.19), but a few will have minimally depressed or normal EEGs.

MAXIMAL DEPRESSION (Fig. 2.20)
The EEG shows only pattern F throughout a recording of sufficient duration. Infants with this abnormality in the first week also show no normal sleep cycle at all. Some spend most of their time awake, some in IS, and some in apparent QS. Serial recordings disclose a progressive improvement in the EEG and sleep cycle, but the former will not become normal in spite of a rapid improvement in the latter.

These graded degrees of background EEG abnormalities are often observed in hypoxic-ischaemic encephalopathy and reflect an increasing degree of brain damage. Each degree of the abnormality is correlated with the degree of disturbance of the sleep cycle (Fig. 2.11), and is also related to the interval after the hypoxic-ischaemic insult. The same EEG abnormality is sometimes associated with different degrees of disturbed sleep cycle. Serial recordings disclose that the sleep cycle is more often affected but normalises more quickly than the background EEG. The relation between sleep states and EEG patterns also has a close correlation with the above classification and is progressively disrupted with increasing EEG severity (Fig. 2.12). In infants less severely affected, the relation is not influenced much (Fig. 2.11) even though the behavioural state cycle and duration are considerably affected. Even in infants whose background EEG is normal, sleep cycle is often abnormal with decrease of QS, the maintenance of which seems to be especially vulnerable in immature brain (Watanabe *et al.* 1980).

The above classification also has an excellent correlation with heart-rate

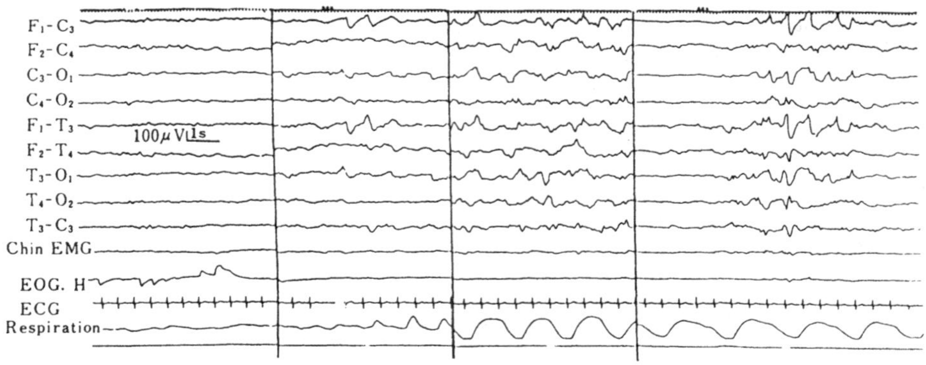

Fig. 2.13. EEG illustrating minimal depression at 40 weeks PCA.

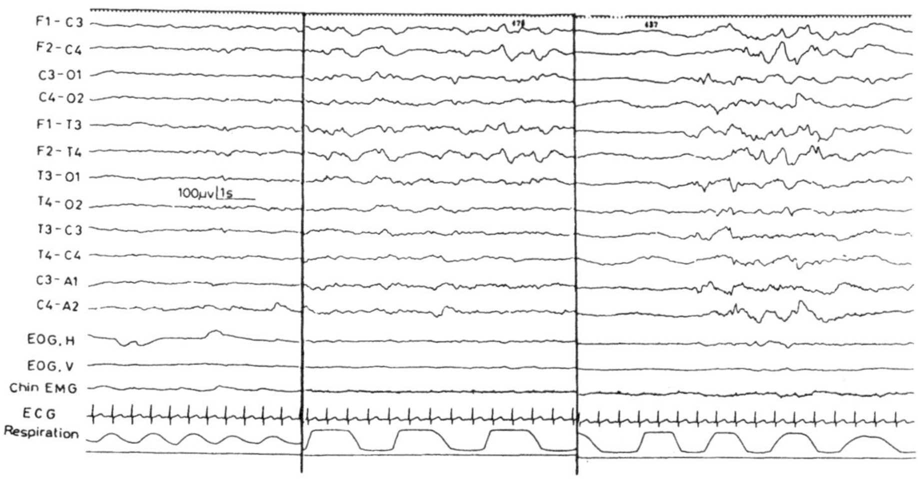

Fig. 2.14. EEG illustrating mild depression at 40 weeks PCA.

variability (Miyazaki *et al.* 1979) and neuroradiological findings (Watanabe *et al.* 1979). It is also correlated with the frequency of body movements during sleep (Hakamada *et al.* 1982).

Abnormalities of cyclic organisation of states have been reviewed by Lombroso (1985, 1987).

OTHER ABNORMALITIES

Low voltage represents background activity of 20 to 30µv or less in AS and 30 to 50µv or less in QS. This pattern is occasionally observed in the subacute stage of severe encephalopathy displaying maximally depressed EEG in the acute stage. Infants with this abnormality in the second week show a disturbed sleep cycle, although the two sleep states can be identified (Fig. 2.11). Low-voltage EEG may

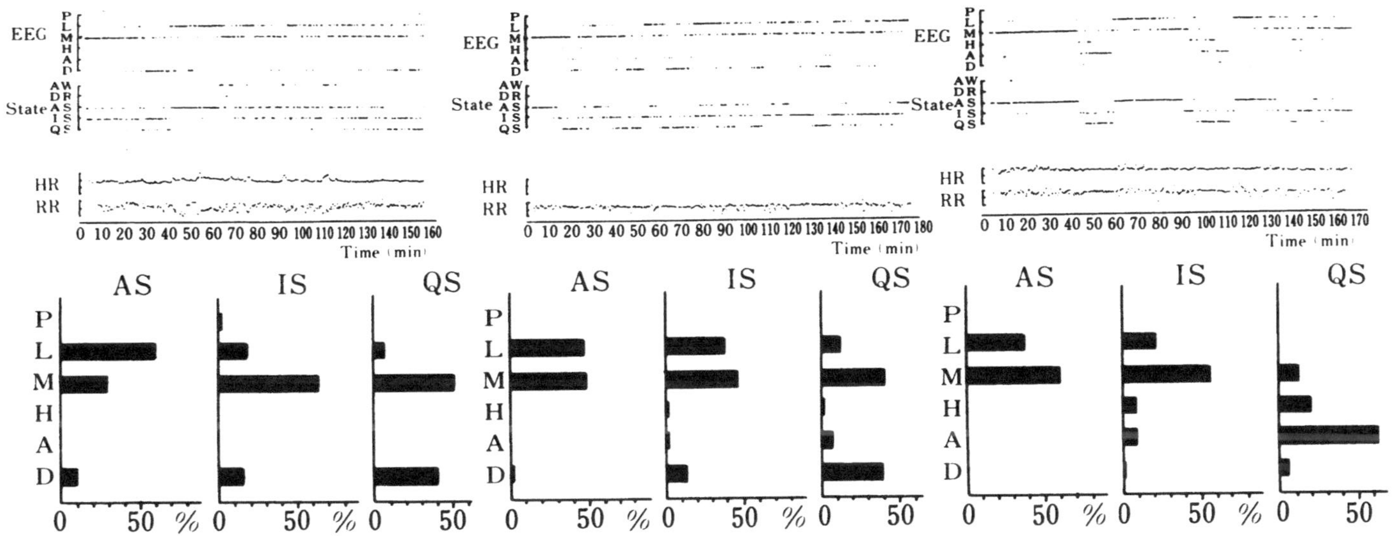

Fig. 2.15. Evolution of EEG and sleep cycles in term newborn infant with mild depression. *Left:* day 1, mild depression; *centre:* day 4, mild depression with slight improvement; *right:* day 7, almost normal. The EEG is classified according to Watanabe *et al.* (1980): F, flat pattern; P, very low-voltage activity; L, low-voltage irregular activity; M, medium-voltage slow activity; H, continuous high-voltage slow activity; A, trace alternant pattern; D, discontinuous pattern. State is classified: AW, awake; DR, drowsiness; AS, active sleep; QS, quiet sleep; IS, indeterminate sleep; HR, heart rate; RR, respiration rate.

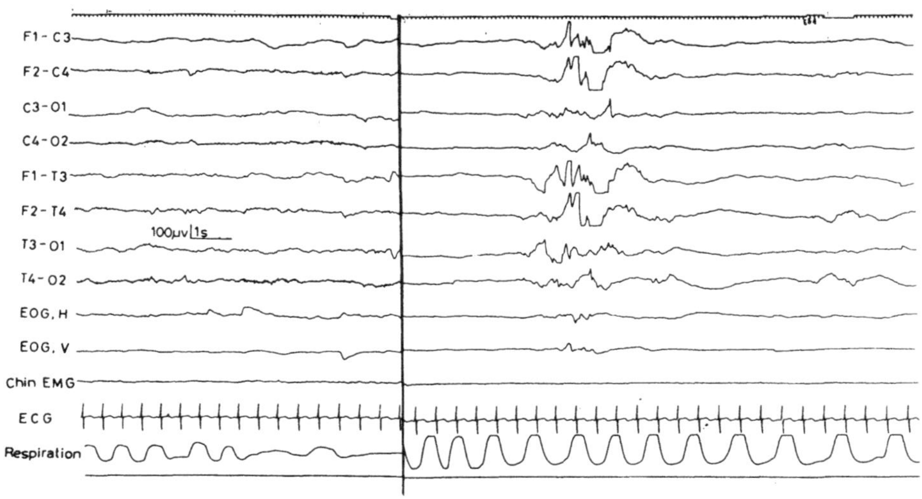

Fig. 2.16. EEG illustrating moderate depression at 40 weeks PCA.

also be observed in bilateral subdural haematoma, cephalhaematoma or iatrogenic causes such as scalp oedema due to leakage from intravenous infusion.

Increased theta and alpha waves and decreased delta waves with variable but mild degrees of background EEG depression are typically seen in hypocalcaemia (Watanabe *et al.* 1982*b*). They are occasionally observed in meningitis (Watanabe *et al.* 1983*b*) or perinatal hypoxia with varying degrees of background EEG depression.

High-voltage rhythmic theta and alpha. Almost continuous high- to medium-amplitude rhythmic alpha/theta activity during wakefulness, becoming discontinuous during QS, is typically seen in holoprosencephaly in the neonatal period (Watanabe *et al.* 1976).

Continuous, intermittent asynchronous delta activity without sleep cycles is observed in marked hydrocephalus (Watanabe *et al.* 1984*c*).

Low- to medium-voltage continuous activity with semirhythmic theta/alpha waves. Almost continuous theta-alpha waves without sleep cycles are infrequently seen in purulent meningitis (Watanabe *et al.* 1983*b*) or intracranial haemorrhage (Watanabe *et al.* 1981). In such cases, subclinical or clinical status epilepticus is often an additional feature.

Periodic bursts of high-amplitude slow waves mixed with sharp waves and of 2 to 4s duration alternate with periods of very attenuated activity of one to three seconds duration. This is characteristic of Ohtahara syndrome (Ohtahara 1978).

Interhemispheric amplitude asymmetry is an invariant voltage asymmetry of more than 50 per cent between hemispheres, and is observed in underlying structural lesions such as an infarct, haemorrhage, or porencephalic cyst. Cephalhaematoma, iatrogenic scalp oedema and technical faults should be excluded.

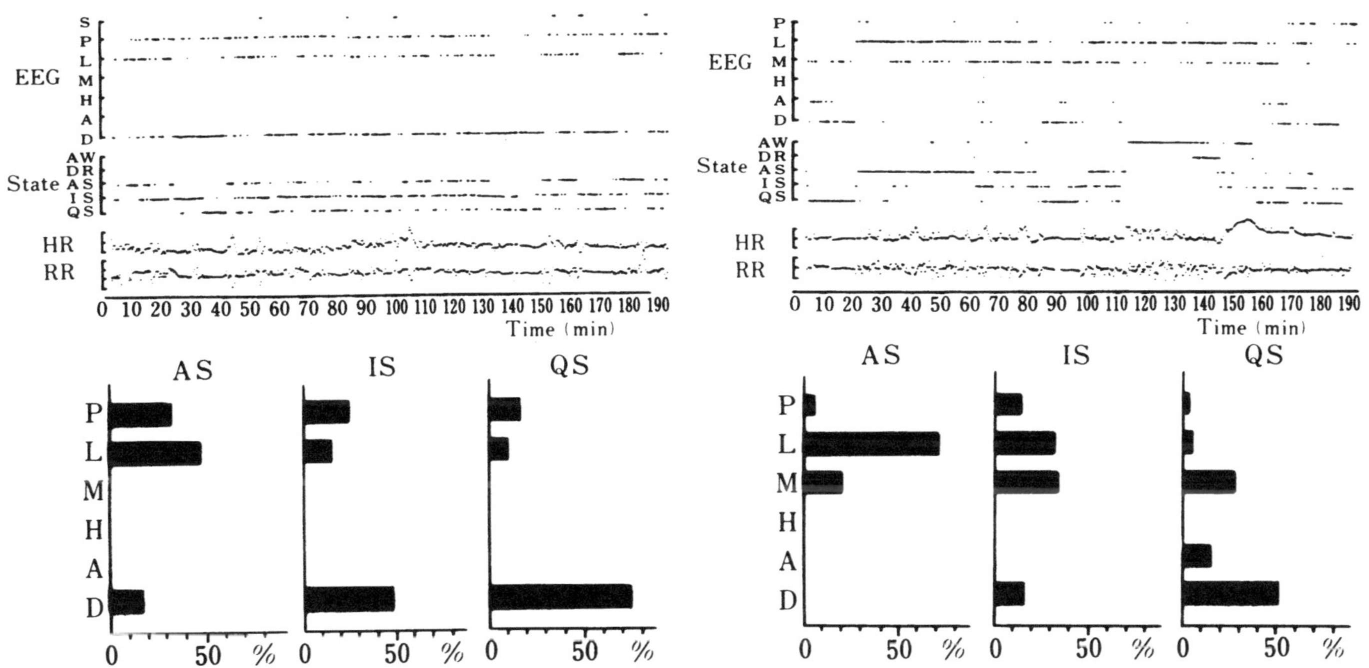

Fig. 2.17. Evolution of EEG and sleep cycles in a term newborn infant with moderate depression. *Left:* day 4, moderate depression; *right:* day 7, mild depression. The EEG is classified according to Watanabe *et al.* (1980): F, flat pattern; P, very low-voltage activity; L, low-voltage irregular activity; M, medium-voltage slow-wave activity; H, continuous high-voltage slow-wave activity; A, trace alternant pattern; D, discontinuous pattern. Sleep state is classified: AW, awake; DR, drowsiness; AS, active sleep; QS, quiet sleep; IS, indeterminate sleep; HR, heart rate; RR, respiration rate.

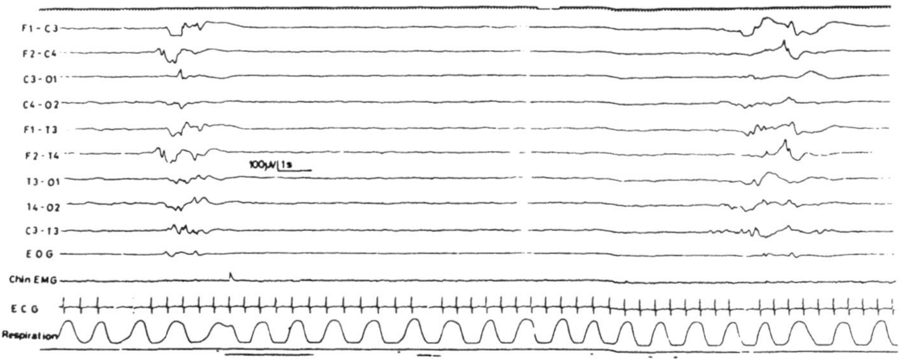

Fig. 2.18. EEG illustrating marked depression at 40 weeks PCA.

Interhemispheric asynchrony is often a feature of hydrocephalus (Watanabe *et al.* 1984*c*), but is seen in other pathological conditions such as hypoxic-ischaemic encephalopathy together with other features.

Dysmature pattern, where the term dysmaturity is used to denote the presence of EEG features inappropriate for a baby's PCA: EEG features immature for PCA in certain stages of sleep are usually observed in prenatal encephalopathy or the chronic stage of hypoxic-ischaemic encephalopathy of the preterm newborn infant. The significance of this pattern has been extensively reviewed by Lombroso (1985) and stressed by Tharp (1989). Transient dysmaturity is usually associated with good neurological outcome but persistence with poor outcome. The presence of immature EEG in all states usually indicates miscalculation of PCA because of a mother's irregular menstrual cycle.

Diffusely slow pattern, which is rare, consists of diffuse and continuously slow activity without reactivity. Persistence beyond two weeks indicates a poor neurological outcome for the infant (Coen and Tharp 1985).

Paroxysmal abnormalities

Interictal spikes or sharp waves are not as significant as in older children in the diagnosis of seizure disorders in neonates. They are often observed in normal newborn infants (Statz *et al.* 1982, Rowe *et al.* 1985). Their frequency may be of some help in the confirmation of seizures (Hughes *et al.* 1983*a*,*b*). Transient spikes or sharp waves seen in term infants are sporadic in appearance, non-repetitive in nature and occur mostly multifocally with parietal predominance (Statz *et al.* 1982). They are more frequent in QS (1/2.3min on average) than in AS (1/18min on average) and are rare in IS (1/hr).

Ictal discharges are more important for the diagnosis of subtle, atypical or subclinical seizures (Staudt *et al.* 1981; Coen *et al.* 1982; Eyre *et al.* 1983; Clancy *et al.* 1987, 1988; Scher *et al.* 1989) and usually display a progressive evolution of discharges (Lombroso 1985, Clancy 1989) except in myoclonic seizures and brief

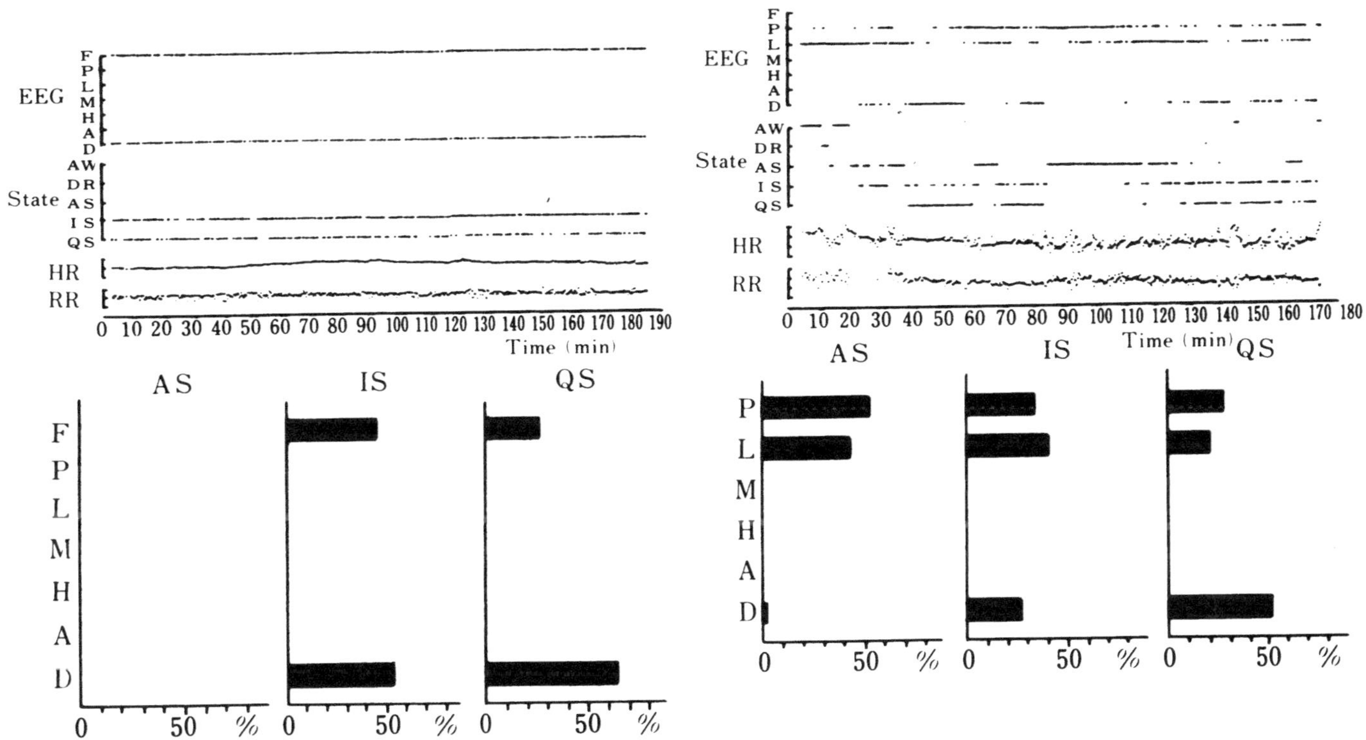

Fig. 2.19. Evolution of EEG and sleep cycle in a term newborn infant with marked depression. *Left:* day 4, marked depression; *right:* day 12, moderate depression. The EEG is classified according to Watanabe *et al.* (1980): F, flat pattern; P, very low-voltage activity; L, low-voltage irregular activity; M, medium-voltage slow-wave activity; H, continuous high-voltage slow-wave activity; A, trace alternant pattern; D, discontinuous pattern. Sleep state is classified: AW, awake; DR, drowsiness; AS, active sleep; QS, quiet sleep; IS, indeterminate sleep; HR, heart rate; RR, respiration rate.

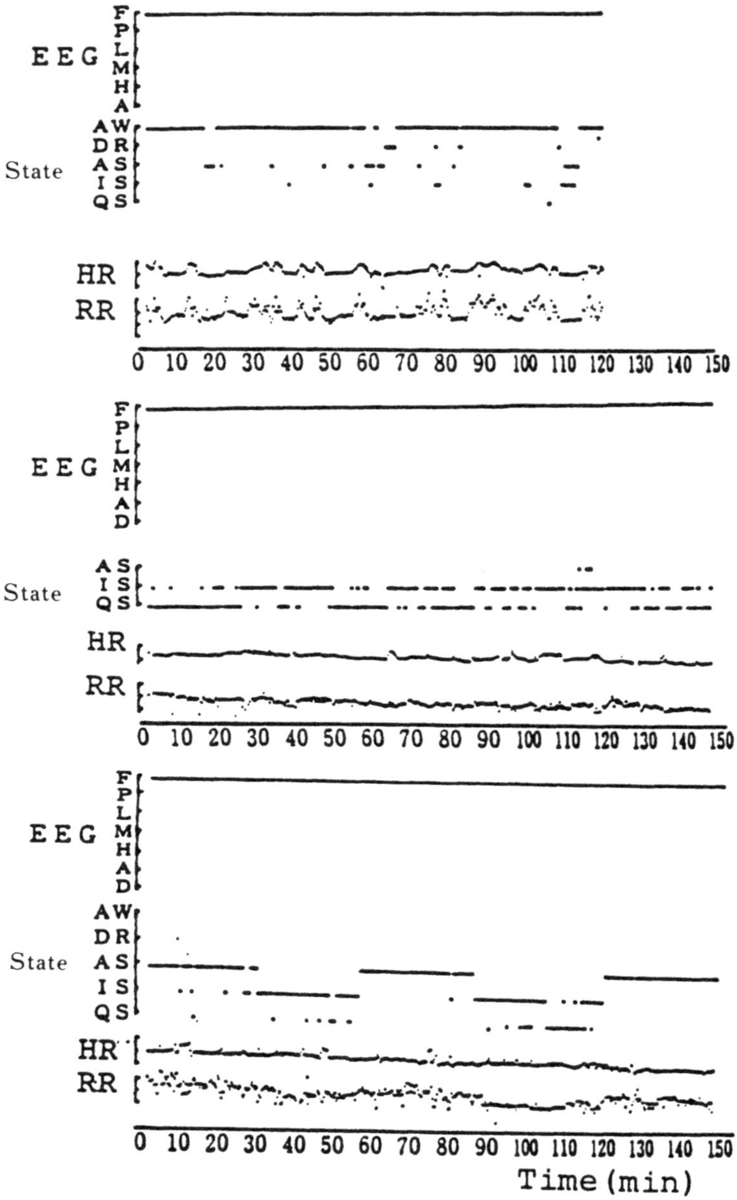

Fig. 2.20. Evolution of EEG and sleep cycles in a term newborn infant with maximal depression. *Top:* day 1, maximal depression; *centre:* day 8, maximal depression; *bottom:* day 15, maximal depression with return of sleep cycles. The EEG is classified according to Watanabe *et al.* (1980): F, flat pattern; P, very low-voltage activity; L, low-voltage irregular activity; M, medium-voltage slow-wave activity; H, continuous high-voltage slow-wave activity; A, trace alternant pattern; D, discontinuous pattern. Sleep state is classified: AW, awake; DR, drowsiness; AS, active sleep; QS, quiet sleep; IS, indeterminate sleep; HR, heart rate; RR, respiration rate.

tonic spasms. They usually begin as low-voltage, rhythmic or sinusoidal waveforms, spikes or sharp waves, and increase in amplitude and decrease in frequency (Clancy 1989), but the frequency of the discharges increases when they begin as slow waves. Rhythmic delta, theta or alpha activities are frequently seen (Watanabe *et al.* 1977, 1982*a*, 1984*b*; Lombroso 1985). On the basis of EEG/polygraphic/video monitoring, Mizrahi and Kellaway (1987) concluded that focal clonic seizures, some form of myoclonic seizures, and focal tonic seizures were consistently associated with electrical seizure activity; but most subtle seizures, all generalised tonic seizures and some forms of myoclonic seizures were either not associated with seizure activity or had an inconsistent relationship with such activity. The significance of EEG in the diagnosis of neonatal seizures has been extensively reviewed recently by Shewmon (1990).

Neonatal EEG and neurological prognosis in the term newborn infant

In perinatal encephalopathy, the background EEGS are closely correlated with the degree of later neurological sequelae (Monod *et al.* 1972, Watanabe *et al.* 1980, Holmes *et al.* 1982, Lombroso 1985, Pezzani *et al.* 1986, Takeuchi *et al.* 1987*b*, Grigg-Damberger *et al.* 1989) but have a different prognostic significance depending on the time of EEG recording (Takeuchi and Watanabe 1989). Normal background EEG before the seventh day, minimal depression before the fourth day, and mild depression before the second day are associated with favourable outcome. On the other hand, marked or maximal depression on any day, moderate depression after the seventh day and mild depression after the 12th day are associated with unfavourable outcome. Neonatal background EEGS are also correlated with the evolution of the EEG in infancy (Hakamada *et al.* 1980). The presence of paroxysmal activities is often correlated with adverse outcomes but is not as highly significant as background EEGS (Rowe *et al.* 1985). Periodic lateralised epileptiform discharges lack diagnostic specificity, but when associated with neonatal asphyxia, may carry a poor prognosis (McCutchen *et al.* 1985).

Abnormal EEGS in the preterm newborn infant

Various classification systems have been reported for abnormal EEGS of the preterm infant (Clancy *et al.* 1984, Lacey *et al.* 1986, Radvanyi-Bouvet *et al.* 1987, Ellison *et al.* 1989), but they all have inherent difficulties. The absolute definition of normality is difficult because preterm delivery itself is an abnormal event. The classification of abnormal EEGS of the preterm infant must cover a long period of postnatal life during which the EEG undergoes a rapid maturational change, and various types of acute and chronic postnatal brain insult may occur in addition to prenatal and perinatal ones. It should also take into consideration not only EEG alterations in the acute stage of brain damage but also those of the subacute and chronic stage. Serial recordings are even more useful in preterm infants than in term infants.

Background EEG *abnormalities mainly seen in the acute stage*

The EEG abnormality of the acute stage of brain insults is usually assessed by the degree of increased discontinuity, which is evaluated by visual inspection (Watanabe *et al.* 1983*a*, Clancy *et al.* 1984) or quantitative analysis (Watanabe *et al.* 1984*a*; Takeuchi *et al.* 1987*a*; Tharp 1987; Connell *et al.* 1987*b*, 1988; Benda *et al.* 1989).

MINIMAL DEPRESSION

Superimposed alpha/beta activities such as delta brushes are attenuated, although the continuity is not affected.

MILD DEPRESSION

This shows a slight increase of discontinuity before 32 weeks PCA, an increase of discontinuous patterns in AS and a slight increase of discontinuity in QS after 31 weeks PCA.

MODERATE DEPRESSION

This displays a moderate increase of discontinuity with decreased continuous pattern before 32 weeks PCA. After 31 weeks both continuous and discontinuous patterns are seen, with the latter more predominant than the former, and the sleep cycle is moderately disrupted with poor correlation between sleep states and EEG patterns.

MARKED DEPRESSION

This exhibits a burst-suppression pattern with very long interburst intervals and loss of sleep cycles and reactivity.

MAXIMAL DEPRESSION

This shows a flat EEG without sleep cycles and reactivity.

OTHER FINDINGS

Delta activities only exhibit loss of alpha/beta and theta activities leaving only delta waves. The EEG also shows increased discontinuity but this is more severe than when increased discontinuity occurs alone.

A hypoactive pattern is a poorly organised low-voltage activity of less than 20 to 50μv with some 50 to 100μv delta waves. This is a severe abnormality.

Relatively low-voltage delta activities show delta waves less than 200μv in infants younger than 30 weeks PCA and less than 150μv in infants older than 29 weeks PCA.

Background EEG *abnormalities seen mainly in subacute and chronic stage*

DISORGANISED PATTERN (Fig. 2.21)

This denotes decomposition of normal background EEG and deformation of normal

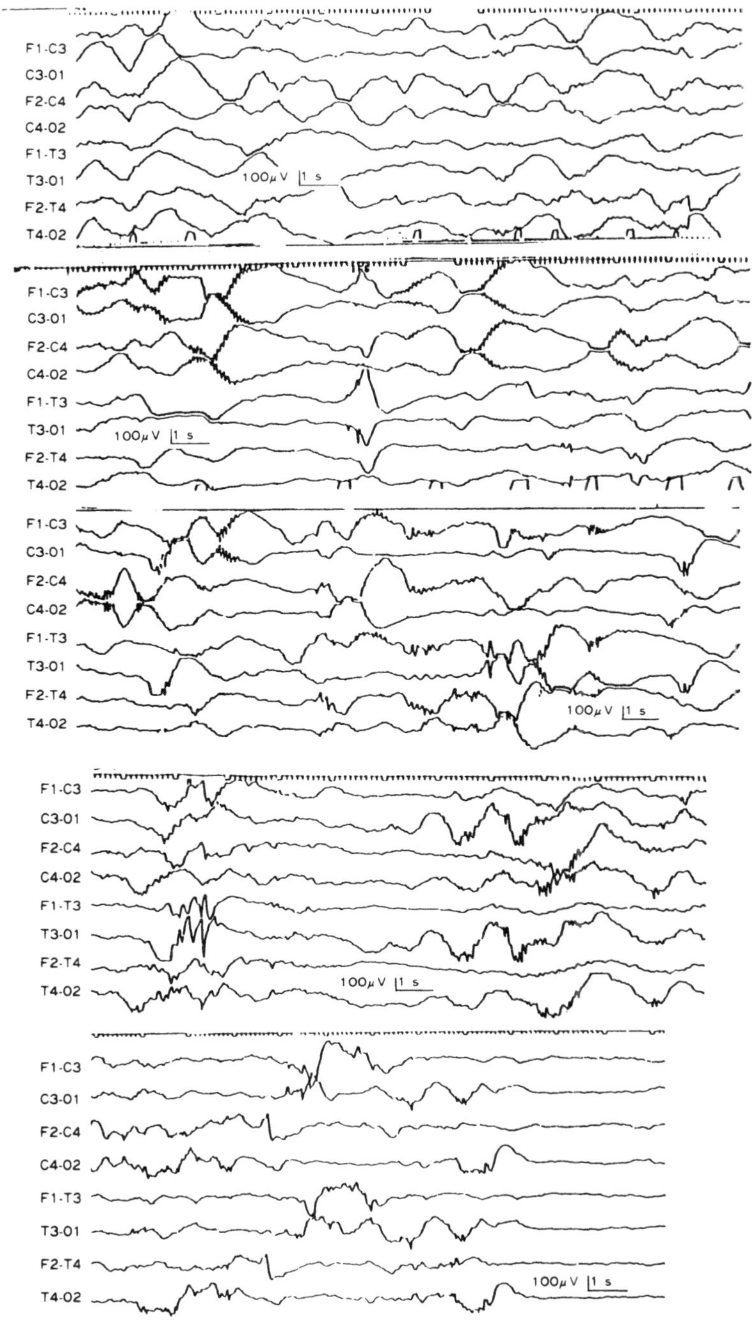

Fig. 2.21. EEGs illustrating disorganised patterns at (*top to bottom*): 30 weeks, 31 weeks, 34 weeks, 36 weeks and 40 weeks PCA.

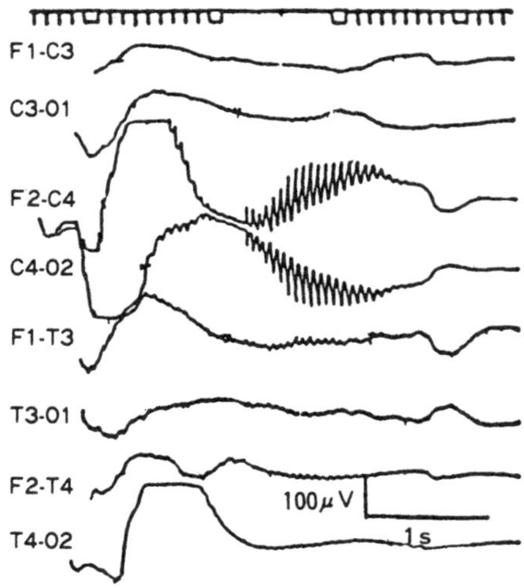

Fig. 2.22. EEG illustrating mechanical brushes on leads F_2–C_4 and C_4–O_2.

waveform without gross abnormality in continuity (Hayakawa *et al.* 1992). This pattern often follows severe depression of background EEG, and is closely associated with deep white matter injury and later occurrence of cerebral palsy.

DYSMATURE PATTERN

This is the presence of patterns immature for PCA, *i.e.* the presence of very high-voltage ultraslow waves and high-voltage temporal theta bursts after 33 weeks, delta brushes after 39 weeks, discontinuous tracing after 39 weeks, or a poor development of mature HVS pattern after 39 weeks PCA. This pattern often follows prolonged mild depression (Hayakawa *et al.* 1991), and is often associated with bronchopulmonary dysplasia (Hahn and Tharp 1990) and later occurrence of mental impairment (Hayakawa *et al.* 1992).

POSITIVE ROLANDIC SHARP WAVES

Since the first description by Cukier *et al.* (1972), there have been many studies on this waveform which was initially thought to be associated with intraventricular haemorrhage (Blume 1982, Clancy and Tharp 1984, Lombroso 1985, Marret *et al.* 1986, Novotny *et al.* 1987, Scher 1988). They are now known to be characteristic in infants with periventricular leukomalacia and usually appear several days or longer after the hypoxic-ischaemic event. They are highly specific but not sensitive for white matter lesions (Aso *et al.* 1989).

Background EEG abnormalities seen in any stage

INTERHEMISPHERIC ASYMMETRY AND ASYNCHRONY

Asynchrony is not necessarily associated with asymmetry, whereas asymmetry often occurs with asynchrony. In the acute stage, both are often associated with

TABLE 2.II
Abnormal background EEGs in the preterm infant

	Acute stage	*Subacute, chronic stage*
Mildly abnormal	Minimal depression Mild depression Relatively low-voltage delta waves	Mildly disorganised pattern in subacute stage Mild dysmaturity
Moderately abnormal	Moderate depression	Mildly disorganised pattern in chronic stage Moderate dysmaturity Mild interhemispheric asynchrony/asymmetry
Markedly abnormal	Marked depression Maximal depression Delta activity only Hypoactive pattern Definite interhemispheric asynchrony/asymmetry	Markedly disorganised pattern Marked dysmaturity Marked interhemispheric asynchrony/asymmetry Positive Rolandic sharp waves

other abnormalities such as varying degrees of depression, and in the chronic stage with disorganised or dysmature patterns.

MECHANICAL BRUSHES (Fig. 2.22)
These waves resemble cogs and are superimposed on slow waves, and are considered to be deformed delta brushes. They are usually associated with severe abnormalities such as moderate depression, positive Rolandic sharp waves, or disorganised pattern. A neonate with this pattern has a poor neurological prognosis.

Serial recordings
Serial recordings from soon after birth until around term may enable one to determine the time of brain insult (Tharp 1987, Connell *et al.* 1988, Tharp *et al.* 1989, Watanabe *et al.* 1989).

Prenatal onset of brain damage may be suspected when the EEG soon after birth already shows findings suggestive of chronic brain damage such as disorganised pattern without displaying signs of acute depression.

Perinatal injury may be most likely if the EEG soon after birth exhibits signs of acute depression without findings suggestive of chronic brain damage.

In postnatal brain damage, the EEG initially displays no signs of acute depression nor of chronic brain damage, but demonstrates those of acute depression during the postnatal course. EEG findings suggestive of a chronic stage of brain damage appear later when signs of acute depression begin to disappear.

Mild but sustained brain insults such as those due to chronic lung disease may not produce definite signs of acute brain damage, but may result in the insidious occurrence of findings suggestive of chronic brain damage in the follow-up EEGS, especially a dysmature pattern.

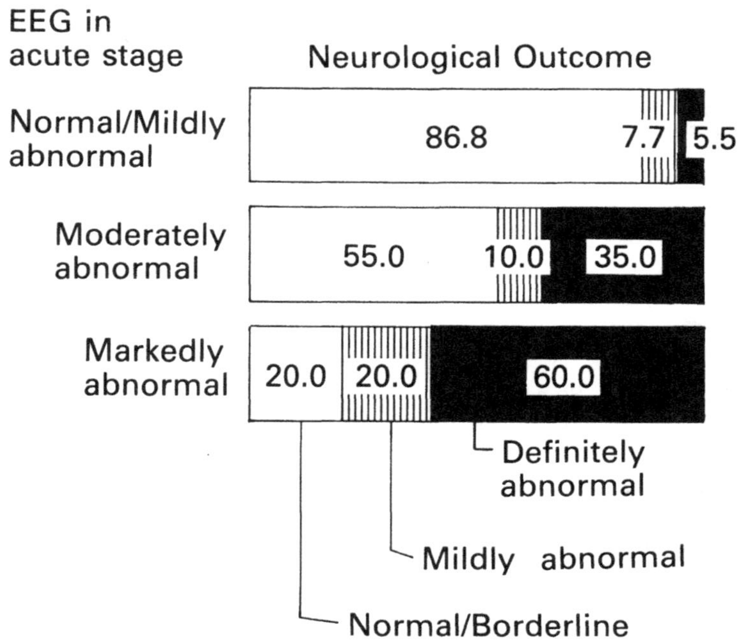

Fig. 2.23. The relationship between EEG in the acute stage of the illness in preterm babies and neurological outcome in surviving infants.

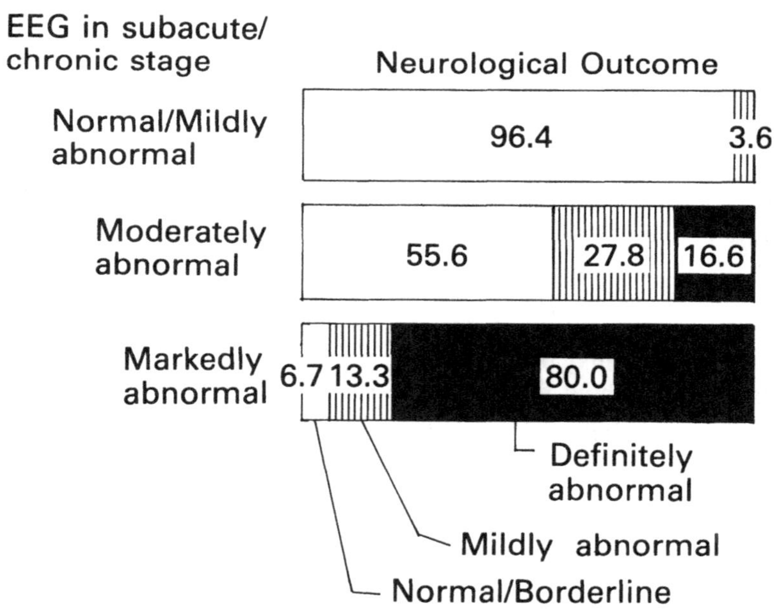

Fig. 2.24. The relationship between the EEG in the subacute and chronic stage of the illness in preterm babies and neurological outcome in surviving infants.

Neonatal EEGs and neurological prognosis in the preterm newborn infant

Serial EEG recordings are a useful prognostic tool (Hayakawa *et al.* 1988, Tharp *et al.* 1989, Watanabe *et al.* 1989). The above EEG abnormalities were categorised into three grades for prognostic purposes (Table 2.II). Most neonates whose worst EEG during the whole postnatal period (birth to full term) showed normal or mild abnormalities, more than half of those whose worst EEG displayed moderate abnormalities, but only a few of those whose worst EEG demonstrated marked abnormalities, developed normally or nearly normally. For the preterm infant, abnormal EEG findings in the subacute and chronic stage were of more prognostic significance than those in the acute stage of brain insult (Figs 2.23, 2.24). This is in contrast to the situation in term neonates in whom the EEG in the first week of life is the most useful.

The effect of delivery and medication on the EEG

The EEG on day 0 may show transient depression, but soon recovers to display normal background on day 1. This may be due to stress associated with delivery.

There has been no systematic study on the effect of medication on the neonatal EEG. Some anticonvulsant drugs evoke fast-wave activity in older children but not in the newborn infant. Usual therapeutic doses of anticonvulsants are not considered to produce definite alteration of EEG (Staudt *et al.* 1982, Bjerre *et al.* 1983, Radvanyi-Bouvet *et al.* 1985), although phenobarbitone was shown to prolong QS (Gabriel and Albani 1977). Intravenous administration of diazepam or phenobarbitone may produce transient suppression of the EEG. We observed that intravenous administration of 10 to 20mg/kg of phenobarbitone for the purpose of prevention of intraventricular haemorrhage in the preterm infant resulted in increased discontinuity lasting 60 to 90 minutes (Fig. 2.9).

Paroxysmal abnormalities in the preterm newborn infant

Paroxysmal abnormalities of the preterm neonate are not basically different from those of the term neonate (Radvanyi-Bouvet *et al.* 1985). There are many sharp transients in the interictal EEGs of the preterm infant and the value of interictal EEG in the confirmation of seizures is not high. The presence of definite ictal discharges usually indicates a severe abnormality.

REFERENCES

American Electroencephalographic Society (1986) 'Guidelines in EEG, 1–7 (Revised 1985).' *Journal of Clinical Neurophysiology*, **3**, 131–168.

Anders, T., Emde, R., Parmelee, A.H. (1971) *A Manual of Standardised Terminology, Techniques, and Criteria for Scoring States of Sleep and Wakefulness in Newborn Infants.* Los Angeles: UCLA Brain Information Service/ BRI Publications Office.

Anderson, C.M., Torres, F., Faoro, A. (1985) 'The EEG of the early premature.' *Electroencephalography and Clinical Neurophysiology*, **60**, 95–105.

Archbald, F., Verma, U.L., Tejani, N.A., Handwerker, S.M. (1984) 'Cerebral function monitor in the neonate. II: Birth asphyxia.' *Developmental Medicine and Child Neurology*, **26**, 162–168.

Aso, K., Scher, M.S., Barmada, M.A. (1989) 'Neonatal electroencephalography and neuropathology.' *Journal of Clinical Neurophysiology*, **6**, 103–123.

Benda, G.I., Engel, R.C.H., Zhang, Y. (1989) 'Prolonged inactive phases during the discontinuous pattern of prematurity in the electroencephalogram of very-low-birthweight infants.' *Electroencephalography and Clinical Neurophysiology*, **72**, 189–197.

Bjerre, I., Hellstrom-Westas, L., Rosen, I., Svenningsen, N. (1983) 'Monitoring of cerebral function after severe asphyxia in infancy.' *Archives of Disease in Childhood*, **58**, 997–1002.

Blume, W.T., Dreyfus-Brisac, C. (1982) 'Positive rolandic sharp waves in neonatal EEG: types and significance.' *Electroencephalography and Clinical Neurophysiology*, **53**, 277–282.

Bridges, S.L., Ebersole, J.S., Ment, L.R., Ehrenkrantz, R.A., Silva, C.G. (1986) 'Cassette electroencephalography in the evaluation of neonatal seizures.' *Archives of Neurology*, **43**, 49–51.

Clancy, R.R. (1989) 'Neonatal seizures.' *In* Stevenson, D.K., Sunshine, P. (Eds) *Fetal and Neonatal Brain Injury*. Toronto: B.C. Decker. pp. 123–140.

—— Tharp, B.R. (1984) 'Positive rolandic sharp waves in the electroencephalograms of premature neonates with intraventricular hemorrhage.' *Electroencephalography and Clinical Neurophysiology*, **57**, 395–404.

—— —— Enzman, D. (1984) 'EEG in premature infants with intraventricular hemorrhage.' *Neurology*, **34**, 583–590.

—— Legido, A. (1987) 'The exact ictal and interictal duration of electroencephalographic neonatal seizures.' *Epilepsia*, **28**, 537–541.

—— —— Lewis, D. (1988) 'Occult neonatal seizures.' *Epilepsia*, **29**, 256–261.

Coen, R.W., McCutchen, C.B., Werner, D., Snyder, J., Gluck, F.E. (1982) 'Continuous monitoring of the electroencephalogram following perinatal asphyxia.' *Journal of Pediatrics*, **100**, 628–630.

—— Tharp, B.R. (1985) 'Neonatal electroencephalography.' *Advances in Perinatal Medicine*, **4**, 267–297.

Connell, J.A., Oozeer, R., Dubowitz, V. (1987*a*) 'Continuous 4-channel EEG monitoring: a guide to interpretation, with normal values, in preterm infants.' *Neuropediatrics*, **18**, 138–145.

—— —— Regev, R., de Vries, L.S., Dubowitz, L.M.S., Dubowitz, V. (1987*b*) 'Continuous 4-channel EEG monitoring in the evaluation of echodense ultrasound lesions and cystic leucomalacia.' *Archives of Disease in Childhood*, **62**, 1019–1024.

—— —— (1988) 'Neonatal electro-encephalography.' *In* Levene, M.I., Bennett, M.J., Punt, J. (Eds) *Fetal and Neonatal Neurology and Neurosurgery*. Edinburgh: Churchill Livingstone. pp. 177–190.

—— de Vries, L., Oozeer, R., Regev, R., Dubowitz, L.M.S., Dubowitz, V. (1988) 'Predictive value of early continuous electroencephalogram monitoring in ventilated preterm infants with intraventricular hemorrhage.' *Pediatrics*, **82**, 337–343.

—— Oozeer, R., de Vries, L., Dubowitz, L.M.S., Dubowitz, V. (1989*a*) 'Continuous EEG monitoring and prognostic considerations.' *Archives of Disease in Childhood*, **64**, 452–458.

—— —— —— —— —— (1989*b*) 'Clinical and EEG response to anticonvulsants in neonatal seizures.' *Archives of Disease in Childhood*, **64**, 459–464.

Cukier, F., Andre, M., Dreyfus-Brisac, C. (1972) 'Apport de l'EEG au diagnostic des hemorragies intra-ventriculaires du premature.' *Revue d'Electroencephalographie et de Neurophysiologie Clinique*, **2**, 318–322.

Curzi-Dascalova, L., Peirano, P., Morel-Kahn, F. (1988) 'Development of sleep states in normal premature and full-term newborns.' *Developmental Psychobiology*, **21**, 431–444.

Dreyfus-Brisac, C. (1979) 'Neonatal electroencephalography.' *Reviews in Perinatal Medicine*, **3**, 397–471.

Ellingson, R.J., Peters, J.F. (1980) 'Development of EEG and daytime sleep patterns in normal fullterm infants during the first three months of life: longitudinal observations.' *Electroencephalography and Clinical Neurophysiology*, **49**, 112–124.

Ellison, P., Franklin, S., Brown, P., Jones, M.G. (1989) 'The evolution of a simplified method for interpretation of EEG in the preterm neonate.' *Acta Paediatrica Scandinavica*, **78**, 210–216.

Engel, R. (1975) *Abnormal Electroencephalograms in the Neonatal Period*. Springfield, IL: C.C. Thomas.

Eyre, J.A., Oozeer, R.C., Wilkinson, A.R. (1983) 'Diagnosis of neonatal seizures by the continuous recording and rapid analysis of the electroencephalogram.' *Archives of Disease in Childhood*, **58**, 785–790.

—— Nanei, S., Wilkinson, A.R. (1988) 'Quantification of changes in normal neonatal EEGs with gestation from continuous five-day recordings.' *Developmental Medicine and Child Neurology*, **30**,

599–607.
Gabriel, M., Albani, M. (1977) 'Rapid eye movement sleep, apnea and cardiac slowing influenced by phenobarbital administration in the neonate.' *Pediatrics*, **60**, 426–430.
Greisen, G., Hellstrom-Westas, L., Lou, H., Rosen, I., Svenningsen, N.W. (1987) 'EEG depression and germinal layer hemorrhage in the newborn.' *Acta Paediatrica Scandinavica*, **76**, 519–525.
—— Pryds, O. (1989) 'Low CBF, discontinuous EEG activity, and periventricular brain injury in ill, preterm neonates.' *Brain and Development*, **11**, 164–168.
Grigg-Damberger, M.M., Coker, S.B., Halsey, C.L., Anderson, C.L. (1989) 'Neonatal burst suppression: its developmental significance.' *Pediatric Neurology*, **5**, 84–92.
Hakamada, S., Watanabe, K., Hara, K., Miyazaki, S. (1980) 'The evolution of some EEG features in normal and abnormal infants.' *Brain and Development*, **2**, 373–377.
—— —— —— —— Kumagai, T. (1982) 'Body movements during sleep in full-term newborn infants.' *Brain and Development*, **4**, 51–55.
Hayakawa, F., Watanabe, K., Hakamada, S., Kuno, K., Aso, K. (1987) 'Fz theta/alpha bursts: a transient EEG pattern in healthy newborns.' *Electroencephalography and Clinical Neurophysiology*, **67**, 27–31.
—— Kuno, K., Watanabe, K. (1988) 'Intracranial lesions and outcome of very low-birthweight infants. Clinical significance of EEG.' *Shonika Rinsho*, **41**, 1801–1805.
—— Watanabe, K., Kuno, K. (1991) 'Evaluation of serial EEG recordings and auditory brainstem responses in early preterm infants.' *No To Hattatsu*, **24**, *in press.*
Holmes, G., Rowe, J., Hafford, J., Schmidt, R., Testa, M., Zimmerman, A. (1982) 'Prognostic value of the electroencephalogram in neonatal asphyxia.' *Electroencephalography and Clinical Neurophysiology*, **53**, 60–72.
—— —— —— (1983) 'Significance of reactive burst suppression following asphyxia in full term infants.' *Clinical Electroencephalography*, **14**, 138–141.
Hughes, J.R., Fino, J., Gagnon, L. (1983*a*) 'Periods of activity and quiescence in the premature EEG.' *Neuropediatrics*, **14**, 66–72.
—— —— —— (1983*b*) 'The use of electroencephalogram in the confirmation of seizures in premature and neonatal infants.' *Neuropediatrics*, **14**, 213–219.
—— —— Hart, L.A. (1987) 'Premature temporal theta (PTθ).' *Electroencephalography and Clinical Neurophysiology*, **67**, 7–15.
Inokuma, K., Watanabe, K., Negoro, T. (1984) 'Developmental changes of topographic EEG features in the newborn.' *No To Hattatsu*, **16**, 371–380.
Karbowski, K., Nencka, A. (1980) 'Right mid-temporal sharp EEG transients in healthy newborns.' *Electroencephalography and Clinical Neurophysiology*, **48**, 461–469.
Karch, D., Rothe, R., Jurisch, R., Heldt-Hildebrandt, R., Lubbesmeier, A., Lemburg, P. (1982) 'Behavioral changes and bioelectric brain maturation of preterm and fullterm newborn infants: a polygraphic study.' *Developmental Medicine and Child Neurology*, **24**, 30–47.
Lacey, D.J., Topper, W.H., Buckwald, S., Zorn, W.A., Berger, P.E. (1986) 'Preterm very-low-birthweight neonates: relationship of EEG to intracranial hemorrhage, perinatal complications, and developmental outcome.' *Neurology*, **34**, 1084–1087.
Lombroso, C.T. (1985) 'Neonatal polygraphy in full-term and premature infants: a review of normal and abnormal findings.' *Journal of Clinical Neurophysiology*, **2**, 105–155.
—— (1987) 'Neonatal electroencephalography.' *In* Niedermeyer, E., Lopes da Silva, F. (Eds) *Electroencephalography: Basic Principles, Clinical Applications, and Related Fields. 2nd Edn.* Baltimore, MD: Urban & Schwarzenberg. pp. 725–762.
Marret, S., Parain, D., Samson-Dollfus, D., Jeannot, E., Fessard, C. (1986) 'Positive rolandic sharp waves and periventricular leucomalacia in the newborn.' *Neuropediatrics*, **17**, 199–202.
McCutchen, C.B., Coen, R., Iragui, V.J. (1985) 'Periodic lateralized epileptiform discharges in asphyxiated neonates.' *Electroencephalography and Clinical Neurophysiology*, **61**, 210–217.
Miyazaki, S., Watanabe, K., Hara, K., Iwase, K. (1978) 'Quantitative analysis of the development of trace alternant in the EEGs of newborn infants.' *Rinsho Noha*, **20**, 38–42.
—— —— —— (1979) 'Heart rate variability in full-term normal and abnormal newborn infants during sleep.' *Brain and Development*, **1**, 57–60.
Mizrahi, E.M. (1986) 'Neonatal electroencephalography: clinical features of the newborn, techniques of recording, and characteristics of the normal EEG.' *American Journal of EEG Technology*, **26**,

81–103.
—— Kellaway, P. (1987) 'Characterization and classification of neonatal seizures.' *Neurology*, **37**, 1837–1844.
Monod, N., Pajot, N., Guidasci, S. (1972) 'The neonatal EEG: statistical studies and prognostic value in full-term and pre-term babies.' *Electroencephalography and Clinical Neurophysiology*, **32**, 529–544.
Nolte, R., Haas, G. (1978) 'A polygraphic study of bioelectric brain maturation in preterm infants.' *Developmental Medicine and Child Neurology*, **20**, 167–182.
Novontny, E.J. Jr., Tharp, B.R., Coen, R.W., Bejar, R., Enzmann, D., Vaucher, Y.E. (1987) 'Positive rolandic sharp waves in the EEG of the premature infant.' *Neurology*, **37**, 1481–1486.
Nowack, W.J., Janati, A., Angtvaco, T. (1989) 'Positive temporal sharp waves in neonatal EEG.' *Clinical Electroencephalography*, **20**, 196–201.
O'Brien, M.J., Lems, Y.L., Prechtl, H.F.R. (1987) 'Transient flattenings in the EEG of newborns—a benign variation.' *Electroencephalography and Clinical Neurophysiology*, **67**, 16–26.
Ohtahara, S. (1978) 'Clinico-electrical delineation of epileptic encephalopathies in childhood.' *Asian Medical Journal*, **21**, 7–17.
Parmelee, A.H., Schulte, F.J., Akiyama, Y., Wenner, W.H., Stern, E. (1968) 'The maturation of EEG activity during sleep in premature infants.' *Electroencephalography and Clinical Neurophysiology*, **24**, 319–329.
—— Akiyama, Y., Stern, E., Harris, M.A. (1969) 'Periodic cerebral rhythm in newborn infants.' *Experimental Neurology*, **25**, 575–584.
—— Stern, E. (1972) 'Development of states in infants.' *In* Clemente, C.D., Purpura, D., Mayer, F.E. (Eds) *Sleep and the Maturing Nervous System.* New York: Academic Press. pp. 199–215.
Pezzani, C., Radvanyi-Bouvet, M-F., Relier, J.P., Monod, N. (1986) 'Neonatal electroencephalography during the first twenty-four hours of life in full-term newborn infants.' *Neuropediatrics*, **17**, 11–18.
Radvanyi-Bouvet, M-F., Vallecalle, M.H., Morel-Kahn, F., Relier, J.P., Dreyfus-Brisac, C. (1985) 'Seizures and electrical discharges in premature infants.' *Neuropediatrics*, **16**, 143–148.
—— de Bethmann, O., Monset-Couchard, M., Fazzi, E. (1987) 'Cerebral lesions in early prematurity: EEG prognostic value in the neonatal period.' *Brain and Development*, **9**, 399–405.
Rowe, J.C., Holmes, G.L., Hafford, J., Baboval, D., Robinson, S., Philipps, A., Rosenkrantz, T., Raye, J. (1985) 'Prognostic value of the electroencephalogram in term and preterm infants following neonatal seizures.' *Electroencephalography and Clinical Neurophysiology*, **60**, 183–196.
Scher, M.S. (1988) 'Midline electrographic abnormalities and cerebral lesions in the newborn brain.' *Journal of Child Neurology*, **3**, 135–146.
—— Painter, M.J., Bergman, I., Barmada, M.A., Brunberg, J. (1989) 'EEG diagnoses of neonatal seizures: clinical correlations and outcome.' *Pediatric Neurology*, **5**, 17–24.
Shewmon, D.A. (1990) 'What is a neonatal seizure? Problems in definition and quantification for investigative and clinical purposes.' *Journal of Clinical Neurophysiology*, **7**, 315–368.
Statz, A., Dumermuth, G., Mieth, D., Duc, G. (1982) 'Transient EEG patterns during sleep in healthy newborns.' *Neuropediatrics*, **13**, 115–122.
Staudt, F., Roth, J.G., Engel, R.C. (1981) 'The usefulness of electroencephalography in curarised newborns.' *Electroencephalography and Clinical Neurophysiology*, **51**, 205–208.
—— Scholl, M.L., Coen, R.W., Bickford, R.W. (1982) 'Phenobarbital therapy in neonatal seizures and the prognostic value of the EEG.' *Neuropediatrics*, **13**, 24–33.
Takeuchi, T., Aso, K., Watanabe, K. (1987*a*) 'A semiquantitative analysis of the EEG of extremely premature newborns.' *No To Hattatsu*, **19**, 184–189.
—— Watanabe, K. (1987*b*) 'Background EEGs and neurological prognosis of newborns.' *No To Hattatsu*, **19**, 281–286.
—— —— (1989) 'The EEG evolution and neurological prognosis of neonates with perinatal hypoxia.' *Brain and Development*, **11**, 115–120.
Tharp, B.R. (1987) 'The electroencephalographic aspects of ischemic hypoxic encephalopathy and intraventricular hemorrhage.' *In* Yabuuchi, H., Watanabe, K., Okada, S. (Eds) *Neonatal Brain and Behavior.* Nagoya: Nagoya University Press. pp. 71–85.
—— (1989) 'Electroencephalography in the assessment of the premature and full-term infant.' *In* Stevenson, D.K., Sunshine, P. (Eds) *Fetal and Neonatal Brain Injury.* Toronto: B.C. Decker. pp. 123–140.

—— Scher, M.S., Clancy, R.R. (1989) 'Serial EEGs in normal and abnormal infants with birth weights less than 1200 grams—a prospective study with long-term follow-up.' *Neuropediatrics*, **20**, 64–72.

Torres, F., Anderson, C. (1985) 'The normal EEG of the human newborn.' *Journal of Clinical Neurophysiology*, **2**, 89–103.

Verma, U.L., Archbald, F., Tejani, N.A., Handwerker, S.M. (1984) 'Cerebral function monitor in the neonate. I: Normal patterns.' *Developmental Medicine and Child Neurology*, **26**, 154–161.

Viniker, D.A., Maynard, D.E., Scott, D.F. (1984) 'Cerebral function monitor studies in neonates.' *Clinical Electroencephalography*, **15**, 185–192.

Watanabe, K. (1978) 'Neurophysiological approaches to the normal and abnormal development of CNS in early life.' *Asian Medical Journal*, **21**, 421–450.

—— Iwase, K. (1972) 'Spindle-like fast rhythms in the EEGs of low-birthweight infants.' *Developmental Medicine and Child Neurology*, **14**, 373–381.

—— —— Hara, K. (1974) 'Development of slow-wave sleep in low-birthweight infants.' *Developmental Medicine and Child Neurology*, **16**, 23–31.

—— Hara, K., Iwase, K. (1976) 'The evolution of neurophysiological features in holoprosencephaly.' *Neuropädiatrie*, **7**, 19–41.

—— —— Miyazaki, S., Kuroyanagi, M., Asano, S., Kondo, K., Kuno, K., Jose, H., Iwase I.S. (1977) 'Electroclinical studies of seizures in the newborn.' *Folia Psychiatrica et Neurologica Japonica*, **31**, 383–392.

—— Miyazaki, S., Hara, K., Kuroyanagi, M., Yamamoto, T., Ito, M., Nakamura, S., Yamada, H. (1979) 'Neonatal EEG and computerized tomography.' *Neuropädiatrie*, **10**, 348–360.

—— —— —— Hakamada, S. (1980) 'Behavioral state cycles, background EEGs and prognosis of newborns with perinatal hypoxia.' *Electroencephalography and Clinical Neurophysiology*, **49**, 618–625.

—— Hara, K., Miyazaki, S. Hakamada, S., Kuroyanagi, M., Nakamura, S., Yamada, H. (1981) 'The value of EEG and cerebral evoked potentials in the assessment of intracranial hemorrhage.' *European Journal of Pediatrics*, **137**, 177–184.

—— —— —— —— (1982*a*) 'Rhythmic alpha discharges in the EEGs of the newborn.' *Clinical Electroencephalography*, **13**, 245–250.

—— —— —— —— (1982*b*) 'Neurophysiological study of newborns with hypocalcemia.' *Neuropediatrics*, **13**, 34–38.

—— Hakamada, S., Kuroyanagi, M., Yamazaki, T., Takeuchi, T. (1983*a*) 'Electroencephalographic study of intraventricular hemorrhage in the preterm newborn.' *Neuropediatrics*, **14**, 225–230.

—— Hara, K., Hakamada, S., Kuroyanagi, M., Kuno, K., Aso, K. (1983*b*) 'The prognostic value of EEG in neonatal meningitis.' *Clinical Electroencephalography*, **14**, 67–77.

—— Inokuma, K., Takeuchi, T., Aso, K. (1984*a*) 'Neurophysiology of neonates and sequelae of early brain damage.' *In* Arima, M., Suzuki, Y., Yabuuchi, H. (Eds) *The Developing Brain and its Disorders*. Tokyo: University of Tokyo Press. pp. 265–278.

—— Negoro, T., Inokuma, K., Yamazaki, T. (1984*b*) 'Subclinical delta status in the newborn—an unfavourable prognostic sign.' *Clinical Electroencephalography*, **15**, 125–131.

—— Yamada, H., Hara, K., Miyazaki, S., Nakamura, S. (1984*c*) 'Neurophysiological evaluation of newborns with congenital hydrocephalus.' *Clinical Electroencephalography*, **15**, 22–31.

—— Takeuchi, T., Hayakawa, F. (1987) 'Neonatal EEG and outcome.' *Rinshou Noha*, **29**, 19–24.

—— Hayakawa, F., Takeuchi, T. (1989) 'The evolution of EEG features before onset of childhood symptomatic epilepsy due to perinatal brain damage.' *In* Suzuki, J., Seino, M., Fukuyama, Y., Komai, S. (Eds) *Art and Science of Epilepsy*. Amsterdam: Elsevier. pp. 127–134.

Werner, S.S., Stockard, J.E., Bickford, R.G. (1977) *Atlas of Neonatal Electroencephalography*. New York: Raven Press.

3
MONITORING OF THE ELECTROENCEPHALOGRAM DURING INTENSIVE CARE

D. Murdoch Eaton, J. Connell, V. Dubowitz and L. Dubowitz

Continuous monitoring of various physiological functions (heart rate, respiratory rate and blood pressure) has become routine practice in neonatal intensive care. In contrast, cerebral activity is rarely adequately assessed. Continuous monitoring of cerebral function can help the early detection of impending abnormalities. The functional integrity of the brain is often compromised in sick neonates either because of primary neurological lesions or as a consequence of unstable physiology. There is no ideal method for cerebral surveillance in the neonatal intensive care situation. Despite limitations, the most direct and easily recorded information about neuronal function is still provided by electrophysiological techniques, including the electroencephalogram (EEG), which can provide a continuous and noninvasive means of recording neuronal function.

Methods available

Conventional multichannel EEG recording

This provides simultaneous recordings from multiple cerebral foci to provide information not only about general background activity but also about topographical distribution and characteristics of focal discharges. The technique is well described and evaluated in standard references (Werner *et al.* 1977) and in the previous chapter. Prolonged polygraphic EEG recordings at the cotside, with simultaneous video monitoring, have been performed to characterise and classify neonatal seizures (Shewmon 1983, Mizrahi and Kellaway 1987). However, despite its acknowledged value, a number of factors have limited its prolonged application in neonatal intensive care.

1. There is a high propensity to electrical interference encountered from other multiple electronic monitoring devices present.

2. The application of a large number of electrodes to the relatively small scalp area available requires prolonged handling of those infants least able to tolerate it, and may impede access for scalp vein infusions or ultrasonographic investigation.

3. Its relative bulk can impede access to the acutely ill neonate.

4. The generation of so many bulky EEG recordings makes interpretation an overwhelming task for the trained interpreter required.

Continuous ambulatory cassette EEG *monitors (Medilog)*

The Medilog was designed for continuous EEG monitoring of adults and young children and comprises a small battery-powered four- or eight-channel tape recorder, two channels of which can be allocated to electrocardiogram (ECG) and a time signal or thoracic impedance. Eyre *et al.* (1983) demonstrated that it was easily applicable to neonatal intensive care units. This allows monitoring of the EEG from selected areas, usually comparing one cerebral hemisphere to another with the four-channel monitor (positions F_3–P_3, F_4–P_4, international 10 to 20 system). The eight-channel system allows monitoring of other areas or other physiological variables, with better definition of sleep states. Silver/silver chloride electrodes are fixed to the scalp with collodion, the electrode cups filled with conducting gel and the hole resealed with collodion to prevent evaporation of the conducting gel. Impedances are measured at least daily and kept below 5kOhm and, if necessary, the collodion seal dissolved with acetone to allow insertion of more conducting gel and then resealed. The short distance between electrodes and preamplifiers minimises electrical interference particularly in those systems where attachment of the preamplifiers to the scalp with collodion reduces movement artefact. In our experience, no adverse effects of such fixative have been noted, although great care must be taken to minimise abrasion of the scalp when reducing the impedances. Twenty-four hours of data are recorded onto a standard c120 cassette tape, which can then be displayed visually on the rapid playback system. Twenty-four hours of data can be reviewed in 24 minutes, and can also be printed for more detailed analysis at a later date via a standard EEG machine. The Medilog is not marketed with a cotside display monitor; but this can be obtained by connecting the output signal from the recorder to a monitor while the tape recording is in progress.

The Medilog thus provides a compact and noninvasive method of monitoring the EEG continuously in sick and immature babies. It allows recording of the 'raw' EEG from at least two channels of EEG so that it can assess interhemispheric symmetry and synchrony. The Medilog permits visualisation of the 'raw' EEG on a time-scale comparable with conventional recording, and thus allows more detailed inspection not only of amplitude changes and the detection of the intermittent periods of low-amplitude discontinuous activity which are a common feature of the neonatal EEG, but also the detection of other types of activity, especially short-duration transients such as spikes and sharp waves which would not be detected by the cerebral function monitor (CFM). With a limited number of EEG electrodes, however, it provides little information about focal activity. Seizures are displayed in exactly the same way as on conventional recording. The continuous monitoring, though, allows recognition not only of these abnormal discharges and quantification of the duration of seizure activity, but also of their effect on background activity and thus useful prognostic information.

Computerised system for neonatal EEG *analysis*

The development of the Oxford Medilog recorder overcame many of the difficulties of continuous EEG recording during neonatal intensive care. However, the immediate value of the data was limited by the need for retrospective visual analysis of large quantities of information. A computerised system of analysis was developed in order to make use of the information provided from such continuous EEG recording that was both automated and on-line (Wertheim *et al.* 1989). Two channels of the four-channel Oxford Medilog recorder, recording EEG, are connected via filters and optical isolation amplifiers to a 12-bit analogue-to-digital converter in a computer which can be placed at the cotside. The filters enable the predominant frequencies of the neonatal EEG below 3Hz to be within the bandwidth, and also provide a high degree of rejection of mains frequency artefact. The two channels of EEG are displayed on the computer screen over 15s epochs, and the computer analyses the mean of the square of the amplitude and continuity in one-minute epochs. In the program, a discontinuous interval is recorded if the amplitude of the EEG remains below 25μv for a period of at least 6s. These values were chosen primarily to detect bursts in preterm infants who have peak amplitudes in the range of 200 to 400μv. Similar thresholds have been used in visual analysis techniques (Connell *et al.* 1987*a*, Eyre *et al.* 1988). The lengths of the intervals so detected in each epoch are summed to give the total discontinuous interval duration per one-minute epoch. In addition, the computer allocates intervals that are below 6s in duration in one epoch to the following epoch if the 6s criterion is met. In this way, intervals occurring over two epochs are not ignored. The total interval duration is expressed as a percentage of the epoch; the mean of the square amplitude and the number of intervals in each epoch for each channel being recorded are displayed and stored on hard disk. The interval duration can be examined on a print-out at the cotside, to assess trends in discontinuity and symmetry. The system also incorporates a number of markers which enable the EEG to be linked in time with clinical events or drug administration. The data are stored on hard disk and can be printed out retrospectively in a compressed fashion, for more detailed analysis of changes. This is the only form of analysed EEG developed specifically for newborn infants, and has allowed recognition of changes associated with drug administration (Murdoch Eaton *et al.* 1989, 1992) and acidosis (Connell *et al.* 1989*c*).

Cerebral function monitor

The CFM was first designed for use in adults (Maynard *et al.* 1969) and reported as applicable to neonates by Bjerre *et al.* (1983). This monitor heavily filters EEG data recorded from biparietal electrodes to limit frequencies below 2Hz and above 15Hz; it amplifies higher frequencies more than lower ones in order to flatten the EEG spectrum; it compresses amplitude logarithmically, then rectifies the signal and traces it as a single-line recording of variable thickness and height, which correlate with amplitude and frequency respectively. A high wide tracing indicates a relatively high EEG voltage with considerable variability in peak-to-peak amplitude, whereas a low, narrow tracing results from a low-voltage tracing with unchanging amplitude. The CFM plots cerebral activity against time. Cerebral activity may be either 'too high' or 'too low' for a specific circumstance. It is not readily apparent how much activity is due to high voltage or frequency (Prior *et al.* 1973, Viniker *et al.* 1984, Borel and Hanley 1985, Talwar and Torres 1988). An additional development to the CFM has been the cerebral function analysing monitor (CFAM), which produces a more detailed plot of the amplitude distribution and also gives an analysis of the frequencies of the EEG waveform (Maynard and Jenkinson 1984). The CFM has been regarded as relatively free of interference; nonetheless it is very important that impedance should be constantly monitored, as the CFM will analyse all artefacts in the same way as true EEG activity and display this as a change in amplitude. Since the CFM provides only a processed signal, a simultaneous standard EEG recording data is advisable when interpretation is in doubt. The monitor displays activity from only one channel, which represents the entire head; thus regional changes are hard to assess unless multiple units are attached to different areas. The CFM is particularly good at detecting changes in amplitude. Seizures are distinguished only by their amplitude characteristics, having a characteristic profile against that of the background activity, and are seen most clearly when they are prolonged, with a distinctive onset and termination. However, we do not know whether the CFM can detect the shorter, less organised seizures seen in preterm infants, or distinguish them from short bursts of high-voltage slow waves which are a normal feature of their background activity. Many neonatal seizures are of very low frequency (1HZ or less) and may not be detected by CFM recorders which have a low-frequency filter of 2HZ. In addition, since it provides a processed EEG signal from only one channel, it is unable to detect other types of activity: especially the short-duration transients such as spikes and sharp waves.

Compressed spectral array

Bickford *et al.* (1972) introduced compressed spectral array (CSA), which records filtered EEG signal predominantly in the frequency domain as a function of time. Two recording channels are available and two pairs of recording electrodes are attached symmetrically on the scalp. Spectral analysis is performed with the fast Fourier transform. A digital computer transforms EEG frequencies present during sequential sampling epochs into a linear representation of the amount of power (amplitude^2) at each of the different EEG frequencies during the sample. The duration of each epoch may be from two seconds to four minutes. These 'power spectra' are then plotted, and the plots are stacked vertically to give a three-dimensional 'mountains-and-valleys' representation for trend analysis. Each line of data represents a single epoch, plotting a power against frequency; power is displayed vertically, frequency is represented by the position of the various peaks on the horizontal axis, and the z axis represents time. Although the CSA readily demonstrates background EEG data, transient changes in EEG signals may be squeezed into the spectral line and not be recognisable as distinct events. EEG patterns such as burst suppression would not be easily seen in CSA because a given spectrum would probably contain some of the burst and some of the suppression, smoothing the patterns together. A shorter averaging period can help to resolve these patterns more easily (Borel and Hanley 1985, Talwar and Torres 1988). CSA resolves only epileptiform discharges of longer duration because signal-averaging reduces resolution of transient electrical events. Recognising seizures can be difficult, though electrical epileptic events with a frequency clearly distinct from the background can be fairly easily recognised. Aziz *et al.* (1986) obtained simultaneous EEGS using the Medilog and spectral array and reported that clinical seizures were easily confirmed by high power in the low frequencies and that subclinical ones were detected in the high-frequency range (20 to 30HZ). In the preterm infant, seizure discharges were distinguishable from normal bursts of activity by their stereotyped nature. However, seizures that were associated with paroxysmal decreases in amplitude were difficult to distinguish from those of amplitude suppression due to any cause. As with the CFM, isolated spike discharges and other abnormal transients would not be detectable.

Sensitivity of CFM and CSA in practice

Monitoring devices such as the CFM and CSA display synthesised and often markedly reduced data, eliminating a major part of the analog signal. Since the CFM is a single-channel recording it does not provide interhemispheric comparison, whereas the CSA records data derived from two channels and allows interhemispheric comparisons. Amplification of frequencies below 2HZ, where a major proportion of the power of the EEG exists in newborn infants, is considerably reduced on CFM. Therefore the lack of distinct changes on CSA and CFM does not exclude the presence of neonatal seizures. These changes may be overlooked because (i) the frequency and amplitude characteristics may not be sufficiently different from the background activity, or (ii) the area of origin may be different from that of electrode placement, or (iii) there may be a shifting focus (*e.g.* neonatal seizures). Care must be taken not to misinterpret changes that may reflect normal fluctuation and variation, response to stimulation, or artefact. Monitoring devices may not be adequate for other diagnostic purposes. For example, they are not capable of demonstrating spikes, sharp waves, or short-term paroxysmal or other types of electrical abnormalities. It has been suggested that the CFM and CSA may be used to indicate when a repeat polygraphic EEG should be done, and that initial and sequential EEGS enhance its utility and should be used in conjunction with continuous monitoring for appropriate interpretation of data. Technical limitations of these instruments can cause problems because of the inevitable interference problems faced in intensive care units. False alarms and increasing electrode impedances can annoy staff who are unfamiliar with the particular instrument.

Normal development of EEG patterns from continuously recorded data

The background EEG in the preterm neonate can be difficult to interpret because it changes with increasing gestational age. Cyclical changes in the EEG depend not only on the infant's sleep state but also on the length of the preceding sleep epoch (Roffward *et al.* 1966, Eyre 1984). Using prolonged recording by standard techniques, well defined criteria of EEG maturation have been established in term and preterm infants (Parmelee *et al.* 1968, Prechtl *et al.* 1969, Werner *et al.* 1977, Dreyfus-Brisac 1979). More recently Anderson *et al.* (1985) extended the work to the very immature infants now surviving.

Two recent studies have analysed continuous four-channel EEG recordings in low-risk preterm infants with no medical problems (Connell *et al.* 1987*a*, Eyre *et al.* 1988). They provided normative data against which to assess high-risk infants. Continuous and prolonged EEG recording ensured adequate sampling, asleep and awake, and enabled quantification of changes.

Method of analysis

Neonatal EEGs were analysed using the playback system of the Medilog. The tapes were transcribed with ink-jet recorders to provide compressed recordings. Connell *et al.* (1987*a*) divided the first 24 hours of recording into five-minute epochs which were allocated to one of five categories of continuity or discontinuity defined as follows:

(1) continuous: complete continuity of activity throughout the epoch
(2) mixed, predominantly continuous with continuous activity for at least 80 per cent of the epoch but with at least one interval of activity attenuated to 10 to 20μv for at least 5s
(3) mixed: both types of activity present with no clear dominance of one over the other
(4) mixed, predominantly discontinuous: a mainly discontinuous epoch which nevertheless contained activity for at least 20 per cent of the time duration, or
(5) discontinuous: activity for less than 20 per cent of the epoch.

The total of each of these five categories during the whole recording period was expressed as a percentage of the total recording time. Connell *et al.* (1987*a*) also measured the interburst intervals from the most discontinuous 60 minutes of recording.

Eyre *et al.* (1988) subdivided their recordings for each of five days into two categories: continuous activity, and trace alternant activity, defined as a discontinuous pattern occurring for more than one minute. For each 24-hour recording they randomly selected 100 burst-suppression units (defined as a single burst of high-voltage slow waves and the following period of attenuated or suppressed activity) and measured the duration of the bursts and of suppressed activity. They also measured the total duration of continuous activity per 24 hours.

Correlation of activity with gestational age

With increasing gestational age, there was a clear and consistent increase in continuous activity, with a concomitant reduction in the amount of discontinuous activity (Fig. 3.1). Connell *et al.* (1987*a*) showed a reduction in completely

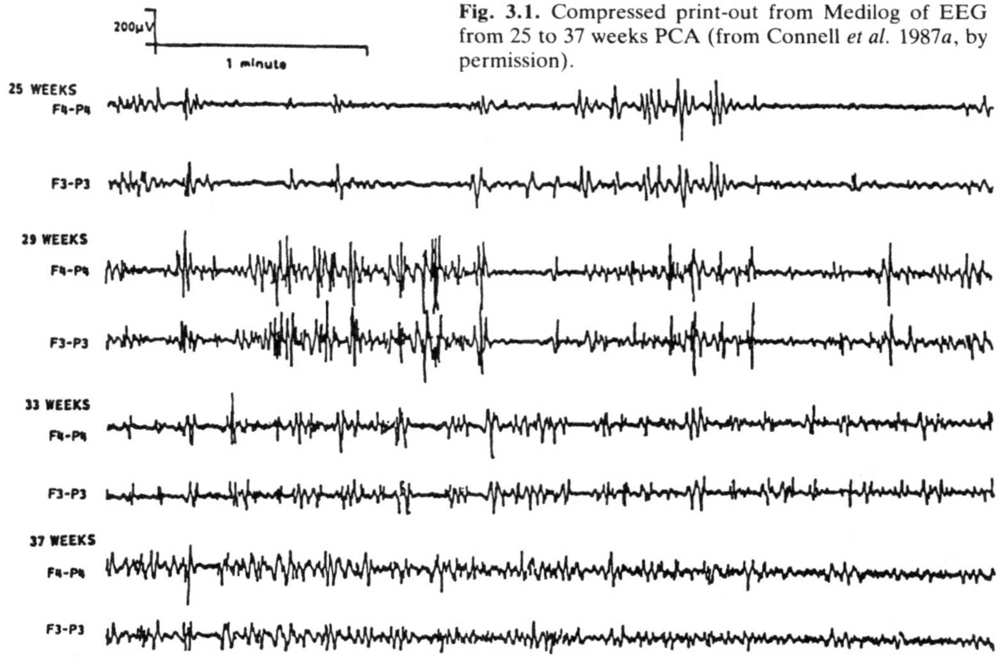

Fig. 3.1. Compressed print-out from Medilog of EEG from 25 to 37 weeks PCA (from Connell *et al.* 1987*a*, by permission).

discontinuous activity from 32 per cent to 11 per cent of total recording time in their population between 26 and 37 weeks, and an increase in completely continuous activity from just under 10 per cent to over 70 per cent. The mixed transitional grades followed a similar trend, reflecting the progressive increase in completely continuous activity. Eyre *et al.* (1988) similarly showed a median value of 10.1 hours per 24 hours of trace-alternant activity at 26 weeks decreasing to 1.6 hours per 24 hours at 42 weeks, and an increase in the duration of epochs of continuous activity from 13 minutes at 26 weeks to 62 minutes at 42 weeks.

Both studies showed a progressive decrease in the duration of the suppressed interval between bursts, and there was much greater variability in the duration of these suppressed intervals in the more immature infants and a significant reduction in this variability with increasing gestational age. Intervals longer than 60s were not seen after 31 weeks; after 35 weeks there were no intervals longer than 30s. However, the duration of each burst of activity was between 2 and 5s and no relationship was found with gestational age.

The dominant frequency at less than 31 weeks was 0.5 to 1.0Hz with a peak amplitude of between 300 and 400μv, and this altered nearer term with an increase in frequencies seen to predominantly 1 to 3Hz and a decrease in peak amplitude to 200 to 300μv.

Connell *et al.* (1987*a*) detected no seizure discharges or isolated spike or sharp waves in this population of low-risk infants. No infant had an asymmetrical

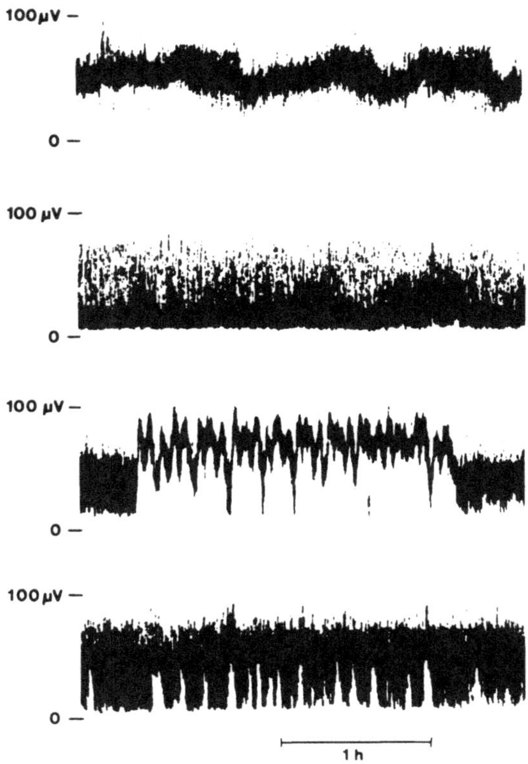

Fig. 3.2. Representative sample of different patterns of EEG activity as displayed by the CFM. *Top to bottom:* normal pattern, suppression-burst activity, repeated ictal epileptogenic activity as shown by a 'sawtooth' pattern in the CFM record (from Hellström-Westas *et al.* 1985, by permission).

recording and at least 95 per cent of bursts were synchronous in all infants.

In these studies the data were obtained from only two channels of EEG. This method allowed prolonged study of well preterm babies without disturbing their care, and enabled quantification of the changes in the cyclical pattern of the EEG with maturation; it would be difficult to make such prolonged recordings of normal preterm infants if multiple channels were used. There was much greater variability in the patterns of the normal preterm baby's EEG, and in fact a lack of variability could be seen as a sign of abnormality. These studies confirm that certain types of activity are not found in low-risk neonates and provide a standard range for normal changes with maturation, against which to assess the integrity of cerebral function in acutely ill preterm infants.

Cerebral function monitor studies

Normal patterns of CFM change in the neonate were described by Verma *et al.* (1984). They differentiated sleep states on physiological characteristics and evaluated the CFM tracings for the general form of the pattern. CFM patterns were described as waveform, flat or spiky. The voltages during the sleep-wake states were recorded as a range, using the lower limits of the range in each sleep-wake state for statistical calculations. CFM activity in sleep states S_1, S_2 and S_6 (quiet sleep, active sleep, and awake and crying respectively) was found to be a direct function of post-conceptional age (PCA). Correlation was best seen in the minimum level of activity, and maximum activity was not a good predictor of PCA. Verma *et al.* (1984) demonstrated that the CFM activity of the newborn infant had a characteristic wave-like pattern and was a direct function of gestational maturity. With increasing PCA, there was a progressive increase in minimum voltage in each sleep-wake state and an increased response to evoked stimuli. CFM patterns in the preterm infant were also described by Viniker *et al.* (1984), who also demonstrated maturational changes in sleep patterns for CFM tracings over the age range 30 to 43 weeks. When they considered tracings from neonates of less than three weeks chronological age, they found significant correlations with weight at the time of recording. In the preterm neonates, where tracings were obtained at a mean chronological age of six weeks, a relationship was found between the EEG measures and Apgar scores at one and five minutes (Fig. 3.2).

Compressed spectral array studies

There are no published data on the normal patterns of development in the preterm infant as detected by spectral analysis. Aziz *et al.* (1986) described two-hour recordings in 10 normal term infants as showing patterns characteristic of quiet sleep (QS) and active sleep (AS) that are easily recognisable by abrupt increases in the power spectra on entering quiet sleep (Fig. 3.3).

Continuous EEG monitoring in specific cerebral pathology

Haemorrhage

Periventricular/intraventricular haemorrhage (PVH/IVH) is common in preterm infants. Its incidence after birth is directly related to maturity. For infants at 30 weeks PCA it is about 50 per cent, increasing with lower PCA (De Vries *et al.* 1988). Continuous monitoring of the EEG has provided information on the timing of the relative development of ultrasound and electrical changes. Recent studies have demonstrated that it is sometimes possible to observe the emergence of EEG abnormality before ultrasound changes occur, suggesting that the EEG is sensitive to the fundamental insult that precipitates the haemorrhage rather than just the effects of the bleed itself. Connell *et al.* (1988) evaluated early continuous EEG recordings with the Medilog in a prospective study, and assessed their value in association with early serial cranial ultrasound scans. They monitored 54 preterm infants of less than 34 weeks PCA who were ventilated for respiratory distress syndrome. All these infants had prospective EEG monitoring within the first 72 hours of birth, which continued for at least 48 hours or until death, as well as daily ultrasound scanning during this period. The EEGs were classified as normal or abnormal, and the abnormal EEGs were then further classified into categories designating increasing severity of abnormalities. They demonstrated a clear trend for EEG abnormalities to be more frequent and severe with increasing grades of

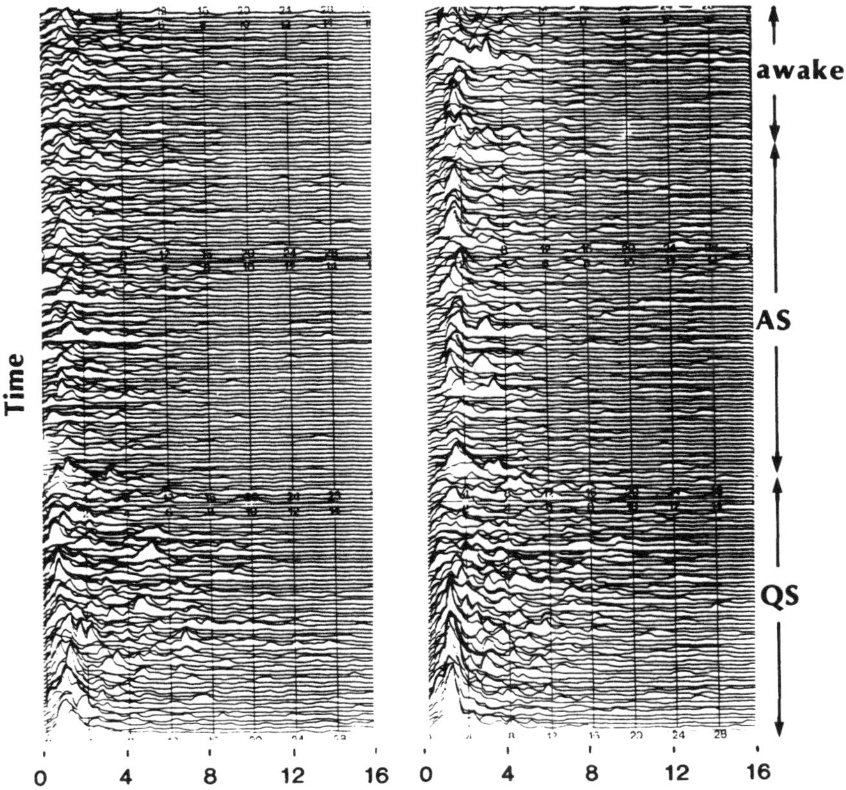

Fig. 3.3. Compressed spectral analysis (left and right hemispheres) of sequential 16s epochs of EEG recorded over one hour in a normal term neonate (from Aziz *et al.* 1986, by permission).

haemorrhage on ultrasound. A normal EEG was not found in any infant with parenchymal extension of the haemorrhage, and this group also contained six of the eight infants who showed seizures on a severely abnormal background EEG. The relative timing of early EEG abnormalities with ultrasound abnormality could be established in 22 infants; EEG abnormalities preceded the ultrasound abnormality in 15 infants; in the remaining seven, further deterioration of an initially abnormal ultrasound was preceded by deterioration of the EEG abnormality. There were no infants in whom abnormality on ultrasound preceded abnormal EEG. This study confirmed the prognostic value of the EEG previously established mainly by studies using standard recording technique. Both the nature of a particular EEG abnormality and its duration were of prognostic value. Of 13 infants with normal EEG, nine had normal outcome and two transient dystonia only. None had major neurological abnormality. With increasing abnormalities of EEG there were fewer normal survivors, and of eight infants with severe background abnormality only one survived but with major neurological abnormality. EEG abnormalities lasting less than 24 hours were associated with normal outcome in seven out of nine infants; the remaining two had only transient abnormalities. In those infants with EEG abnormalities lasting more than seven days, none were normal on follow-up. Some types of EEG abnormality were consistently good predictors of neurological abnormality. For example, seizures on persistently low-amplitude or asymmetrical backgrounds and maximal amplitude depression with or without seizures were consistently associated with major neurological abnormality or death. Lower degrees of abnormality and normal EEGs were still significant but were less effective in distinguishing those with minor neurological abnormality. Duration of abnormality was of particular value in determining prognosis in these infants. However, EEG abnormalities were rarely extremely prolonged and even quite severe abnormalities might resolve within a week. This emphasises the importance of early recording if adequate prognostic data are to be acquired.

Greisen *et al.* (1987) monitored amplitude-integrated EEG using the CFM from high-risk infants of less than 32 weeks PCA within 24 hours of birth and continued for at least 50 hours. Infants who developed germinal layer haemorrhages developed depression of background activity, particularly distinct in the presence of severe haemorrhages. Four infants developed germinal-layer haemorrhages after 30 hours of age and all had depressed activity before the development of the haemorrhage. The authors did not comment on the prognostic relevance of their findings.

Cystic and non-cystic leukomalacia

Recent refinements in ultrasound techniques have permitted diagnosis of ischaemic lesions. These initially present as areas of increased echogenicity on ultrasonography; some resolve but others proceed to extensive cyst formation, with a very poor prognosis. Although prognosis based on the presence of extensive cysts seems to be reliable, the cysts are not present initially and may take two to four weeks to develop. Marret *et al.* (1986) reported the significance of positive Rolandic sharp waves on standard EEGs in periventricular ischaemia. Continuous monitoring with the Medilog assessed the prognostic value of early and sequential EEG recording in infants with echodense ultrasound lesions and subsequent extensive cystic leukomalacia (Connell *et al.* 1987*b*). Thirty-one preterm infants (mean PCA 31 weeks) with persistent echodensities were prospectively studied with continuous EEG recordings, commenced within 48 hours of birth, and sequential recordings were made for 24-hour periods at intervals of two to four weeks until term or discharge. EEGs were graded for abnormalities similarly to their haemorrhage study (Connell *et al.* 1988), taking into account the degree of abnormality, background activity and seizures. Eighteen infants had normal EEG recordings: 16 did not develop cysts, one presented with periventricular leukomalacia and one developed it subsequently. The most severe EEG abnormalities were seen in four infants with subcortical leukomalacia, and five of eight infants with less abnormal EEGs had periventricular leukomalacia at presentation or subsequently developed it. The EEG again showed a close correlation with the functional severity of the ultrasonographic lesion, showing much more frequent and serious abnormalities in infants with cystic leukomalacia than in those whose densities resolved without cysts. A normal initial EEG recording was not always associated with a normal outcome; two survivors had normal initial recordings but abnormal outcome. However, if the sequential EEG recordings were persistently abnormal, so was the outcome. Seizures (which were present in four infants) were also associated with an abnormal outcome. Maximal background depression, which was seen in the four infants with subcortical leukomalacia, and not in any other group, identified the exceptional severity of associated functional damage. The advantage of EEG monitoring is that it supplies prognostically relevant information from the first day of recording, whereas that derived from ultrasonography was not available for two to four weeks, when the densities had resolved or cysts had formed.

There are no published data available on the changes seen with CFM monitoring in infants with leukomalacia.

Hypoxic-ischaemic encephalopathy

Extensive studies with polygraphic EEG recordings have established the important principle that the degree of EEG abnormality, and the rate at which it recovers, are reliable indicators of the functional severity of the asphyxial insult and the prognosis for the neurological outcome of the infant concerned. A normal EEG between the first and third days of life (Dreyfus-Brisac 1979) is associated with a good prognosis in most cases. A severely abnormal EEG is usually associated with a poor prognosis (Dreyfus-Brisac 1979, Watanabe 1980, Holmes 1982). Persistently low-amplitude, discontinuous or unreactive traces are associated with a poor outcome. While seizures are also a significant abnormality, the degree of background EEG abnormality is more important for determining prognosis.

Our own experience supports the significance of EEG abnormalities in birth asphyxia. The most severe background abnormalities, found in those infants with diffuse echogenicity on the cranial ultrasound scans, were associated with very poor prognosis. Continuous monitoring has shown that the duration of background abnormality is also related to prognosis; abnormalities lasting more than 24 hours were usually associated with major neurological abnormalities.

Prognostic sensitivity of the EEG in asphyxia has also been reported in studies using the CFM. Bjerre *et al.* (1983) studied infants with severe asphyxia between 12 hours and 49 days, and found that a persistently interrupted CFM trace was always associated with abnormal outcome. Of 18 infants with interrupted background activity in CFM tracings, none were healthy at follow-up when aged eight months to three years: 15 had died and the other three had signs of brain damage. A continuous trace was not always related to a good outcome; of eight infants with such a trace, four were healthy at follow-up, two had neurological abnormalities and two died. They also showed that in the nine infants whose CFM tracings changed from interrupted to continuous, four were normal at follow-up and three of these had had reversal of the CFM tracing within two days. In the study by Archbald *et al.* (1984), using the CFM in asphyxiated infants, a normal pattern was associated with favourable outcome in 18 out of 20 infants. A severely abnormal background (*i.e.* a flat pattern with low voltage, with or without spikes) indicated a grave prognosis and all eight showing this pattern died, while all three infants with persistence of a preterm pattern beyond the first seven days had long-term neurological problems.

There are no published data on spectral analysis of the EEG in relation to haemorrhagic or ischaemic cerebral lesions.

Seizures

The EEG is very valuable in the primary diagnosis of seizures, and in monitoring the response to therapy. The EEG of very sick babies in intensive care should be monitored continuously, because of the high incidence of seizures, the difficulty of making a diagnosis and the increasing use of paralysis to facilitate artificial ventilation. Mizrahi and Kellaway (1987) designed a cribside EEG/polygraphic-video monitor and performed prolonged recordings of infants clinically suspected to be having fits. They recorded 415 clinical seizures in 71 infants; 11 other infants had electrical seizure activity without clinical accompaniments. They found that seizures that were consistently and coherently related to focal EEG seizure activity had a high correlation with focal brain lesions, and had a favourable short-term outcome. Seizures that were inconsistently related to EEG seizure activity were correlated with diffuse processes such as hypoxic-ischaemic encephalopathy and had a poor short-term outcome. The clinical and background EEG features of infants whose seizures were not accompanied by EEG seizure activity suggested that these seizures may not be epileptic in character. Most 'subtle' seizures, all generalised tonic seizures, and some forms of myoclonic seizures, were either not associated with EEG seizure activity or had an inconsistent relationship with such EEG activity.

Eyre *et al.* (1983) detected EEG seizures in 20 of 25 preterm infants, only 11 of whom had clinical manifestations, suggesting an important role for this investigation in the detection of subclinical seizures. Bridges *et al.* (1986) monitored continuously with the Medilog only if a standard EEG failed to detect seizures, and this could account for their lower incidence of EEG seizures detected in seven of 37 infants. The most comprehensive study of neonatal seizures detected by continuous EEG monitoring was by Connell *et al.* (1989*a*,*b*), who monitored 275 term and preterm infants as part of their prospective evaluation of this form of monitoring. EEG seizure activity was found in 55 infants (25 per cent); clinical signs were simultaneous in only 12 of these, and completely absent in another 23. In the remaining 20 infants, EEG seizure activity either preceded or outlasted the clinical signs; six of these infants were paralysed. EEG seizure activity was never seen in low-risk infants. This study also stressed the significance of the background EEG in prognosis, particularly in seizures associated with haemorrhage or hypoxic-ischaemic insults. Normal background activity between seizures was usually associated with normal neurological outcome. Excessively discontinuous background EEG activity as an isolated abnormality was associated mainly with transient dystonia, and the outcome was worse with increasing severity of background EEG abnormality. All those with persistently asynchronous, asymmetrical or low-amplitude traces either died or had a major neurological abnormality. This study also allowed quantification of the duration of seizure activity, and showed the worst prognosis to be associated with a peak frequency of more than 25 seizures a day, or a total daily duration of seizure activity of more than 30 minutes, or persistence of seizure activity for more than 48 hours.

Eyre *et al.* (1983) reported cases in which EEG seizure activity persisted after clinical seizures had apparently ceased in response to therapy. There are no clear guidelines as to how far clinical management should be determined by the EEG, and in particular whether continuing anticonvulsant therapy is warranted and would affect prognosis. Connell *et al.* (1989*b*) looked at the clinical and EEG response to anticonvulsants in their population of 55 infants with neonatal seizures, 31 of whom received anticonvulsants on clinical grounds. EEG and clinical response were complete in only two and equivocal in six infants. Clinical response with persistent EEG seizures occurred in 13, and there was neither clinical nor EEG response in 10. They also found no significant improvement in the generally poor neurological outcome compared with that in the 24 infants whose seizures were not treated because of limited or absent clinical manifestations. The background EEG abnormality was a guide to potential lack of response to anticonvulsant drugs, and was also predictive of subsequent clinical outcome irrespective of treatment. Anticonvulsants are not generally thought to interfere significantly with the prognostic function of the EEG, but there is concern about the EEG depressant effects of very high barbiturate levels found in anaesthesia. Staudt *et al.* (1982) compared the degree of background EEG depression, plasma phenobarbitone levels and clinical outcome in 26 infants with seizures. The EEG abnormalities correlated well with outcome, but bore no relation to the anticonvulsant level and thus concluded that the EEG depression was related to the underlying cerebral pathology and not to therapy. In the CFM study of Bjerre *et al.* (1983), high phenobarbitone concentrations were deliberately aimed for, to produce brain protection in asphyxiated infants. They found that even at concentrations as high as 130μmol/l, CFM traces did not change from continuous to discontinuous. Since many neonates with seizures are already being treated with anticonvulsants at the time of EEG recording, these studies are important in establishing that anticonvulsant therapy does not appear to restrict the prognostic value of the EEG.

Hellström-Westras *et al.* (1985) used the CFM to monitor 87 high-risk newborns in their intensive care unit, and found the typical saw-tooth pattern representative of seizure activity in 26 infants, 24 of whom had clinical convulsions. However, they reported periods of silent seizures lasting for one hour or more in 14 of these 26 infants, and confirmed that long periods of electrographical seizure activity may pass undetected even by the skilled clinical observer. Aziz *et al.* (1986) reported that with the exception of the identification of isolated spike discharges, seizure activity was as readily recognisable with the CSA as with simultaneous Medilog EEG recording; seizure discharges tended to be stereotyped and stood out as fairly high-power bursts in a restricted number of frequencies. However, where seizures were associated with paroxysmal decreases in amplitude of the conventional EEG, reduced power was evident on the CSA but it was difficult to distinguish these changes from those of suppression due to any cause. Hakeem and Wallace (1990), using the CSA in infants from 28 to 42 weeks gestation, confirmed that clinical observation was not only unreliable in detecting seizures in the newborn, but was also a poor indicator of the effectiveness of anticonvulsant therapy.

Computerised system for neonatal EEG analysis

Preliminary results with this new system, which is specifically designed for analysis of the neonatal EEG, indicate that it may be a useful tool to assess changes at the cotside, and to allow close correlation with drug administration and changes in physiological parameters including blood pressure, acid-base status and blood gases. Previously undescribed EEG suppression with pethidine administration (a commonly used drug in neonatal practice for sedation of ventilated infants) has important implications for interpretation of intermittently recorded EEGs (Murdoch Eaton *et al.* 1989). EEG changes have also been seen with acidosis (Connell *et al.* 1989) and the EEG changes preceded any abnormality detected in routine monitoring of some of the infants. The potential value of a computerised on-line system of neonatal EEG analysis to the clinician is very considerable. This system may also provide information on the effects of other drugs in routine neonatal use on cerebral function, and important information on the relationship between EEG changes and changes in physiological parameters that are known to precede the development of detectable intracerebral pathology.

Conclusions and recommendations for monitoring

The main diagnostic contribution of continuous EEG monitoring during intensive care lies in its capacity for greatly increasing the rate of detection of neonatal seizures and providing a method of assessment of response to therapy. In combination with ultrasound scanning, the EEG can contribute to diagnostic evaluation of the severity of lesions, and EEG changes can even precede those seen on ultrasound. Valuable prognostic information is provided by the background activity of the EEG in that a normal EEG is highly predictive of normal outcome, whereas certain abnormal EEG features are constantly associated with subsequent major neurological abnormality or death. These EEG features are readily available from a very early stage and may both precede and be prognostically more sensitive than information obtained from ultrasound.

It is impossible to monitor every infant admitted to a neonatal intensive care unit. The greatest return from limited resources may be achieved by restricting prospective monitoring to high-risk infants during the first 48 to 72 hours after birth or after later acute illness, as these are the most likely times of onset of haemorrhagic, hypoxic or ischaemic cerebral lesions and of seizure disorders. For purposes of seizure detection, priority may further be given to infants less likely to exhibit clinical manifestations: *i.e.* those of less than 32 weeks PCA and those paralysed for mechanical ventilation. Infants in whom clinical seizures have been diagnosed may still gainfully be monitored in view of the frequent persistence of EEG seizures long after clinical manifestations have ceased. In all these infants, observations of therapeutic response to anticonvulsants may also be made during this time. In those infants with significant background abnormalities, recording may be continued for prognostic purposes at intervals determined by the degree of abnormality and its rate of resolution.

The ideal method of monitoring has not yet been achieved, and each of those currently available has its own advantages. Ideally, it should be simple to apply and maintain, be easy to interpret and make available clinically useful information. The Medilog cassette method has the advantage of providing the raw EEG data, but its analysis is retrospective and requires some skill and knowledge of EEG. Probably the most practical and easy to apply is the CFM, which provides recognisable patterns for interpretation at the cotside by a relatively untrained interpreter. Unfortunately it has limited use in the very small preterm infant. Though it is a simple practical system, clinically easy to interpret and good for seizure detection, its filters are inappropriate for the very immature infant and many of the slow frequencies dominant at these PCAS are filtered out, which may give false impressions of the degree of cerebral activity. CSA has the advantage of recording information from both cerebral hemispheres, and gives good pictures at the cotside. However, in very preterm infants, data must be interpreted carefully because of the monitors' inappropriate filters. There are also no published normative data on the application of this system to the preterm infant. The information provided by any method of neurological surveillance is important, but it remains to be determined whether its contribution to diagnosis and therapeutic monitoring can actually lead to significant improvements in clinical management and outcome.

REFERENCES

Anderson, C.M., Torres, F., Faoro, A. (1985) 'The EEG of the early premature.' *Electroencephalography and Clinical Neurophysiology*, **60**, 95–105.

Archbald, F., Verma, U.L., Tejani, N.A., Handwerker, S.M. (1984) 'Cerebral function monitor in the neonate. II: Birth asphyxia.' *Developmental Medicine and Child Neurology*, **26**, 162–168.

Aziz, S.S., Wallace, S.J., Murphy, J.F., Sainsbury, C.P.Q., Gray, O.P. (1986) 'Cotside EEG monitoring using computerised spectral analysis.' *Archives of Disease in Childhood*, **61**, 242–246.

Bickford, R.G., Billinger, T.W., Fleming, N., Stewart, L. (1972) 'The compressed spectral array (CSA): a pictorial EEG.' *Proceedings of San Diego Biomedical Symposium*, **11**, 365–370.

Bjerre, I., Hellström-Westas, L., Rosen, L., Svenningsen, N. (1983) 'Monitoring of cerebral function after severe asphyxia in infancy.' *Archives of Disease in Childhood*, **58**, 997–1002.

Borel, C., Hanley, D. (1985) 'Neurologic intensive care unit monitoring.' *Critical Care Clinics*, **1**, 223–239.

Bridges, S.L., Ebersole, J.S., Ment, L.R., Ehrenkranz, R.A., Silva, C.G. (1986) 'Cassette electroencephalography in the evaluation of neonatal seizures.' *Archives of Neurology*, **43**, 49–51.

Connell, J.A., Oozeer, R., Dubowitz, V. (1987*a*) 'Continuous 4-channel EEG monitoring: a guide to interpretation, with normal values, in preterm infants.' *Neuropediatrics*, **18**, 138–145.

—— —— Regev, R., De Vries, L.S., Dubowitz, L.M.S., Dubowitz, V. (1987*b*) 'Continuous four-channel EEG monitoring in the evaluation of echodense ultrasound lesions and cystic leucomalacia.' *Archives of Disease in Childhood*, **62**, 1019–1024.

—— De Vries, L., Oozeer, R., Regev, R., Dubowitz, L.M.S., Dubowitz, V. (1988) 'Predictive value of early continuous electroencephalogram monitoring in ventilated preterm infants with intraventricular hemorrhage.' *Pediatrics*, **82**, 337–343.

—— Oozeer, R., De Vries, L.S., Dubowitz, L.M.S., Dubowitz, V. (1989*a*) 'Continuous EEG monitoring of neonatal seizures: diagnostic and prognostic considerations.' *Archives of Disease in Childhood*, **64**, 452–458.

—— —— —— —— —— (1989*b*) 'Clinical and EEG response to anticonvulsants in neonatal seizures.' *Archives of Disease in Childhood*, **64**, 459–464.

—— Dubowitz, L., Dubowitz, V., Murdoch Eaton, D., Oozeer, R., Wertheim, D., Willetts, R., Wootton, R. (1989*c*) 'A computerized system for on-line monitoring and analysis of the human neonatal electroencephalogram.' *Journal of Physiology*, **417**, 24P.

De Vries, L.S., Larroche, J-C., Levene, M.I. (1988) 'Germinal matrix haemorrhage and intraventricular haemorrhage.' *In* Levene, M.I., Bennett, M.J., Punt, J. (Eds) *Fetal and Neonatal Neurology and Neurosurgery*. Edinburgh: Churchill Livingstone. pp. 312–326.

Dreyfus-Brisac, C. (1979) 'Neonatal electroencephalography.' *Reviews in Perinatal Medicine*, **3**, 397–471.

Eyre, J.A. (1984) 'A method of assessing consciousness in the newborn.' Oxford University: D. Phil. thesis. pp. 146–160.

—— Oozeer, R.C., Wilkinson, A.R. (1983) 'Diagnosis of neonatal seizure by continuous recording and rapid analysis of the electroencephalogram.' *Archives of Disease in Childhood*, **58**, 785–790.

—— Nanei, S., Wilkinson, A.R. (1988) 'Quantification of changes in normal neonatal EEGs with gestation from continuous five-day recordings.' *Developmental Medicine and Child Neurology*, **30**, 599–607.

Greisen, G., Hellström-Westas, L., Lou, H., Rosen, I., Svenningsen, N.W. (1987) 'EEG depression and germinal layer haemorrhage in the newborn.' *Acta Paediatrica Scandinavica*, **76**, 519–525.

Hakeem, V.F., Wallace, S.J. (1990) 'EEG monitoring of therapy for neonatal seizures.' *Developmental Medicine and Child Neurology*, **32**, 858–864.

Hellström-Westas, L., Rosen, I., Svenningsen, N.W. (1985) 'Silent seizures in sick infants in early life.' *Acta Paediatrica Scandinavica*, **74**, 741–748.

Holmes, G., Rowe, J., Hafford, J., Schmidt, R., Testa, M., Zimmerman, A. (1982) 'Prognostic value of the electroencephalogram in neonatal asphyxia.' *Electroencephalography and Clinical Neurophysiology*, **53**, 60–72.

Marrett, S., Parain, D., Samson-Dollfus, D., Jeannot, E., Fessard, C. (1986) 'Positive Rolandic sharp waves and periventricular leukomalacia in the newborn.' *Neuropediatrics*, **17**, 199–202.

Maynard, D., Prior, F., Scott, F.D. (1969) 'Device for continuous monitoring of cerebral activity in resuscitated patients.' *British Medical Journal*, **4**, 545–546.

—— Jenkinson, J.L. (1984) 'The cerebral function analysing monitor.' *Anaesthesia*, **39**, 678–690.

Mizrahi, E.M., Kellaway, P. (1987) 'Characterization and classification of neonatal seizures.' *Neurology*, **37**, 1837–1844.

Murdoch Eaton, D., Wertheim, D., Oozeer, R., Dubowitz, L.M.S., Dubowitz, V. (1989) 'The pethidine effect on the neonatal EEG.' *Early Human Development*, **19**, 217.

—— —— —— —— —— Royston, P. (1992) 'The effect of pethidine on the neonatal EEG.' *Developmental Medicine and Child Neurology*, **34**, 155–163.

Parmelee, A.H., Schulte, F.J., Akiyama, Y., Wenner, W.H., Stern, E. (1968) 'The maturation of EEG activity during sleep in premature infants.' *Electroencephalography and Clinical Neurophysiology*, **24**, 319–329.

Prechtl, H.F.R., Weinmann, H., Akiyama, Y. (1969) 'Organisation of physiological parameters in

normal and neurologically abnormal infants.' *Neuropädiatrie*, **1**, 101–129.
Prior, P.F., Virden, R.S.M., Maynard, D.E. (1973) 'An EEG device for monitoring seizure discharges.' *Epilepsia*, **14**, 367–372.
Roffwarg, H.P., Muzio, J.N., Dement, W.C. (1966) 'Ontogenetic development of the human sleep-dream cycle.' *Science*, **152**, 604–619.
Shewmon, D. (1983) 'Brief interictal rhythmic discharges in newborns.' *Electroencephalography and Clinical Neurophysiology*, **56**, 24P.
Staudt, F., Scholl, M.L., Coen, R.W., Bickford, R.W. (1982) 'Phenobarbital therapy in neonatal seizures and the prognostic value of the EEG.' *Neuropediatrics*, **13**, 24–33.
Talwar, D., Torres, F. (1988) 'Continuous electrophysiologic monitoring of cerebral function in the pediatric intensive care unit.' *Pediatric Neurology*, **4**, 137–147.
Verma, U.L., Archbald, F., Tejani, N., Handwerker, S.M. (1984) 'Cerebral function monitor in the neonate. I: Normal patterns.' *Developmental Medicine and Child Neurology*, **26**, 154–161.
Viniker, D.A., Maynard, D.E., Scott, D.F. (1984) 'Cerebral function monitor studies in neonates.' *Clinical Electroencephalography*, **15**, 185–192.
Watanabe, K., Miyazaki, S., Hara, K., Hakamada, A. (1980) 'Behavioural state cycles, background EEGs, and prognosis of newborns with perinatal hypoxia.' *Electroencephalography and Clinical Neurophysiology*, **49**, 618–625.
Werner, S.S., Stockhard, J.E., Bickford, R.G. (1977) *Atlas of Neonatal Electroencephalography*. New York: Raven Press.
Wertheim, D., Connell, J., Oozeer, R., Brydon, J., Dubowitz, L.M.S., Dubowitz, V. (1989) 'A new computerized method of analysis of continuous neonatal EEG recordings.' *In* Gennser, G., Marsal, K., Svenningsen, N., Lindstrom, K. (Eds) *Fetal and Neonatal Measurements III. Proceedings of the Third International Conference on Fetal and Neonatal Physiological Measurements*. Malmo: Ronneby.

4
SOMATOSENSORY EVOKED POTENTIALS

R. W. I. Cooke

The somatosensory evoked potential (SEP) is the sequence of voltage changes generated in the brain and the pathway from a peripheral nerve following a transient stimulus, usually electrical, of a peripheral sensory nerve. It is unique among evoked potentials in that the peripheral receptor organ is usually bypassed. While there is an argument for a more physiological stimulus such as a pinprick or tap (Pratt *et al.* 1981), the advantage with electrical or magnetic stimulation of the nerve is that most of the larger diameter fibres are stimulated simultaneously, and a more coherent volley is sent to the CNS. Unless an electrical impulse is very strong, it will only stimulate the largest and fastest fibres which for sensory nerves are responsible in the main for touch and proprioception. The interpretation of the resulting cortical responses is thus more straightforward, although its clinical use is restricted.

The median or digital nerves, and the posterior tibial or popliteal nerves, are usually stimulated to produce SEPS. With other nerves, such as the trigeminal, the responses are smaller and rather ill defined, and have not to date been used in investigating the newborn infant. In mixed nerves of the upper limb, selective stimulation techniques show that the major contribution to the SEP response is derived from the sensory fibres (Halonen *et al.* 1988). Sensitive amplification and averaging techniques enable discrimination between the evoked response and other larger and more random physiological potentials with which the signal is mixed.

There is no universal agreement about the origin of SEPS. In adult man, the origins of the potentials observed in normal subjects are deduced by their absence in subjects with sensory loss due to lesions at various known levels in the pathway. This is more difficult to do in children as there are fewer model cases with strictly localised lesions in the brain which allow analytical investigation. Extrapolation from the adult is made difficult by the very different latencies and amplitudes of the responses in immature individuals.

Evoked potentials are recorded at a distance from the nerve axon or synapse that generates them, and are conducted to the detecting electrode through the surrounding tissues which act as a volume conductor. The depolarisation of an axon will be observed as a positive potential field in advance of the direction of propagation with the amplitude inversely proportional to the square of the distance from the generator and proportional to the angle subtended by the cross-section of the nerve trunk. An intense negative and less directional potential is observed in a plane perpendicular to the depolarised region of the nerve. The distribution, polarity and latency of the evoked potential may be obtained from simultaneous observations from different electrodes, and the likely anatomical origin of the various components of the response may be hypothesised.

Nomenclature of SEPS

Naming the components of the SEP is confusing, as different authors have used different names. Individual components are identified by their latency, *i.e.* the time at which they occur following the peripheral stimulus, their polarity, the position at which they are observed to be maximal and to a lesser extent by the amplitude and shape of waveform. While in the adult the latencies of the components are reasonably consistent from one normal individual to another, the rapid changes in central nervous system (CNS) maturation and body size in the newborn infant makes such identification more difficult. Differences in equipment characteristics from one laboratory to another, and particularly in the selection of filtering of the signals, may make the final appearances of the response very different. Individual components are referred to by a letter and number. The letter (N for negative or P for positive) refers to the polarity of the wave, and the number either to the latency in milliseconds (ms) from the time of the stimulus (*e.g.* N_{20}) or alternatively, especially when newborn infants are being considered, the order in which the component was observed (*e.g.* N_1, P_2).

Median nerve SEPS

In the adult, following stimulation of the median nerve, the first major component of the response noted is N_9. It is most easily detected from an electrode placed over the brachial plexus (Erb's point). Although it represents activity just outside the spinal cord, it is easily recorded and therefore a convenient marker for the entry of the afferent volley to the CNS. It is preserved but with loss of subsequent responses in traction injury to the brachial plexus. Sensory axons in the dorsal roots of the spinal cord, 2 or 3ms later, give rise to P_{12} detected over the scalp. Further presynaptic and postsynaptic events in the dorsal horn near root entry give rise to N_{13}/P_{14}, and N_{13}/P_{15} may be detected over the scalp representing activity in the medial lemniscus and cuneate nucleus. After P_{15}, at least 19 other components have been described. The best known of these is N_{20} (also known as N_1), which represents the arrival of the volley at the post-Rolandic cortex. This component begins at about 18ms, and the earlier parts of the wave are thought to represent thalamic activity. Prominent waves are seen at P_{30}, N_{35}, and P_{45}. Activity between N_{20} and P_{30} arises probably within the area of representation of the hand in the sensory cortex. P_{30} is thought to originate from a dipole in the central sulcus. After P_{45} (middle latency), components probably represent early activity outside the somatic sensory receiving area and their appearance is dependent on the integrity of that area. Much later components such as P_{100} (somatic late response) and N_{200} represent the so-called cognitive evoked potential components and are very variable. They are also seen in the ipsilateral cortex where they arrive via association pathways (Nakanishi *et al.* 1983, Tomita *et al.* 1988).

Posterior tibial nerve SEPS

Stimulation of the posterior tibial nerve (PTN) above the ankle, or more usually in the popliteal fossa in adults, results in a triphasic wave which travels up the spinal cord. With electrodes placed at S_1, two potentials at N_9 and N_{12} are noted. Over L_1/T_{12} the initial potential is N_{12} (also referred to as N_1) and thought to be predominantly of postsynaptic origin, with contributions from the cauda equina and spinal cord. It is comparable with N_{13} from median nerve stimulation. From electrodes over the cervical spine, an N_{30} may be obtained which is of brainstem origin, possibly from activity evoked in the lemniscal pathway. Cortical responses to PTN stimulation in the popliteal fossa are nearly all maximal on the midline of the scalp, 2cm posterior to the vertex, which corresponds to the primary sensory area for the leg and foot. The initial cortical potential P_{34}, maximal at P_{38}, is thought to be the primary response of the sensory motor cortex. It is followed by subsequent peaks at N_{45}, P_{56}, N_{74}, P_{99}, N_{126}, and P_{204} due to cortical activity. The lack of an initial negative peak, analogous to the N_{20} from median nerve stimulation, is probably due to difficulty in detecting the cortical generator on the medial surface of the contralateral gyrus in the interhemispheric fissure. P_{38} itself is best seen slightly lateral to the midline on the ipsilateral cortex, a position which 'sees' this area best (Seyal and Gabor 1985).

The components of the responses to median and posterior tibial nerve stimulation in the fullterm and preterm infant are much simpler than in the older individual. The responses are generally later and of greater amplitude. Most clinical studies have simply looked for the latency of N_1 following median nerve stimulation and P_1 for PTN stimulation with or without simultaneous recording of Erb's potential or spinal potential over L_1 (spL_1) so that these latencies may be subtracted to derive a central conduction time, and also act as a confirmation that a volley has entered the CNS. Late waves in the newborn infant are very variable and often poorly defined, making comparisons between subjects difficult.

Technical considerations

The techniques for recording SEPS and the ensuing results have varied widely. While most workers have used electrical stimulation of the median nerve, some have used electrical stimuli to the fingers (Desmedt *et al.* 1976) and even mechanical stimuli (Hrbek *et al.* 1968, Pratt *et al.* 1981). There is variation in the rate of stimulation and the number of stimuli averaged, and although the positions of the principal scalp electrodes are standard, those of additional electrodes are not. Filter settings vary from 2 to 100HZ to 30 to 3000HZ, the latter used to record early faster components of the SEP response. Averaging times vary from 50 to 5000ms when early or late components of the response have been studied. A 50 or 60HZ notch filter, which is sometimes employed to remove mains interference, often alters the response characteristics. For cortical SEPS, electrodes are usually positioned according to the Picton modification of the international 10 to 20 electrode system, based on percentage distances from four standard points on the head: the nasion, inion, left and right preauricular points. For median nerve SEPS, the active electrodes are positioned at pc3 and pc4, and referenced to the mid-frontal position. The site of maximal response (*i.e.* the contralateral parietal hand focus) has been determined by Manil *et al.* (1967), and in the term infant lies 50 to 75mm from the midline and 20mm behind the biauricular frontal plane. The measurements in the preterm infant are correspondingly smaller.

Electrodes are applied to skin cleaned with surgical spirit. It is not necessary to shave the scalp. Attachment can be with collodion and gauze, or with adhesive rings and tape. Gentle scarification of the skin with a blunt needle allows the electrode impedance to fall below 3kOhm. Impedances need to be rechecked during a recording session (Klimach and Cooke 1988*a*).

For PTN SEPS, scalp electrodes are placed at PCZ-L/R, *i.e.* just lateral to PCZ (Picton's modification) on the same side as the stimulating electrodes. To record the spinal volley, an electrode is placed over the spinous process of L_1 (spL_1), with a reference electrode over the ipsilateral iliac crest (ic-L/R). A filter of 20 to 2000HZ, with averaging time of 50ms, is used (White and Cooke 1989*a*).

Peripheral nerve conduction time in the upper limb can be calculated from a recording from an electrode placed at Erb's point in the mid-clavicular line referenced to a mid-frontal electrode. A sharp negative deflection signals the arrival of the volley at the brachial plexus. A filter of 20 to 2000HZ is used, with an averaging time of 20ms.

For SEPS in general, a stimulus frequency of 0.5HZ is used. Some workers have used a faster stimulation rate but this may not allow an adequate recovery time, and may modify the response. The stimulus is a short square-wave pulse of 0.1ms duration, and of an intensity just sufficient to produce a muscle twitch (about 5 to 15mA). Stimulation is usually unilateral, although bilateral stimulation of the PTN produces a larger response cortically.

To date most SEP responses have been displayed after averaging as the output of a single- or four- to eight-channel recorder. The response of the cortex, however, may be viewed as a whole, rather than that at one or more single points on the surface, especially if the later or association responses are of interest. 'Maps' of cortical activity can be generated by averaging simultaneously from 20 or more channels, and by using suitable algorithms. This technique has been used mostly to 'map' electroencephalographic (EEG) activity, but may as easily be used for displaying SEP data (Duffy *et al.* 1978, Desmedt and Bourguet 1985). The value of this technique in the newborn infant has not been fully evaluated.

SEP latencies and age

SEP latencies decrease with age until well into childhood (Desmedt *et al.* 1976, Tomita *et al.* 1986). Normative age-specific data are a prerequisite if SEPS are to

TABLE 4.I
Representative values for N_1 peak median SEP latency (pC4–Fz) in ms (SD)

	Birth	*2 mths*	*4 mths*	*6 mths*	*12 mths*
Desmedt and Manil (1970)	33.9				
Hrbek *et al.* (1973)	35 (8)				
Willis *et al.* (1984)	24.3 (2.1)	20.2 (1.6)	19.1 (1.3)	17.4 (1.1)	17.2 (1.7)
Bartel *et al.* (1987)					15.9 (1)
Zhu *et al.* (1987)	24.9 (2.7)	21.8 (2)	◄ - - - -	18.8 (1.6)	- - - - ►
Klimach and Cooke (1988*a*)	40 (6)				
Laureau *et al.* (1988)	25 (2)	20.4 (1.1)		17.5 (0.8)	
Taylor and Fagan (1988)				17.7 (0.8)	15.7 (0.9)

TABLE 4.II
Representative values for P_1 peak posterior tibial SEP latency in ms (SD)

	Preterm newborn infant	*Term newborn infant*
Cindro *et al.* (1985)		37.5 (2.5)
Gilmore *et al.* (1987)	54.9 (8.9)	
White and Cooke (1989*a*)		43.6 (8)

assess progress or delay in maturation in the developing infant. The maturation with growth of SEPs is mainly associated with cell-growth processes such as myelination, and with cell differentiation and synaptic development. These changes would be expected to provide at least two time courses for change, conduction velocity changes due to myelination and the synaptic changes which dominate cortical potential latencies.

Desmedt *et al.* (1973), using median nerve stimulation, compared the contribution of the 'peripheral conduction' up to the dorsal column nuclei with the 'central conduction' time from the dorsal column to the latency of N_1 (a cortical generator). Soon after birth the peripheral latency comprised one third of the total N_1 latency, at seven months it comprised one half, and at 20 years it comprised three quarters. Peripheral nerve conduction velocities hardly change after three years of age, so the later increase in contribution is mainly due to an increase in the length of the peripheral pathway. This varying contribution of peripheral and central latency makes the practice of correcting latencies for body length somewhat questionable (Chu and Hong 1985, Bartel *et al.* 1987).

Because of these maturational changes, a number of attempts have been made to fit curves relating SEP latencies to age. These have ranged from simple linear functions, to single exponential curves, hyperbolic functions and the sum of three decaying exponentials. While each of these curve-fits serves as a means of data reduction, it has yet to be determined if they can be based on developmental models. Eggermont (1988) argued that his three exponential model comprising a

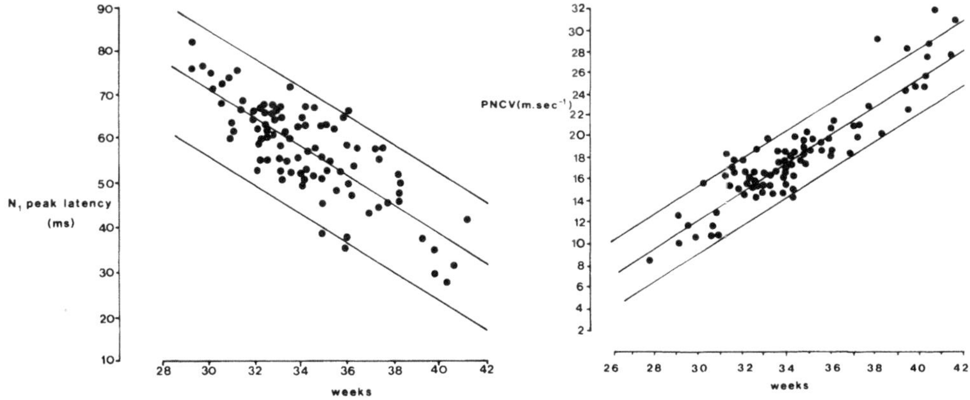

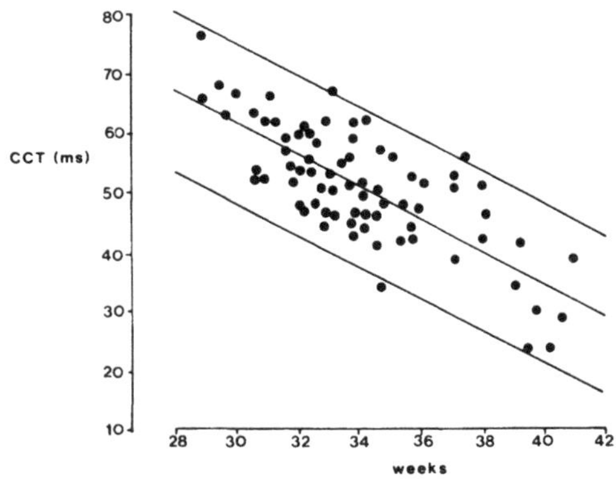

Fig. 4.1. *Above left*: graph of N_1 peak latency of SEP against PCA. *Above right*: graph of peripheral nerve conduction velocity against PCA. *Left*: graph of central conduction time (CCT) against PCA. (From Klimach and Cooke 1988*a*.)

short time-constant process ($\tau = 3\frac{1}{2}$ weeks), a medium speed process ($\tau = 26$ weeks), and a slow process ($\tau = 4.7$ years), described not only the maturation of SEPs but auditory and visual evoked potentials as well, thus providing a unified hypothesis. The three processes are suggested to represent initial rapid increases in synaptic density, myelination, and either later, slower myelination of distal tracts or an increasing concentration of galactolipids in the brainstem which parallels it.

Many workers have published normative data for newborn and older infants, but comparison between results remains difficult because of the variety of methodologies and age groups used. Tables 4.I and 4.II illustrate the range of values seen for the important short latency peaks N_1 (median SEP) and P_1 (PTN SEP) cortical responses. Those authors publishing data on preterm infants by gestational age (GA) or post-conceptional age (PCA) have usually described their results in terms of a linear regression of latency on age (Hrbek *et al.* 1973; Klimach and Cooke 1988*a*; White and Cooke 1989*a*,*b*). Such an approximation is a useful approach for this short period of rapid change, although the relationship does not hold outside this range (Figs 4.1 to 4.3).

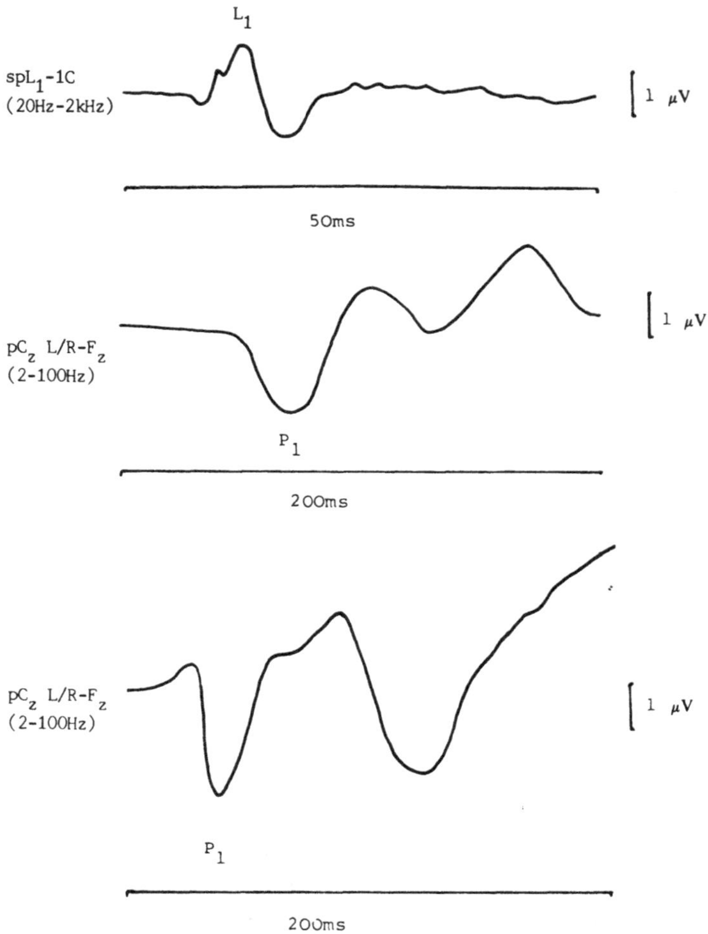

Fig. 4.2. *Top*: representative recording of lumbar spinal potential—L_1. *Centre*: representative cortical recording from preterm infant at 31 weeks. *Bottom*: representative cortical recording from preterm infant at 39 weeks, following posterior tibial nerve stimulation.

Sleep state and SEPS

In adults the sleep state does not appear to alter the latency or amplitude of early SEPS, but the later 'cognitive' waves vary considerably. Similar observations have been made for median nerve SEPS in the newborn infant (Desmedt and Manil 1970). Gilmore *et al.* (1987) reported that the infant's state of alertness appeared to alter the morphology of P_1 after PTN stimulation, but this may have been due to a reduction in muscle artefact. The effect of sleep state on N_1 morphology following median nerve stimulation was first examined by Hrbek *et al.* (1969) who found larger responses during quiet sleep. It has been suggested that these findings were artefactual. Most workers record SEPS during quiet sleep in infants since this yields a

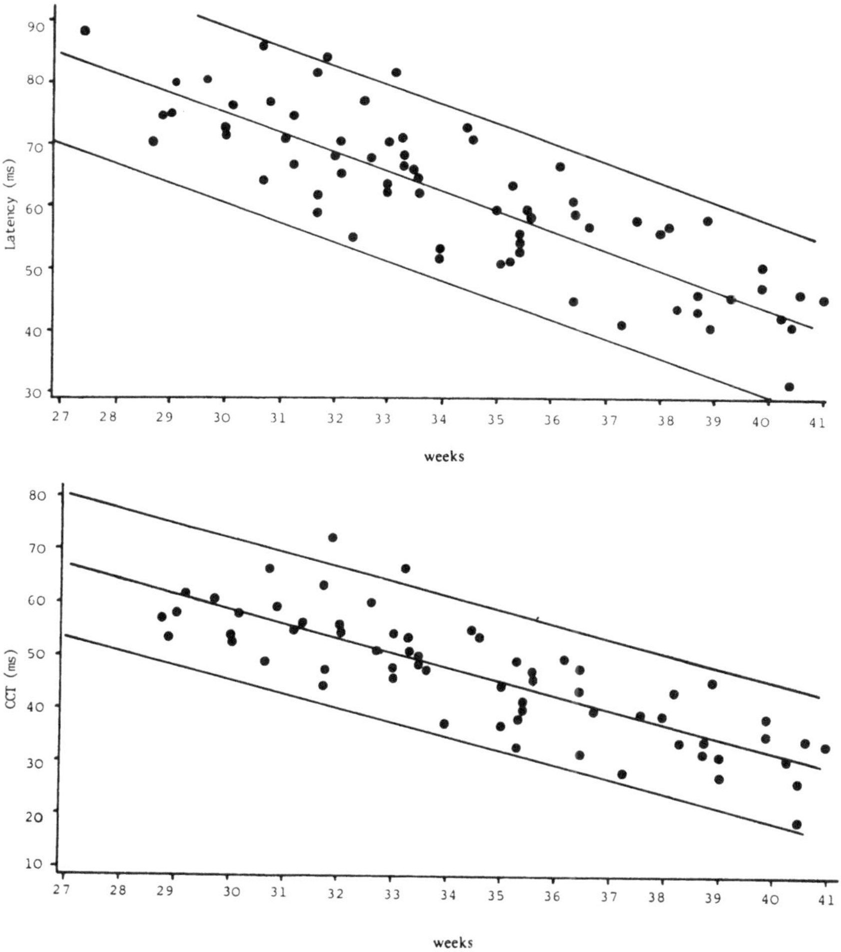

Fig. 4.3. *Top*: plot of P_1 peak latency following posterior tibial nerve stimulation against PCA. *Bottom*: plot of CCT against PCA.

clearer response due to reduced movement artefact. Reduction of extraneous signals may also affect the averaged response. Nevertheless, Addy *et al.* (1987) and Emerson *et al.* (1988) also observed latency prolongation of N_1 in sleep. Yamada *et al.* (1988) clarified this further by showing that sleep significantly alters short-latency SEP peaks, but differentially affects frontal and parietal responses. However, the differences are small.

An interesting related phenomenon in the sleeping newborn was shown by Wolff *et al.* (1974). The exposure of infants to 'white noise' during sleep did not affect the short-latency peaks, but did enhance the amplitude and increase the latency of the late SEP components in both REM and quiet sleep, showing the interaction of responses from continuous and intermittent stimuli at cortical level.

Clinical applications of SEP in the newborn and young infant

SEP in congenital hypothyroidism

Laureau *et al.* (1986) recorded median nerve SEPS longitudinally in six infants diagnosed as having congenital hypothyroidism (CH) in a neonatal screening programme. Increased wave N_{19} and P_{22} latencies were observed together with increased N_{13} to N_{19}, and N_{19} to N_{22} interpeak latencies (IPL) were observed before treatment. These abnormalities tended to correct following thyroxine therapy, although six months later two infants still showed increased N_{13} to N_{19} IPL. Both had very low serum T_4 levels at diagnosis and were the most severely affected.

Subsequently the same group described a long-term follow-up study of 48 infants with CH (Laureau *et al.* 1987). At 18 months and three years, SEP latencies and IPLS in treated children did not differ significantly from controls, although significant partial correlations were found between SEP IPLS and T_4 levels at the time of diagnosis. Similarly N_{19}–P_{22} IPL correlated with the reasoning scale of the Griffiths test, suggesting that SEP might be used to detect CH children at risk of subsequent developmental abnormalities.

Hypoglycaemia and SEPS

A novel use for the SEP was made recently by Koh *et al.* (1988) to study the effects of hypoglycaemia on CNS function in infants and children. Layer IV of the cortex, which is the site of sensory afferent fibre input to the somatosensory areas of the cortex, has been shown to have a high rate of glucose utilisation. A measure of neural activity in the somatosensory pathways would therefore provide a sensitive index of the lowest blood glucose concentration compatible with normal neuronal function. In one four-month-old child, a fall in blood glucose from 4.2 to 2.3mmol/l caused a prolongation of N_1 latency from 20 to 24ms. A threshold of 2.6mmol/l blood glucose appeared necessary for the maintenance of normal function.

Use of SEP in predicting later motor disability

Although normative data for SEPS have existed for more than two decades, it is only fairly recently that they have been used to predict neuromotor outcome in the newborn and in infants in the first months of life. This interest has been stimulated by the increased survival of very preterm infants, often with ultrasound evidence of ischaemic or haemorrhagic brain lesions. Although ultrasound scans correlate reasonably well with gross motor outcome, notable exceptions have been described, indicating the need for a functional rather than anatomical diagnostic test in early life. Laget *et al.* (1976) studied 43 children with hemiplegic cerebral palsy, and found a positive correlation between median nerve SEPS and the affected side using the amplitude of the responses rather than the latency.

Willis *et al.* (1984) reported two infants with neonatal IVH who had very abnormal median nerve SEPS and who subsequently developed cerebral palsy. Gorke (1986) investigated 120 infants referred between one and 10 months of age because of suspected risk of neurodevelopmental impairment. Forty-seven who subsequently proved normal were used as a control group. Among the remaining 73 patients, 19 had absent or abnormally delayed (>2SD) responses, and all had subsequent motor disability. Klimach and Cooke (1988*b*) recorded median SEPS in 30 preterm infants with cranial ultrasound abnormalities. Of 25 survivors followed up for at least six months, all with normal SEPS in the neonatal period were subsequently normal neurodevelopmentally. The infants in this group were not only those with minor ultrasound abnormalities. The group included two infants with unilateral parenchymal haemorrhages, one with cerebral atrophy, and one with post-haemorrhagic hydrocephalus and a ventriculoperitoneal shunt. All 10 infants with cerebral palsy at follow-up had abnormal SEPS in the neonatal period.

White and Cooke (1989*c*) also described follow-up studies on 84 preterm infants with abnormal cranial ultrasound scans and/or neurological signs in the neonatal period. All had median nerve SEPS and 36 also had posterior tibial nerve SEPS. A prolonged (>2SD) median N_1 peak latency correlated well with abnormal motor outcome, with a specificity of 77 per cent and a sensitivity of 86 per cent. Two of three infants with cerebral palsy but normal SEPS had mild spastic diplegia. Although more difficult to perform, posterior tibial nerve SEPS appear to overcome this failure, and a sensitivity of 93 per cent and specificity of 85 per cent were achieved for the prediction of cerebral palsy. Similarly Willis *et al.* (1989) showed that in 39 very low birthweight infants, studied with short latency median nerve SEPS at two, four and six months, all 12 infants with absent or delayed N_1 responses had motor abnormalities at follow-up. However they also demonstrated that a single normal SEP was of relatively little prognostic value, although two or three normal SEPS made adverse outcome very unlikely.

Asphyxia and SEPS

Many imaging techniques and physiological measurements have been described for use in the prognosis of perinatal asphyxia, though none has proved entirely satisfactory to date. This field was one of the first clinical applications suggested for SEPS in the newborn infant. Hrbek et al. (1977) combined SEPS and VEPS for the purpose, but the duration of follow-up was very short, and other methodological problems made the value of the technique difficult to assess.

Willis *et al.* (1987) studied 10 asphyxiated term infants within the first six months of life, and followed them subsequently to a mean age of 20 months. One or more median SEPS were performed at two, four and six months, and follow-up consisted of an independent neurological and developmental examination. One infant died with severe cerebral palsy at five months, before formal evaluation. SEPS were considered abnormal when an N_1/P_1 was absent or had a latency of >3SD above the mean for prior laboratory norms. Results of SEPS correlated with subsequent outcome in every patient, with normal and abnormal infants at later assessment separable on the basis of the prior SEPS. However, the severity of the later disability could not be inferred from the SEPS.

Conclusion

With modern computerised equipment, SEPs in the newborn and young infant are a simple clinical tool for the evaluation of the sensory pathways. Their close association with motor tracts means that CNS lesions producing motor deficits are likely to be common to both. SEPs can provide specific and sensitive prediction of later impairment, and useful data on neural dysfunction whether from asphyxia or other biochemical or hormonal abnormalities.

REFERENCES

Addy, R.O., Dinner, D.S., Luders, H., Lesser, R.P., Morris, H.H., Wyllie, E. (1987) 'Effect of sleep on median nerve short-latency somatosensory evoked potentials.' *Journal of Clinical Neurophysiology*, **4**, 243–244.

Bartel, P., Conradie, J., Robinson, E., Prinsloo, J., Becker, P. (1987) 'The relationship between median nerve somatosensory evoked potential latencies and age and growth parameters in young children.' *Electroencephalography and Clinical Neurophysiology*, **68**, 180–186.

Chu, N.-S., Hong, C.-T. (1985) 'Erb's and cervical somatosensory evoked potentials: correlations with body size.' *Electroencephalography and Clinical Neurophysiology*, **62**, 319–322.

Cindro, L., Prevec, T.S., Beric, A. (1985) 'Maturation of cortical potentials evoked by tibial-nerve stimulation in newborns, infants and children aged four and eight years.' *Developmental Medicine and Child Neurology*, **27**, 740–745.

Desmedt, J.E., Manil, J. (1970) 'Somatosensory evoked potentials of the normal human neonate in REM sleep, in slow wave sleep and in waking.' *Electroencephalography and Clinical Neurophysiology*, **29**, 113–126.

—— Noel, P., Debecker, J., Nameche, J. (1973) 'Maturation of afferent conduction velocity as studied by sensory nerve potentials and by cerebral evoked potentials.' *In* Desmedt, J.E. (Ed.) *New Developments in Electromyography and Clinical Neurophysiology*. Basel: Karger. pp. 52–63.

—— Brunko, E., Debecker, J. (1976) 'Maturation of the somatosensory evoked potentials in normal infants and children, with special reference to the early N1 component.' *Electroencephalography and Clinical Neurophysiology*, **40**, 43–58.

—— Bourguet, M. (1985) 'Color imaging of parietal and frontal somatosensory potential fields evoked by stimulation of median or posterior tibial nerve in man.' *Electroencephalography and Clinical Neurophysiology*, **62**, 1–17.

Duffy, F.H., Burchfield, J.L., Lombroso, C.T. (1978) 'Brain electrical activity mapping (BEAM): a method for extending the clinical utility of EEG and evoked potential data.' *Annals of Neurology*, **5**, 309–321.

Eggermont, J.J. (1988) 'On the rate of maturation of sensory evoked potentials.' *Electroencephalography and Clinical Neurophysiology*, **70**, 293–305.

Emerson, R.G., Sgro, J.A., Pedley, T.A., Hauser, W.A. (1988) 'State-dependent changes in the N20 component of the median nerve somatosensory evoked potential.' *Neurology*, **38**, 64–68.

Gilmore, R., Brock, J., Hermansen, M.C., Baumann, R. (1987) 'Development of lumbar spinal cord and cortical evoked potentials after tibial nerve stimulation in the preterm newborn: effects of gestational age and other factors.' *Electroencephalography and Clinical Neurophysiology*, **68**, 28–39.

Görke, W. (1986) 'Somatosensory evoked potentials indicating impaired motor development in infancy.' *Developmental Medicine and Child Neurology*, **28**, 633–641.

Halonen, J.-P., Jones, S., Shawkat, F. (1988) 'Contribution of cutaneous and muscle afferent fibres to cortical SEPs following median and radial nerve stimulation in man.' *Electroencephalography and Clinical Neurophysiology*, **71**, 331–335.

Hrbek, A, Hrbekova, M., Lenard, H.-G. (1968) 'Somatosensory evoked responses in newborn infants.' *Electroencephalography and Clinical Neurophysiology*, **25**, 443–448.

—— —— —— (1969) 'Somatosensory, auditory and visual evoked responses in newborn infants during sleep and wakefulness.' *Electroencephalography and Clinical Neurophysiology*, **26**, 597–603.

—— Karlberg, P., Olsson, T. (1973) 'Development of visual and somatosensory evoked responses in preterm newborn infants.' *Electroencephalography and Clinical Neurophysiology*, **34**, 225–232.

—— —— Kjellmer, I., Olsson, T., Riha, M. (1977) 'Clinical application of evoked EEG responses in newborn infants. 1: Perinatal asphyxia.' *Developmental Medicine and Child Neurology*, **19**, 34–44.

Klimach, V.J., Cooke, R.W.I (1988*a*) 'Maturation of the neonatal somatosensory evoked response in preterm infants.' *Developmental Medicine and Child Neurology*, **30**, 208–214.

—— —— (1988*b*) 'Short-latency cortical somatosensory evoked responses of preterm infants with ultrasound abnormality of the brain.' *Developmental Medicine and Child Neurology*, **30**, 215–221.

Koh, T.H.H.G., Aynsley-Green, A., Tarbit, M., Eyre, J.A. (1988) 'Neural dysfunction during hypoglycaemia.' *Archives of Disease in Childhood*, **63**, 1353–1358.

Laget, P., Salbreux, R., Raimbault, J., d'Allest, A.M., Mariani, J. (1976) 'Relationship between changes in somesthetic evoked responses and electroencephalographic findings in the child with hemiplegia.' *Developmental Medicine and Child Neurology*, **18**, 620–631.

Laureau, E., Vanasse, M., Hebert, R., Letarte, J., Glorieux, J., Desjardins, M., Dussault, J.H. (1986) 'Somatosensory evoked potentials and auditory brain-stem responses in congenital hypothyroidism. 1: A longitudinal study before and after treatment in six infants detected in the neonatal period.' *Electroencephalography and Clinical Neurophysiology*, **64**, 501–510.

—— Hebert, R., Vanasse, M., Letarte, J., Glorieux, J., Desjardins, M., Dussault, J.H. (1987) 'Somatosensory evoked potentials and auditory brain stem responses in congenital hypothyroidism. 2. A cross sectional study in childhood. Correlations with hormonal levels and developmental quotients.' *Electroencephalography and Clinical Neurophysiology*, **67**, 521–530.

—— Majnemer, A., Rosenblatt, B., Riley, P. (1988) 'A longitudinal study of short latency somatosensory evoked responses in healthy newborns and infants.' *Electroencephalography and Clinical Neurophysiology*, **71**, 100–108.

Manil, J., Desmedt, J.E., Debecker, J., Chorazyma, H. (1967). 'Les potentiels cérébraux évoqués par la stimulation de la main chez le nouveau-né normal.' *Revue Neurologique*, **117**, 53–61.

Nakanishi, T., Tamaki, M., Ozaki, Y., Arasaki, K. (1983) 'Origins of short latency somatosensory evoked potentials to median nerve stimulation.' *Electroencephalography and Clinical Neurophysiology*, **56**, 74–85.

Pratt, H., Amlie, R.N., Starr, A. (1981) 'Short latency mechanically evoked peripheral nerve and somatosensory potentials in newborn infants.' *Pediatric Research*, **15**, 295–298.

Seyal, M., Gabor, A.J. (1985) 'The human posterior tibial somatosensory evoked potential: synapse dependent and synapse independent spinal components.' *Electroencephalography and Clinical Neurophysiology*, **62**, 323–331.

Taylor, M.J., Fagan, E.R. (1988) 'SEPs to median nerve stimulation: normative data for paediatrics.' *Electroencephalography and Clinical Neurophysiology*, **71**, 323–330.

Tomita, Y., Nishimura, S., Tanaka, T. (1986) 'Short latency SEPs in infants and children: developmental changes and maturational index of SEPs.' *Electroencephalography and Clinical Neurophysiology*, **65**, 335–343.

—— Tanaka, T., Kamimura, N., Shimozawa, N., Takishima, S., Takeshita, K. (1988) 'Origin and clinical significance of subcortical components in short-latency somatosensensory evoked potentials in children.' *Electroencephalography and Clinical Neurophysiology*, **69**, 199–208.

White, C.P., Cooke, R.W.I. (1989*a*) 'Maturation of the cortical evoked response to posterior tibial nerve stimulation in the preterm neonate.' *Developmental Medicine and Child Neurology*, **31**, 657–664.

—— —— (1989*b*) 'Maturation of the early cortical somatosensory evoked potentials in the preterm infant.' *In* Gennser, G., Marsal, K., Svenningsen, N., Lindstrom, K. (Eds) *Fetal and Neonatal Physiological Measurements III. Proceedings of the Third International Conference on Fetal and Neonatal Physiological Measurements.* Malmo: Ronneby.

—— —— (1989*c*) 'The use of somatosensory evoked potentials (SEPs) in the prediction of motor handicap in the preterm infant.' *In* Gennser, G., Marsal, K., Svenningsen, N., Lindstrom, K. (Eds) *Fetal and Neonatal Physiological Measurements III. Proceedings of the Third International Conference on Fetal and Neonatal Physiological Measurements.* Malmo: Ronneby.

Willis, J., Seales, D., Frazier, E. (1984) 'Short latency somatosensory evoked potentials in infants.' *Electroencephalography and Clinical Neurophysiology*, **59**, 366–373.

—— Duncan, C., Bell, R. (1987) 'Short-latency somatosensory evoked potentials in perinatal asphyxia.'

Pediatric Neurology, **3**, 203–207.
——— ——— ——— Pappas, F., Moniz, M. (1989) 'Somatosensory evoked potentials predict neuromotor outcome after periventricular hemorrhage.' *Developmental Medicine and Child Neurology*, **31**, 435–439.
Wolff, I., Matsumiya, Y., Abroms, I.F., Van Velzer, C., Lombroso, C.T. (1974) 'The effect of white noise on the somatosensory evoked response in sleeping newborn infants.' *Electroencephalography and Clinical Neurophysiology*, **37**, 269–274.
Yamada, T., Kameyama, S., Fuchigami, Y. Nakazumi, Y., Dickins, Q.S., Kimura, J. (1988) 'Changes of short latency somatosensory evoked potential in sleep.' *Electroencephalography and Clinical Neurophysiology*, **70**, 126–136.
Zhu, Y., Georgesco, M., Cadilhac, J. (1987) 'Normal latency values of early cortical somatosensory evoked petentials in children.' *Electroencephalography and Clinical Neurophysiology*, **68**, 471–474.

5

THE ASSESSMENT OF HEARING AND BRAINSTEM FUNCTION

C. R. Kennedy

Epidemiology and significance of hearing impairment in infancy

Children with congenital hearing loss of 65dB relative to normal hearing threshold level (NHL) and upwards (severe to profound deafness) will not develop speech and language normally (Sancho *et al.* 1988). The cost of this impairment, with its consequent secondary cognitive deficits, is therefore very high. There is some evidence that early rehabilitation is effective in reducing this impairment (Markides 1986). It is uncertain whether this is due to a 'critical period' for language acquisition in infancy, because systematic study of this question has been hampered by the lack of effective and well applied systems for early detection.

Mild hearing loss may also lead to deleterious effects on language but probably only if it is persistent (Rapin 1979, Haggard and Hughes 1991). The most convincing reports of measurable adverse developmental consequences of mild hearing loss have been in children suffering prolonged periods of otitis media with effusion in the first two years of life (*e.g.* Teele *et al.* 1984). An in-depth review by Haggard and Hughes (1991) concluded that the general cognitive effect of this condition on full-scale verbal IQ amounts to about 0.5 of a population SD unit at five years of age, falling to 0.3 of an SD unit at nine years of age. At this age, even the largest studies do not show statistically significant effects, partly due to the affected children 'catching up'.

The prevalence of severe to profound deafness in infancy has been reported to be 1.5 to three per thousand in several studies reviewed by Peckham (1986). One of the largest cohort studies reported a prevalence estimate of 2.6 per 1000 for severe bilateral hearing impairment judged to require special educational provision at the age of seven years (Peckham *et al.* 1972). If less severe hearing losses (35dB or worse on at least two frequencies in one or both ears) were added, the prevalence rose to 5.7 per cent. Most profound deafness is prenatal in origin. Among such children requiring special education in the UK in the early 1960s, hereditary deafness accounted for 50 to 60 per cent; prenatal infection (especially rubella and cytomegalovirus), 6 to 7 per cent; perinatal causes (mostly associated with preterm birth), 12 per cent; postnatal causes, 20 per cent (including 17 per cent post-meningitis); and no cause identified in the remaining 20 per cent (Fraser 1976). The distribution of aetiologies is remarkably similar if milder degrees of hearing impairment are included (Fraser 1976, Thiringer *et al.* 1984).

Screening for hearing impairment in infancy

Among those affected by a loss of greater than 50dB in the better ear among European Community children born in 1969, hearing impairments were detected in only 10 per cent by the age of one year and 55 per cent by the age of three years (Martin *et al.* 1981). Figures for the USA are similar (Simmons 1978). There is little reason to suppose that age of detection has decreased significantly since then. Thus there is a need to improve the means of detecting such losses. Because severe hearing impairment has much greater potentially reversible effects on communication skills than milder hearing impairment, the aim of an infant screening programme should be to detect severe and profound losses and to reduce the age at which intervention is begun (Sancho *et al.* 1988). Because of the relatively low prevalence of this degree of hearing impairment, the specificity of any screening test has to be high to avoid unacceptably large numbers of unimpaired infants failing the screening test for each case of genuine hearing impairment detected.

Current screening practice

1. TARGETED SCREENING

Many hearing-impaired children come from definable population subgroups at high risk of hearing impairment. Within such groups, the risk of moderate to profound hearing loss is increased 20- to 100-fold (Sancho *et al.* 1988). The American Academy of Pediatrics (1982) recommended that infants at high risk of impairment should be screened by the age of three months and should be receiving habilitation by the age of six months. The risk factors which they specified were:

(1) family history of childhood hearing impairment
(2) congenital perinatal infection (sic)
(3) anatomic malformations involving the head or neck
(4) birthweight of less than 1500g
(5) hyperbilirubinaemia at levels exceeding the indication for exchange transfusion
(6) bacterial meningitis, and
(7) severe asphyxia.

In the USA, current screening practice reflects these guidelines: universal screening has never been widely adopted there and only high-risk infants, as defined above, are likely to be tested by one of several possible neonatal tests (see below). Unfortunately, less than half of the children with severe to profound deafness have such identifiable risk factors. For example, sensorineural hearing loss detected amongst infants who weighed less than 2000g at birth or who spent more than 24 hours in the special care baby unit (SCBU) in a 1984/85 birth cohort in the Oxford region made up only 29 per cent of all infants from the same birth cohort on a regional register of sensorineural deafness detected by the age of three years (Johnson and Ashurst 1990). The 'at-risk population' in that study probably included all the groups specified by the American Academy of Pediatrics other than those with a family history of childhood hearing impairment; so it is apparent that, in practice, hearing tests also have to be applied to those not in identified groups at high risk in order to identify most cases of hearing impairment.

2. UNIVERSAL SCREENING

Universal screening has been the adopted policy throughout the United Kingdom in the form of a behavioural 'distraction test' administered by health visitors at eight months (Stewart-Brown and Haslum 1987). The effects on tested and untested infants have never been compared. The average age of detection of hearing impairment using this test can be reduced by improving health-visitor training and by introducing explicit guidelines to assist parents in their own observations of their child's hearing (McCormick 1983, Scanlon and Bamford 1990). However, the failure rate of the distraction test remains unacceptably high, both at eight and 16 months (16.3 per cent and 6.8 per cent respectively in a cohort of unselected children, and 18.3 per cent and 3.2 per cent respectively in a SCBU population—Brown *et al.* 1989, Johnson and Ashurst 1990). An onward referral rate of 2.6 to 6.6 per cent following failure on distraction testing over an entire health district with sensitivity for severe hearing impairment as low as 50 per cent was reported by Scanlon and Bamford (1990).

This test has three other built-in drawbacks. Firstly, for a variety of reasons, coverage of as little as 80 per cent of the population with the test further reduces its efficacy (Brown *et al.* 1989), especially since infants with hearing impairment are over-represented in the untested group (Johnson and Ashurst 1990). Secondly, in infants who are correctly identified as hearing-impaired, the diagnostic process is rarely complete before the age of one year, delaying intervention beyond the optimum time. Thirdly, because of the high prevalence of middle-ear disorders in the second six months of life, many cases of fluctuating mild or moderate hearing impairment are detected where the benefits of intervention are doubtful and a screening test is therefore inappropriate (Stewart-Brown and Haslum 1987). All three problems could be avoided by a suitable neonatal test.

Neonatal tests of hearing

Comprehensive testing of hearing should include evaluation of the ability to hear sounds at different frequencies within the speech range and to discriminate speech with a soft stimulus. Unfortunately such accurate and reliable measurement of the ability to hear is not yet possible in the newborn infant. Three main types of measure have been used to provide early predictors of an infant's future hearing ability. The most universally accepted method is the auditory brainstem response (ABR), which is a measure of the effect of an auditory stimulus on electroencephalographic (EEG) activity. The two other types of responses which will be considered in turn below are (i) behavioural responses and (ii) the emitted sound or 'echo'—the otoacoustic emission (OAE)—which may be recorded in the ear canal some milliseconds (ms) after an auditory stimulus has been presented in that ear. Automation in measuring all three types of response—ABR, behavioural and

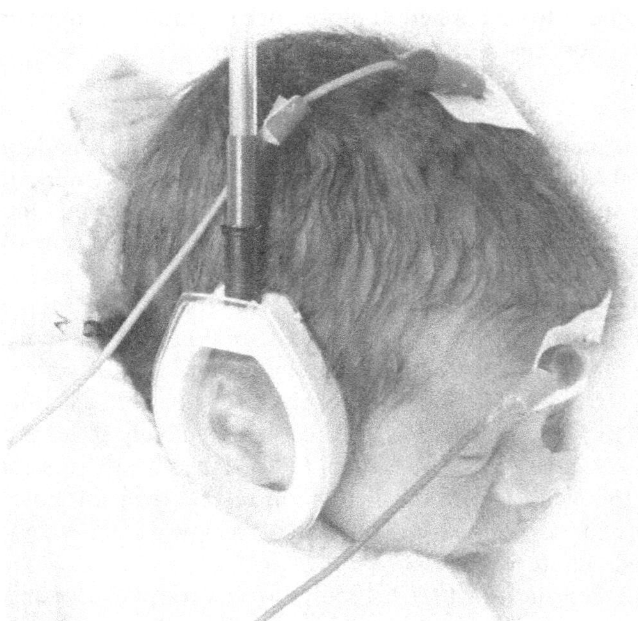

Fig. 5.1. Recording the ABR from an infant for automated ('Algo 1') pass/refer analysis. The auditory stimulus is presented through a sound coupler attached to the ear. Electrode montage is vertex-positive, nape-reference, forehead-ground.

OAE—has also been developed for screening purposes. In the case of ABR, the recorded information has also been used to make inferences about aspects of brainstem function other than hearing, and these will also be touched on.

The auditory brainstem response

The measurement of EEG changes initiated by an auditory stimulus became possible with the introduction of averaging computers in the 1960s. These changes can be divided into responses seen in three phases: early (less than 10ms), middle (10 to 80ms) and late (50 to 400ms). The late (cortical) components are heavily influenced by attention and arousal. However, the early (brainstem) components first described by Jewett and Williston (1971) have been favoured both for the determination of thresholds and for the differentiation of cochlear from retrocochlear disturbance of function. Frye Osier *et al.* (1982) suggested that the middle components could also be of use in neonatal hearing screening.

Morphology and maturation of the ABR

The click-evoked ABR is usually recorded with three or four surface electrodes, with the active electrode at the vertex or high forehead and reference and ground electrodes on ipsilateral and contralateral mastoids/earlobes respectively. The nape of the neck and forehead are alternative sites for reference and ground (Fig. 5.1). The ABR consists of a series of vertex-positive waves designated I to V (Fig. 5.2). The best electrode position for recording varies for each wave (Parker 1981).

Fig. 5.2. The components of the ABR (from Krumholz *et al.* 1985, by permission).

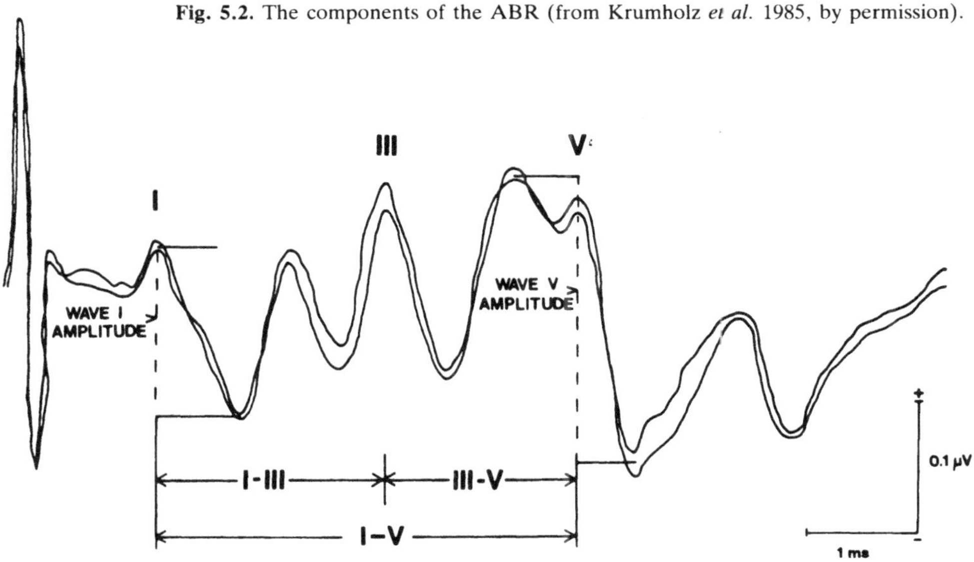

Broad-band 100μs square-wave clicks at less than 20/s will give the clearest responses. Stimulus polarity, bandwidth, masking of the contralateral ear, and bandpass filtration of EEG signal are also important testing variables. Stimulus intensity is measured in peak equivalent sound pressure level (SPL), but usually reported relative to NHL. Intraoperative recordings in adults suggest that waves I and II arise from the eighth nerve, wave III from the cochlear nucleus and wave V from the lateral lemniscus.

Determination of the type and degree of hearing loss may be aided by reference to a number of features of the ABR: absolute latencies of waves I, III and V; I to V inter-peak latency; the ratio of amplitudes of I to wave V; and measurement of differences between latencies of responses to stimuli presented to the left and right ears. These variables may be affected by stimulus intensity and by the maturity of the infant.

An ABR response is first recordable with a high-intensity stimulus in some infants of 26 or 27 weeks post-conceptional age (PCA) and in most by 30 weeks. Latencies and thresholds decrease thereafter. The importance of this effect decreases with increasing age (Fig. 5.3). Maturational norms have been reported by several investigators (Schulman-Galambos and Galambos 1975, Starr *et al.* 1977, Goldstein *et al.* 1979, Fawer and Dubowitz 1982, Weber 1982, Stockard *et al.* 1983*a*). Few if any of these studies can claim to have excluded all infants with either audiological or neurological abnormalities from their 'normal' population. Wave V latency decreases from 9.9ms at 26 weeks to 6.9 to 7.5ms at 40 to 41 weeks PCA. The ABR of preterm infants is far more variable than that of term infants (Krumholz *et al.* 1985). Wave I to V inter-peak interval is 5ms at 40 weeks compared to 4ms in

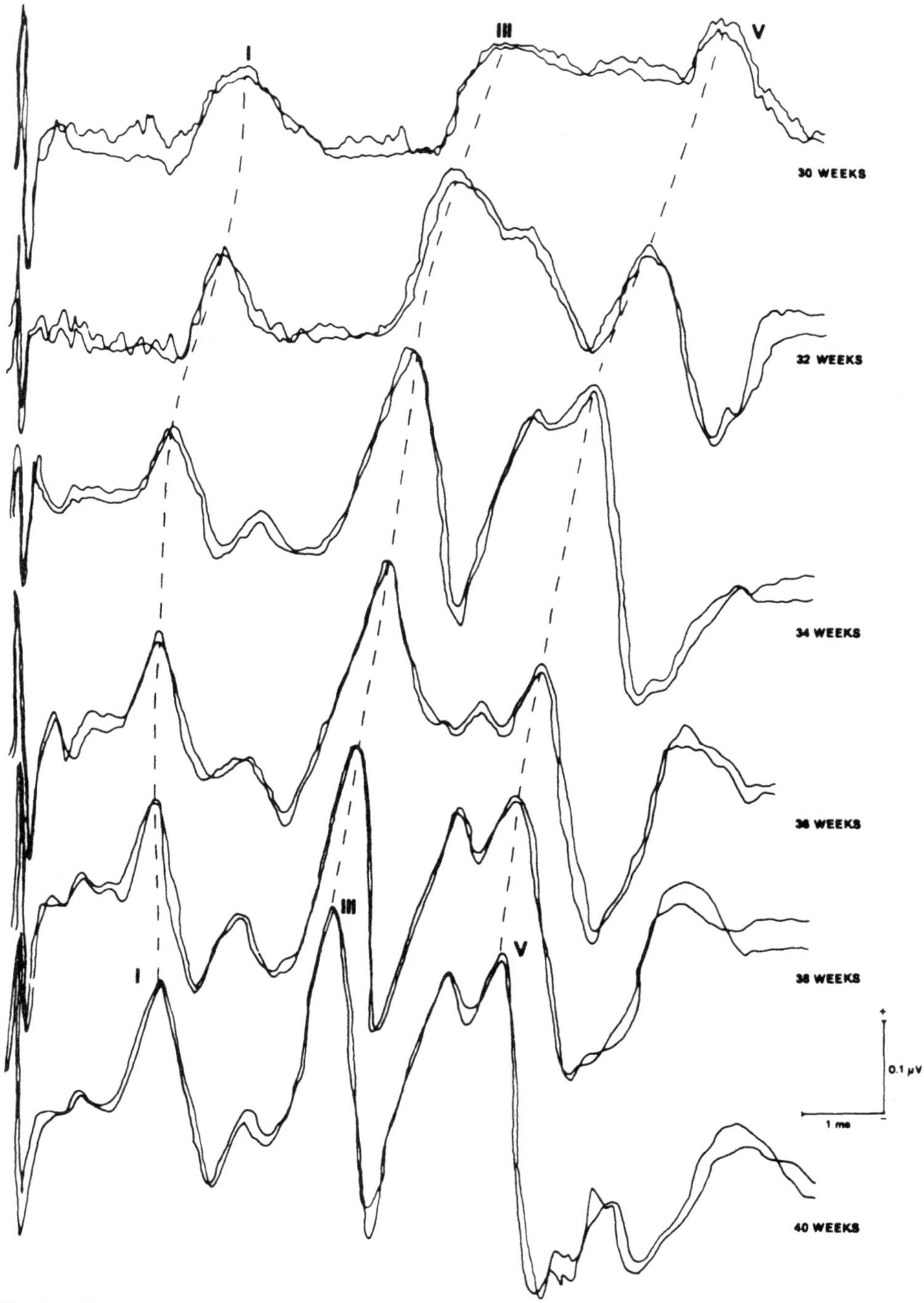

Fig. 5.3. An example of serial ABR studies in an individual preterm infant (from Krumholz *et al.* 1985, by permission).

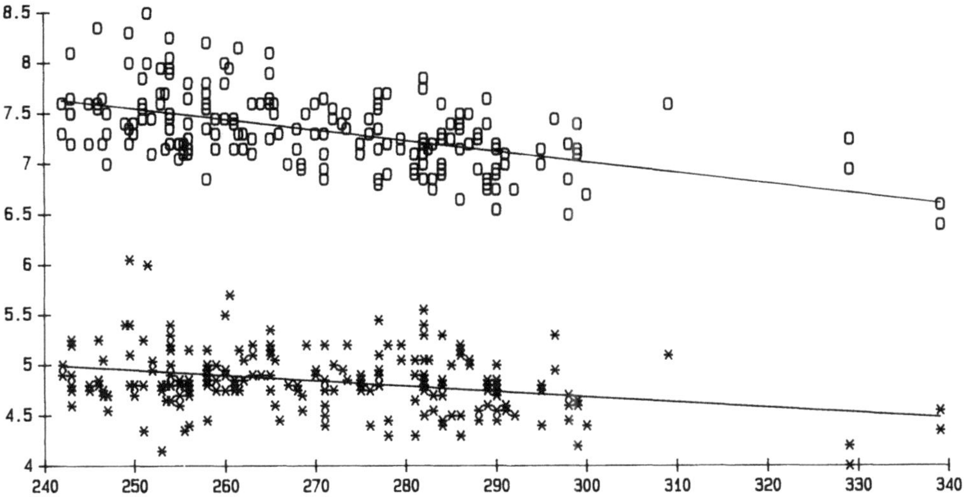

Fig. 5.4. Maturation of ABR with age. Latencies (ms) for wave III (*upper trace*, ◯) and wave V (*lower trace*, ⋇) plotted vertically, PCA at time of testing, plotted horizontally. The population consisted of infants admitted to SCBU for more than 48 hours (N 223); normal term infants on the wards (N 86); and infants at increased risk of hearing impairment because of craniofacial malformation or a family history of childhood deafness (N 61). Any baby with abnormal middle-ear function at the time of testing, or with hearing impairment at follow-up, was excluded. Neurological impairment was not an exclusion criterion (courtesy of Dr R.D. Thornton). ◯ = JV; ⋇ = JIII.

adults. Adult latency values are reached at 12 to 18 months (Hecox and Galambos 1974, Salamy and McKean 1976). Because of the variation in stimulus and recording parameters, each laboratory should establish its own norms (Fig. 5.4).

The ABR *as a predictor of hearing impairment*

Evidence about the ABR as a screening tool may appear to be conflicting. In a review of 32 reports on the subject, Murray *et al.* (1985) reported variations in failure rates from less than 1 per cent to 22.2 per cent on repeat testing of infants at follow-up who failed an initial ABR test. However, the very high failure rate on early ABRS reported in some series included infants who were often still sick or preterm. Inappropriate prediction of hearing impairment has sometimes been made because of failure to appreciate that abnormality of the ABR may arise, not only as a result of hearing impairment but also as a result of other brainstem abnormalities, congenital or acquired. Murray *et al.* (1985) made three recommendations for testing neonatal ABR: (i) ABR testing for hearing impairment should be delayed until the infant is close to term and medically stable; (ii) sufficient ABR measurements (*i.e.* latency of wave I, latency-intensity functions) should be made to exclude abnormalities caused by middle-ear disease or collapsed ear canals; and (iii) when elevated thresholds are accompanied by indications of neuromaturational delay (such as prolonged I to V intervals) they should be interpreted cautiously. An elevated threshold to an auditory stimulus may be due to either a peripheral or a brainstem cause if the I to V interval is also increased. Provided that these points of interpretation are observed, abnormalities of wave I can be used to predict both the presence and the type of hearing impairment (Stockard *et al.* 1983*b*). Two more recent studies have also reported that failure on ABR testing of high-risk infants at term, using a 40 to 45dB stimulus, has a 67 to 73 per cent positive predictive value for moderate to profound hearing loss (Pettigrew *et al.* 1986, Kramer *et al.* 1989).

Automated versions of ABR testing, such as 'Algo 1', have been developed, in which the similarity of the infant's ABR to a stored template is used to designate the response 'pass' or 'refer' (Kileny 1988). Early reports suggest that such devices may at least match the specificity of conventional ABR testing as a neonatal screen for hearing impairment while reducing testing-time and the need for skilled interpretation of the ABR trace (Kileny 1988, Kennedy *et al.* 1991). Such devices are not yet programmed to distinguish between peripheral and central patterns of abnormality.

ABR as a predictor of other neurological abnormality

Neonatal ABR bears no consistent relationship to later ability to hear in *preterm* infants, nor in infants with severe brain-damage. On the other hand, ABR results may be useful in predicting severe brain-damage in term neonates with intact hearing. Stockard *et al.* (1983*b*) reported follow-up audiological and neurological evaluation of 181 high-risk preterm infants. About half had suffered hypoxic-ischaemic encephalopathy, with most of the rest having craniofacial anomalies or hyperbilirubinaemia requiring exchange transfusion. Abnormal patterns of ABR could be divided into either

(1) absence of response, or
(2) a peripheral pattern, consisting of elevation of wave I threshold with or without elevation of wave V threshold, or
(3) a 'central' pattern consisting of prolongation of I to V inter-peak latency or the absence of components of the ABR beyond I.

Overall, of all the subjects with central abnormalities (with or without peripheral changes), 87 per cent had moderate to severe neurodevelopmental abnormality. Unfortunately the frequency of such neurological abnormalities in infants without the ABR abnormalities was not reported, nor was the gestational age at birth.

It must be stressed that these correlations were between the *final pre-discharge* ABR test which was always done beyond 36 weeks PCA; transient abnormalities of no significance are frequently seen in more immature infants. Although these correlations appear high, they are not high enough to be used with confidence in an individual case. For example, four of 13 surviving asphyxiated infants had normal neurodevelopmental outcome in spite of abnormal inter-peak latencies (Stockard *et al.* 1983*b*); one asphyxiated infant with complete absence of the later components of the ABR had minimal neurological sequelae. Hecox and Burkard (1982) and Stockard *et al.* (1983*b*) reported that initially abnormal ABRs in asphyxiated infants may revert to normal over three to four weeks in cases with a favourable neurological outcome.

Several centres have reported ABR abnormalities in preterm infants with intraventricular haemorrhage with or without post-haemorrhagic ventricular dilatation. The presence and degree of ABR abnormality has been reported to show poor correlation with the size of the intracranial haemorrhage, intracranial pressure and neurodevelopmental outcome (Lary *et al.* 1989, Beverley *et al.* 1990). In this context, most abnormalities of the ABR resolve irrespective of subsequent ventricular size (Lary *et al.* 1989). The prognostic value of ABR in the very low birthweight infant is certainly very limited in view of the high incidence of transient abnormalities in preterm infants with a favourable outcome. In general, the presence of abnormalities of the neonatal ABR must be confirmed on retesting at least one month later and should never be used as a justification for withdrawing treatment.

Behavioural tests of hearing

The view held by some developmental paediatricians, that a high-frequency rattle can be used to elicit behavioural responses amenable to reliable assessment by an observer, remains unsubstantiated: specificity of such testing is low, at less than 80 per cent (Bonfils *et al.* 1990), and sensitivity undocumented. Since such testing is cheap and quick, however, it might be useful as a preliminary screen—to be followed immediately in infants failing the test by a more specific test.

Attempts to measure cardiovascular, respiratory and motor responses in infants, to derive an objective automated screening test, have resulted in the Crib-O-Gram in the USA and the Linco-Bennett Auditory Response Cradle in the UK. At a first Auditory Response Cradle test, there was a high rate for failure or abandonment: 7.9 per cent and 10.5 per cent in two reports on both low-risk and SCBU infants (Bhattacharya *et al.* 1984, Hall and Garner 1988), and 21 per cent in a SCBU population (McCormick *et al.* 1984). Failure of the cradle to detect severe bilateral sensorineural hearing-loss was reported by McCormick *et al.* (1984), although the automated pass/fail decision algorithm has since been improved. A quick and simple nonspecific test could still be useful if followed immediately in infants failing the test by a more specific test. However, one full-time tester could screen only 30 or 40 babies a week using the Linco-Bennett Auditory Response Cradle (Hall and Garner 1988) which is no better than could be achieved with a much more specific automated ABR test. Similarly high failure rates were also reported for the Crib-O-Gram as well as low sensitivity with a best estimate of five cases of hearing impairment *missed* per 1000 babies tested (Prager *et al.* 1987)!

Otoacoustic emissions

The cochlea actively produces energy in the audible frequency range in response to an auditory stimulus. Some of this energy passes back through the ossicles into the ear canal, where it may be detected as sound, which is referred to as an OAE (Kemp

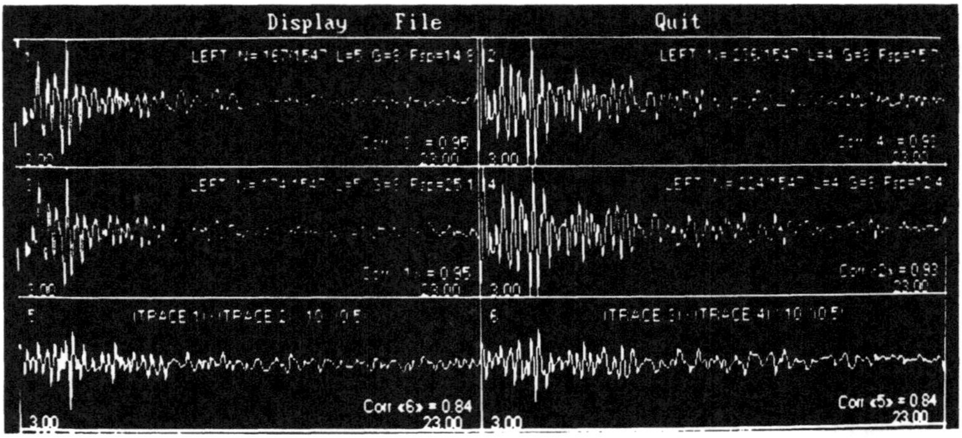

Fig. 5.5. The OAE and information derived from it shown on a computer display screen during testing with the POEMS. In each box an OAE is shown with time plotted horizontally, from 3 to 23ms after the click stimulus, and amplitude plotted vertically. Boxes 1 and 3 show the averaged emission evoked by two series of presentations to the left ear of 46dB nHL clicks (level 5) at 33 clicks per second recorded with the same amplification level (gain level 8) for both series. The F_{SP} shown in each box is the F statistic for sound pressure level in the response, akin to a signal to noise ratio. The correlation between the emissions obtained in the two series is shown in both box 1 and box 3. Boxes 2 and 4 show a similar series of results obtained using a 36dB nHL stimulus (level 4). The trace in box 5 is the non-linear component of the emission obtained by subtracting a multiple of the emission in box 2 from the emission in box 1—this would be equal to zero if the emission increased in proportion to the amplitude of the evoking stimulus in a linear fashion (see text). Box 6 is derived in a similar fashion from boxes 3 and 4. The correlation between the traces in boxes 5 and 6 is shown in both boxes. The patient data are compared with preset pass/fail criteria (*e.g.* pass at a given level if $F_{SP} > 2$ and Corr Coeff > 0.5 between two series of presentations) derived from a population of infants without hearing impairment.

1978). The precise physiology of these emissions is not yet understood but the energy is thought to be produced by outer hair cells in order to enhance the precision of the selectivity of the cochlear response to differing sound frequencies. Stimulated OAEs can be recorded in 98 to 100 per cent of normal term infants (Elberling *et al.* 1985, Stevens *et al.* 1989, Bonfils *et al.* 1990).

The morphology of OAEs stimulated by a click stimulus (Fig. 5.5) varies widely, but forms a consistent 'fingerprint' for any one individual. They can be detected by a microphone inserted in the ear canal and recorded using the same type of computer-averaging techniques employed for the ABR. The amplitude of an OAE is non-linear with respect to the amplitude of the evoking stimulus, the emission having a higher energy than the evoking stimulus at low-stimulus intensity but rapidly saturating at higher-stimulus intensities. This non-linearity of the OAE is useful in helping to distinguish true emissions from artefact (Fig. 5.5).

In adults, emissions are lost early if there is dysfunction of the peripheral auditory system, such as that produced by a high therapeutic blood level of aspirin. OAEs stimulated by clicks or pure tones are in current use as tools in screening for hearing impairment. Distortion product OAEs, produced by two continuous pure

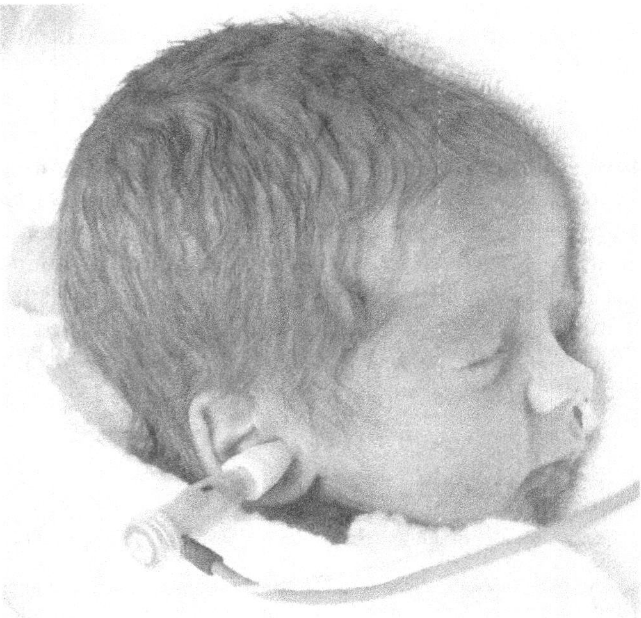

Fig. 5.6. Recording the OAE from a term infant. Both the stimulus presentation and the recording of the evoked emission are carried out by the single probe.

tones separated by a prescribed frequency distance, may have future application in determining objectively frequency-specific hearing thresholds (Martin *et al.* 1990).

OAES may have a role in neonatal hearing screening. The response can be recorded from the same probe used to present the stimulus, obviating the need for time-consuming scalp electrodes (Fig. 5.6). A screening test using two different stimulus intensities may be completed in one minute per ear and with minimal disturbance to the baby.

A study of OAES in a SCBU population (Stevens *et al.* 1989) reported a 19.7 per cent failure rate on the test in one or both ears. However, work in Southampton suggests that automated pass/fail systems such as the programmable otoacoustic emissions systems (POEMS, Fig. 5.5) may decrease this failure rate (Cope and Lutman 1988): in a study of 370 infants, divided into low-risk, SCBU and high-risk (because of positive family history of deafness or of craniofacial deformity), unilateral (bilateral) failure rates were 3.5 per cent (1.2 per cent), 5.6 per cent (1.4 per cent) and 22.9 per cent (11.5 per cent) in the respective groups using POEMS with a 36dB NHL stimulus (Kennedy *et al.* 1991). Failure to detect an OAE is a very sensitive predictor of ABR failure in the first two or three months of life (Stevens *et al.* 1989, Kennedy *et al.* 1991) and is moderately sensitive for even mild hearing impairment confirmed later in the first year of life (Kennedy *et al.* 1991). Although the test is predicted to miss some cases of 'central' deafness, there have been no reports so far of persistent severe congenital sensorineural deafness following detection of neonatal OAES. However, because of the low prevalence of sensorineural hearing loss, reliable estimates of the sensitivity of OAEs for sensorineural hearing impairment must come from larger-scale studies of the technique with longer periods of follow-up.

Future studies

Future studies may establish whether a neonatal screening protocol incorporating OAE detection should replace the eight-month distraction test, or be used as an adjunct to it, or not be used at all. If these studies can demonstrate that such a screen is effective in reducing the age at which intervention for severe to profound deafness is begun, it will still have to be proved that the benefits of such intervention justify the cost of screening. In the more distant future, distortion product OAEs (Martin *et al.* 1990) may be used to derive frequency-specific audiograms in the newborn infant.

REFERENCES

American Academy of Pediatrics, Committee on Infant Hearing (1982) 'Position statement, 1982.' *Pediatrics*, **70**, 496–497.

Beverley, D.W., Smith, I.S., Beesley, P., Jones, J., Rhodes, N. (1990) 'Relationship of cranial ultrasonography, visual and auditory evoked responses with neurodevelopmental outcome.' *Developmental Medicine and Child Neurology*, **32**, 210–222.

Bhattacharya, J., Bennett, M.J., Tucker, S.M. (1984) 'Longterm follow-up of newborns tested with the auditory response cradle.' *Archives of Disease in Childhood*, **59**, 504–511.

Bonfils, P., Dumont, A., Marie, P., Francois, M., Narcy, P. (1990) 'Evoked otoacoustic emissions in newborn hearing screening.' *Laryngoscope*, **100**, 186–189.

Brown, J., Watson, E., Alberman, E. (1989) 'Screening infants for hearing loss.' *Archives of Disease in Childhood*, **64**, 1488–1495.

Cope, C., Lutman, M. (1988) 'Otoacoustic emissions.' *In* McCormick, B. (Ed.) *Paediatric Audiology 0–5 Years*. London: Taylor & Francis. pp. 221–245.

Elberling, C., Parbo, J., Johnsen, N.J., Bagi, P. (1985) 'Evoked acoustic emissions: clinical application.' *Acta Otolaryngologica*, (Suppl. **421**), 77–85.

Fawer, C., Dubowitz, L.M.S. (1982) 'Auditory brainstem response in neurologically normal preterm and full-term newborn infants.' *Neuropediatrics*, **13**, 200–206.

Fraser, G.R. (1976) *The Causes of Profound Deafness in Childhood.* London: Baillière Tindall. pp. 318–320.

Frye-Osier, H.A., Goldstein, R., Hirsh, J.E., Weber, K. (1982) 'Early and middle ear components to clicks as response indices for neonatal hearing screening.' *Annals of Otorhinolaryngology*, **91**, 272–276.

Goldstein, P., Krumholz, A., Felix, J., Shannon, D., Carr, R. (1979) 'Brainstem-evoked responses in neonates.' *American Journal of Obstetrics and Gynecology*, **135**, 622–628.

Haggard, M., Hughes, E. (1991) *Screening Children's Hearing—A Review of the Literature and Implications of Otitis Media.* London: HMSO.

Hall, D.M., Garner, J. (1988) 'Feasibility of screening all neonates for hearing loss.' *Archives of Disease in Childhood*, **63**, 652–653.

Hecox, K., Galambos, R. (1974) 'Brainstem auditory evoked responses in human infants and adults.' *Archives of Otolaryngology*, **99**, 30–33.

—— Burkard, R. (1982) 'Developmental dependencies of the human auditory evoked response.' *Annals of the New York Academy of Sciences*, **388**, 538–556.

Jewett, D.L., Williston, J.S. (1971) 'Auditory evoked far fields averaged from the scalp of humans.' *Brain*, **94**, 681–696.

Johnson, A., Ashurst, H. (1990) 'Screening for sensorineural deafness by health visitors.' *Archives of Disease in Childhood*, **65**, 841–845.
Kemp, D.T. (1978) 'Stimulated acoustic emissions from within the hearing system.' *Journal of the Acoustical Society of America*, **64**, 1386–1391.
Kennedy, C.R., Kimm, L., Cafarelli Dees, D., Evans, P.I.P., Hunter, M., Lenton, S., Thornton, R.D. (1991) 'Otoacoustic emissions and auditory brainstem responses and subsequent hearing impairment.' *Archives of Disease in Childhood*, **66**, 1124–1129.
Kileny, P.R. (1988) 'New insights on infant ABR hearing screening.' *Scandinavian Audiology*, (Suppl. **30**), 81–88.
Kramer, S.J., Vertes, D.R., Condon, M. (1989) 'Auditory brainstem responses and clinical follow-up of high-risk infants.' *Pediatrics*, **83**, 385–392.
Krumholz, A., Felix, J.K., Goldstein, P.J., McKenzie, E. (1985) 'Motivation of the brainstem auditory evoked potential in premature infants.' *Electroencephalography and Clinical Neurophysiology*, **62**, 124–134.
Lary, S., De Vries, L.S., Kaiser, A., Dubowitz, L.M.S., Dubowitz, V. (1989) 'Auditory brainstem responses in infants with post-haemorrhagic ventricular dilatation.' *Archives of Disease in Childhood*, **64**, 17–23.
McCormick, B. (1983) 'Hearing screening by health visitors—a critical appraisal of the distraction test.' *Health Visitor*, **56**, 449–451.
—— Curnock, D.A., Spavins, F. (1984) 'Auditory screening of special care neonates using the auditory response cradle.' *Archives of Disease in Childhood*, **59**, 1168–1172.
Markides, A. (1986) 'Age of fitting of hearing aids and speech intelligibility.' *British Journal of Audiology*, **20**, 165–168.
Martin, G.K., Whitehead, M., Lonsbury-Martin, B.L. (1990) 'Potential of evoked otoacoustic emissions for infant hearing screening.' *Seminars in Hearing*, **11**, 186–204.
Martin, J.A.M., Bentzen, O., Colley, J.R.T. Hennebert, D., Holm, C., Iurato, S., da Jonge, G.A., McCullen, O., Meyer, M.I., Moore, W.J., Morgon, A. (1981) 'Childhood deafness in the European community.' *Scandinavian Audiology*, **10**, 165–174.
Murray, A.D., Javel, E., Watson, C.S. (1985) 'Prognostic validity of auditory brainstem evoked response screening in newborn infants.' *American Journal of Otolaryngology*, **6**, 120–131.
Parker, D.J. (1981) 'Dependence of the auditory brainstem response on electrode location.' *Archives of Otolaryngology*, **107**, 367–371.
Peckham, C.S. (1986) 'Hearing impairment in childhood.' *British Medical Bulletin*, **42**, 145–149.
—— Sheridan, M., Butler, N.R. (1972) 'School of attainment of seven year old children with hearing difficulties.' *Developmental Medicine and Child Neurology*, **14**, 592–602
Pettigrew, A.G., Edwards, D.A., Henderson-Smart, D.J. (1986) 'Screening for auditory dysfunction in high risk neonates.' *Early Human Development*, **14**, 109–120.
Prager, D.A., Stone, D.A., Ross, D.N. (1987) 'Hearing loss screening in the neonatal intensive care unit; auditory brainstem response versus Crib-O-Gram; a cost-effectiveness analysis.' *Ear and Hearing*, **8**, 213–216.
Rapin, I. (1979) 'Conductive hearing loss effects on children's language and scholastic skills.' *Annals of Otology, Rhinology and Laryngology*, **88** (Suppl. 60), 3–13.
Salamy, A., McKean, C.M. (1976) 'Postnatal development of human brainstem potentials during the first year of life.' *Electroencephalography and Clinical Neurophysiology*, **40**, 418–426.
Sancho, J., Hughes, E., Davis, A., Haggard, M.P. (1988) 'Epidemiology of hearing impairments in children and its application to screening.' *In* McCormick, B. (Ed.) *Paediatric Audiology 0–5 Years.* London: Taylor & Francis. pp. 1–35.
Scanlon, P.E., Bamford, J.M. (1990) 'Early identification of hearing loss: screening and surveillance methods.' *Archives of Disease in Childhood*, **65**, 479–484.
Schulman-Galambos, C., Galambos, R. (1975) 'Brainstem auditory evoked responses in premature infants.' *Journal of Speech and Hearing Research*, **18**, 456–465.
Simmons, F.B. (1978) 'Identification of hearing loss in infants and young children.' *Otolaryngology Clinics of North America*, **11**, 19–28.
Starr, A., Amlie, R.N., Martin, W.H., Saunders, S. (1977) 'Development of auditory function in newborn infants revealed by auditory brainstem potentials.' *Pediatrics*, **60**, 831–839.
Stevens, J.C., Webb, H.D., Hutchinson, J., Connell, J., Smith, M.E., Buffin. J.T. (1989) 'Click evoked

otoacoustic emissions compared with brainstem electrical response.' *Archives of Disease in Childhood*, **64**, 1105–1111.
Stewart-Brown, S., Haslum, M.N. (1987) 'Screening for hearing loss in childhood; a study of national practice.' *British Medical Journal*, **294**, 1386–1388.
Stockard, J.E., Stockard, J.J., Coen, R.W. (1983*a*) 'Auditory brainstem response variability in infants.' *Ear and Hearing*, **4**, 11–23.
—— —— Kleinberg, F., Westmoreland, B.F. (1983*b*) 'Prognostic value of brainstem auditory evoked potentials in neonates.' *Archives of Neurology*, **40**, 360–365.
Teele, D.W., Klein, J.O., Rosner, B.A. (1984) 'Otitis media with effusion during the first three years of life and development of speech and language.' *Pediatrics*, **74**, 282–287.
Thiringer, K., Kankkunen, A., Liden, G., Niklasson, A. (1984) 'Perinatal risk factors in the aetiology of hearing loss in preschool children.' *Developmental Medicine and Child Neurology*, **26**, 799–807.
Warren, M.P. (1989) 'The auditory brainstem response in pediatrics.' *Otolaryngology Clinics of North America*, **22**, 473–500.
Weber, B.A. (1982) 'Comparison of auditory brainstem response latency norms for premature infants.' *Ear and Hearing*, **3**, 257–262.

6
VISUAL EVOKED POTENTIALS

Margot J. Taylor

Unlike the evoked potentials in other modalities, the visual evoked potentials (VEPS) have been used in the neonatal population for decades. However, the range of stimuli used and the number and breadth of applications has increased considerably in the last several years. The VEPS offer a window both on visual system function and, more generally, on cerebral or neurological function, and as such are now invaluable aids to neonatologists, ophthalmologists and neurologists in their assessments of neonates. This chapter will review the VEP in the newborn infant: its methodologies, maturational changes and clinical applications.

Methodology

VEPS can be elicited by light flashes (stroboscopic lamps or light-emitting diode—LED—goggles) or by pattern stimuli (reversing, onset/offset, checks, bars or pinwheels). Pattern stimuli are more sensitive measures of visual function and are the only way to estimate visual acuity neurophysiologically. Although transient VEPS are the most commonly used, steady-state VEPS (Atkinson *et al.* 1979, Moskowitz and Sokol 1980, Porciatti 1984) and 'sweep' techniques (Norcia *et al.* 1987) also provide accurate assessment of the visual system: particularly when they are analysed by fast Fourier transform (Norcia and Tyler 1985, Eizenmann *et al.* 1989*a*). Patterned VEPS are not always feasible in the assessment of neonates, however; flash VEPS also yield valuable information.

Flash VEPS

Flash VEPS are now usually recorded in response to red LED goggle stimulation. Goggles are far less cumbersome than the stroboscopic flash, are easily used in intensive care and operating room settings and have no accompanying auditory stimulation. There are differences in the latency, amplitude and distribution of the VEPS elicited by LEDS and stroboscopic flashes (Mushin *et al.* 1984, Taylor and Farrell 1987), and therefore one must have stimulus-specific norms, although in the neonatal population the primary components are similar. The variability of both types of flash VEPS is high, and the range of normal is wide, particularly when there are also rapid maturational changes in the response.

The VEP is recorded from occipital electrodes, typically referenced to either FZ or the earlobes. For flash VEPS a single active electrode at OZ is usually sufficient. Some have found that an electrode over each occipital lobe yields more information (Groth *et al.* 1970, Kurtzberg 1982), while others have reported the intrahemispheric variability to be so large in normals that this measure may not be useful

(Ellingson 1986). Infant VEPS should have a sweep of 1000ms and a stimulus rate of 0.5/s with a bandpass of 1 to 100HZ, and approximately 20 to 60 trials per average are required. Preterm infants usually require fewer trials per average, due to a much larger signal-to-noise ratio. We have found 20 to 30 trials quite adequate. Pryds *et al.* (1988) reported reliable VEPS in preterm infants recording only three trials at a stimulation rate of one flash every 30s. Flash VEPS can be recorded in all normal neonates born from 24 weeks gestational age (GA), as soon after birth as is manageable, although Pryds *et al.* (1988) found significant temperature-related changes in the VEP within the first few hours of life. Subsequently the VEPS were stable in the infants that were stable clinically.

Pattern VEPS

High-contrast reversing checkerboards are the most commonly used pattern stimuli in the assessment of infants, although steady-state VEPS to sinusoidal gratings are also established stimuli for this age (Moskowitz and Sokol 1980, Fiorentini *et al.* 1983). Due to the large VEPS recorded in young infants, only 30 to 50 trials are usually required to obtain a reproducible response; preterm infants require only about 20 (Grose *et al.* 1989). A bandpass of 1 to 100HZ is recommended (although 1 to 30 or 1 to 50HZ are also commonly used), a rate of 2/s and a sweep of 300 to 500ms. Several adaptations to standard pattern VEP testing procedures are necessary to obtain adequate pattern VEPS in babies: (i) the infant is held, seated, in front of the stimulus screen either in a booth or in an area away from distractions; (ii) an observer (screened from view) maintains the infant's attention with sounds and/or small objects in front of the reversing stimuli; (iii) an interrupt switch is used so that trials are averaged only when the infant is looking at the stimuli; and (iv) a large stimulus field is best used so that small changes in gaze do not affect the recorded VEP. Although both binocular and monocular testing can be done in young infants (McCulloch and Skarf 1991), in clinical testing situations, usually only binocular testing is completed because of limited co-operation and attention spans.

Sweep techniques using sinusoidal gratings as the patterned stimuli are also feasible in neonates, and have the advantage of yielding VEPS to a range of spatial frequencies within 10 to 20s (Norcia *et al.* 1987). But even with the short testing time, these authors found that in the early post-term period, no recordable VEPS could be obtained in almost half of the infants, due to technical difficulties in testing very small babies.

In preterm babies, a small hand-held pattern stimulator can be used for testing in incubators or on the wards (Grose *et al.* 1989, Harding *et al.* 1989). Pattern VEPS to two degree checks (reversing at a rate of 1 to 3/s) were recorded in 50 per cent of babies born between 28 and 35 weeks, within the first week of life, although the authors do not say at what age in the cross-sectional data the pattern VEP was reliably found. In terms of post-conceptional age (PCA), however, it was recorded in some infants as young as 30.5 weeks and consistently in those 33 weeks PCA and older (Grose *et al.* 1989, Harding *et al.* 1989). Although this can yield reliable VEPS, this method has not yet been used for assessment of visual acuity, and still only produces VEPS in half of the preterm neonates, when first tested. This method may supersede the use of flash VEPS in normal preterm infants, but as it can only be used in awake, alert neonates, it will not be as likely to become routine for clinical assessment. It is often assumed that pattern VEPS cannot be done in preterm infants until they have reached 40 weeks PCA (Kurtzberg 1982), and they are certainly more easily and reliably recorded after this age.

Effects of state of arousal

The effect of sleep state on the VEPS in neonates has been investigated in several studies (Hrbek *et al.* 1969; Ellingson *et al.* 1973, 1986; Glaze *et al.* 1983). The findings have shown consistently that no significant changes occur with awake or sleep states in term newborn infants. Some of the studies found intrasubject differences in VEP amplitude with sleep states with a term population, in that some infants showed larger responses during wakefulness, and others in regular sleep: but the overall effects were not significant. When collecting normative data in preterm newborn infants we remarked on VEP variability as a function of apparent changes in arousal; as found with the above reports, this did not appear to be a factor in term infants. Thus we looked at the effect of sleep on the VEPS in preterm babies (born at 28 to 36 weeks). The N300 was the only wave present across the sleep states in all the neonates. There was a significant reduction in its amplitude with quiet sleep (Whyte *et al.* 1987) but no significant latency prolongations. There were no significant differences among awake, atypical and active sleep states. Although we have found the effect of sleep to be somewhat variable, as reported by others in the literature, if a distinction is made between quiet sleep and other arousal states, consistent and significant differences in amplitudes emerge in the preterm population. Our findings confirmed those of Watanabe *et al.* (1973), who also reported the VEP amplitude to be greater in rapid eye movement (REM) versus quiet sleep in preterm infants, a comparison similar to our active versus quiet sleep. They also found that latencies did not change significantly, but tended to be shorter during wakefulness. Grose *et al.* (1989) also noted the flash VEP to be attenuated during sleep in preterm infants. We found that the P200 appeared particularly sensitive to sleep state, disappearing completely in both quiet and active sleep in the preterm infants in whom the component could be recorded. Perhaps this is due to less stability with this component, which, when present, is only newly emerged in the preterm population.

These results emphasise the need to test the infants in the same wake-sleep state both in cross-sectional and longitudinal studies of VEP in order to make valid maturational comparisons of latency or amplitude changes. This is critical in preterm infants due to the rapid developmental changes in the VEPS of preterm babies, which may be missed due to the effect of sleep on their VEPS (*i.e.* the presence of an early P200 may not be evident if the baby is tested when in quiet sleep). This is not, however, an effect that has been observed in term or post-term infants. In other than preterm neonates, the VEPS are usually easier to record in a sleeping infant, due to less artefactual interference.

The effects of drugs on the neonatal VEP has not been well investigated, but generally the VEP appears to be very resistant to medication effects, at least in the term population. Sedation should not be required for testing neonates; if the baby is too restless when awake to record VEPS, one should wait until the infant falls into natural sleep. Drugs that may be given in the neonatal period (*e.g.* phenobarbitone) in our experience do not significantly affect routine VEP recordings, provided that the VEPS are not recorded immediately following a bolus drug injection.

Developmental changes

Maturational changes in the VEPS are due to a combination of changes in synaptogenesis and myelination, as reviewed in Chapter 1. The developmental data are necessary for any clinical laboratory, to establish age-related normal limits. These norms must be established for the specific type of stimuli being used in the laboratory. These developmental data are also important for the study of normal maturational changes in the central nervous system (CNS), and can provide unique data on possible generators, or neuro-anatomical correlates, of the VEP components. Within the visual system, the most rapid changes occur in the last trimester of pregnancy and the first months after term birth.

Preterm maturation

Over the last few decades a number of investigators have studied VEPS in term and preterm neonates, noting the markedly different waveforms in infants born at various gestational ages (*e.g.* Hrbek and Mares 1964, Umezaki and Morrell 1970, Watanabe *et al.* 1972). However, the earliest studies did not have signal averagers, required long recording times and only had the use of stroboscopic flash as the stimulus source, which was cumbersome and could not be placed inside an incubator (thus producing variable stimulus intensities). With the advent of LED goggles as a stimulus source, consistency in stimulus parameters could be maintained across infants studied (Mushin *et al.* 1984). Another recent innovation for flash VEPS in the preterm nursery is the use of a light-cable, attached to a flash unit, which can be held in front of the infant's eyes inside the incubator (Pryds *et al.* 1988). Although different studies of preterm maturation have used different stimuli, the general pattern of development is similar, and from now on stimulus type will be mentioned only when relevant.

We studied cross-sectional and longitudinal VEPS in preterm neonates that demonstrated the maturation of the waveform with increasing GA and provided electrophysiological evidence of differences in intrauterine versus extrauterine maturation of the visual system (Taylor *et al.* 1987). VEPS were recorded from OZ, referenced to FZ, using the standard recording paradigm outlined above. LED goggles are held lightly over the infant's eyes and at least two averages of 40 to 60 trials each were collected to binocular stimulation. All the babies were tested in an

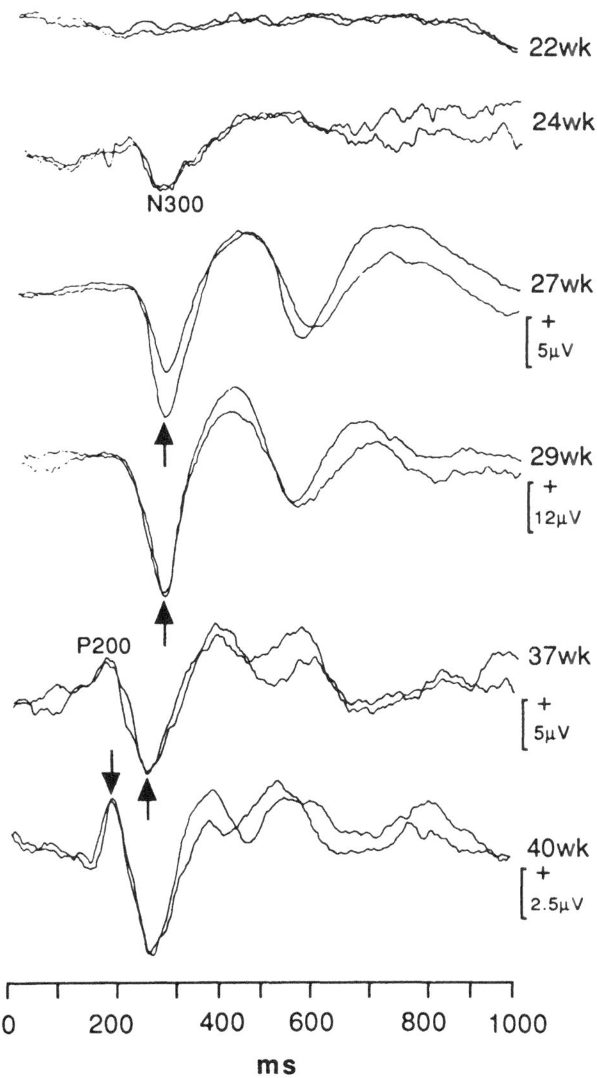

Fig. 6.1. VEPs to LED stimulation from newborn infants, showing no recordable response at 22 weeks PCA, the emergence of N300 at 24 weeks PCA, the late positivity following the N300 (usually around 450ms), which is evident from about 26 weeks onwards, and then little change until closer to term, when the P200 emerges, and becomes the most prominent wave in the normal term neonate's VEP.

awake or active sleep state. Replicable waveforms could be recorded in all infants of 24 weeks PCA and older; infants who were 22 to 23 weeks PCA had no recordable VEPS (Fig. 6.1). In the neonates 24 to 26 weeks PCA there is only a single monophasic negative peak with a latency of about 300ms (N300). The N300 is followed by a large positive peak at about 450ms but more variable in latency than N300. This biphasic waveform is found consistently from 27 to 32 weeks GA, and, until term, both N300 and P450 are remarkably stable in their occurrence and latencies. We did not find that the latencies of these waves changed significantly with increasing GA, although such age-related changes have been reported.

In some infants born between 30 and 35 weeks GA, an earlier positive peak is seen at around 200ms (P200) (Fig. 6.1). This wave is present in all normal neonates of 37 weeks PCA and older. Peaks earlier than the P200 (*i.e.* the N70, which has a mean latency of 155ms in term infants) were not seen in the preterm infants and were not seen reliably in the infants until close to term. The amplitude of the waves was variable, as is typically found with evoked potentials (EPS), although P200 was usually smaller than N300 or P450. There was no notable variation in the amplitude of N300 or P450 with GA; P200 was smaller, however, in the less mature neonates.

In neonates followed longitudinally the same waveforms are seen, but there are differences in the age at which they are first seen. The most remarkable difference between cross-sectional and longitudinal data is found with P200. This wave is seen consistently only in infants born at 37 weeks GA or older, yet it is seen as early as 26.5 weeks in longitudinal studies. It can emerge from 1.5 to seven weeks after birth, at an average PCA of 30.5 weeks (range 26.5 to 35 weeks PCA). The appearance of P200 in the preterm infants born at 30 to 32 weeks was not accelerated as much as was seen in some born at 22 to 26 weeks. The emergence of the earlier positivity preceding P200, the P100, was present in virtually all preterm infants by the time they were at term PCA. The presence of these two quite distinct positive components is seen in some newborn term infants, but is the pattern seen consistently in those past term.

The results of our cross-sectional studies are largely consistent with those found by other investigators, although the literature shows considerable variability in the reported VEPS in preterm neonates, probably due to methodological and technical differences. Umezaki and Morrell (1970) and Watanabe *et al.* (1972, 1973) found the large negative wave to be bifid in most of the preterm neonates, and several studies thought this to be age specific (*e.g.* Stanley *et al.* 1987). The bifid N300 could be attributed in part to the use of stroboscopic light as the stimulus, as it can produce a more complex waveform, as well as the use of bipolar montages (*e.g.* Hrbek and Mares 1964, Watanabe *et al.* 1972, Pryds *et al.* 1989) which, due to the widespread distribution of the flash VEP, could also contribute to a more complex waveform. Our data do not demonstrate a bifid N300 being specific to a certain age, as it was seen sporadically from 27 weeks to term in both longitudinal and cross-sectional data. N300 was bifid in a number of infants, sometimes within the same recording session (Fig. 6.2), and sometimes at widely spaced intervals in longitudinal studies. We found that there was no consistent pattern of this waveform in the preterm infants studied, and we consider it a variant of normal, probably a function of arousal level (Whyte *et al.* 1987).

Kurtzberg and Vaughan (1986) found that the predominant surface-negativity of the early preterm period (26 to 32 weeks) is replaced by an initial surface-positivity between 36 and 38 weeks PCA. The P200, N300 and P400 are comparable to the three components that Kurtzberg (1982) considered mandatory for a normal-term VEP. Stanley *et al.* (1987) also found the dominant negative waves of 28 to 31 weeks PCA to include an earlier positive component by 34 weeks PCA, and an earlier

Fig. 6.2. VEPs recorded consecutively (*i.e.* no more than a few minutes apart) showing a bifid N300 in one average and a more typical N300 in the other average. These kinds of studies, which we have seen at various ages in the preterm population, suggest that the bifid N300 is due to arousal level rather than a maturational change.

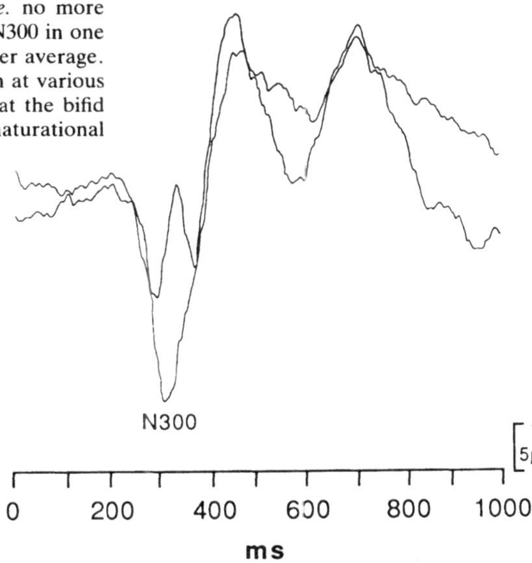

negativity (the N70) by 37 weeks PCA. These studies are consistent with earlier literature, which also found a slow negative wave to be the main component in neonates younger than 30 weeks PCA, with an earlier positive wave appearing between 30 and 35 weeks PCA.

Other investigators have reported age-related decreases in N300 or N1 component latency (Watanabe *et al.* 1972, Kurtzberg and Vaughan 1986, Pryds *et al.* 1989). Watanabe *et al.* (1972) commented that their labelling of one and then two negatives (much like the bifid N300) was arbitrary; age-related and arousal-related changes could therefore be arbitrary too. Stanley *et al.* (1987) also had what we would consider clearly bifid N300 waves, and labelled the earlier aspect the N1, again yielding apparent latency decreases. Alternatively, however, the differences between various studies are related to stimulus type; all those reporting decreases in N300 latency with age over the preterm population used white stroboscopic stimuli. Using red LED goggle stimuli, we have not seen any age-related latency decreases in over 120 preterm infants tested.

Some studies have failed to distinguish GA and PCA in preterm infants. Stanley *et al.* (1987) chose to ignore the postnatal age of the preterm infants, assuming that problems associated with immaturity may in fact delay maturation in the visual system. Placzek *et al.* (1985) investigated the maturation of the VEP and although they followed some infants longitudinally (born at 27 to 35 weeks GA), they also did not differentiate between GA and PCA in terms of the emergence of components, and thus may not have noted the early appearance of the P200 in some of the more preterm babies. They did find that visual maturation is delayed in abnormal preterm infants, consistent with reports from others (*e.g.* Guthkelch *et al.* 1984). Their normal data were consistent with our cross-sectional data.

The rapid change in the VEP in the longitudinal studies, with waveforms emerging earlier than they do in the cross-sectional data, suggests that development in the visual cortex may be accelerated in the extrauterine versus intrauterine environment. Accelerated maturation has been postulated in the visual system by others investigating pattern VEPs in infants, comparing those born at term and those born preterm but tested post-term PCA (Sokol and Jones 1979, Fiorentini *et al.* 1983, Norcia *et al.* 1987). Our longitudinal data during the early preterm period offer electrophysiological indication of accelerated neuronal development. Maturation of the auditory and somatosensory systems, as reflected by brainstem auditory and somatosensory evoked potentials, do not appear to be altered by preterm birth, probably because these sensory systems (unlike the visual system) receive stimulation *in utero*. Testing infants as soon as possible after birth appears to be critical for obtaining an accurate neurophysiological assessment of visual system function at a particular GA.

The changing VEP waveform (with the components emerging at particular latencies, in a fixed order) probably reflects stages in the physiological development of the visual system (Kurtzberg and Vaughan 1986, Stanley *et al.* 1986, Taylor *et al.* 1987). Takashima *et al.* (1980) presented detailed analyses of neuronal development in the visual cortex in preterm neonates, and neuro-anatomical changes appear to coincide with VEP maturational changes. Between 24 and 35 weeks the depth of the visual cortex doubles and the neurons of the primary visual cortex undergo maximal phases of dendritic differentiation and development. Only after 24 weeks GA, when neuronal migration is complete and basilar dendritic development is well under way in layer V, are any VEPs seen. Apical dendrites are developing after 30 weeks GA and P200 is seen with increasing frequency from 30 to 32 weeks until 36 weeks GA, after which time it is always present in normal neonates. Also near term, the waveform loses its simple biphasic pattern of the preceding 10 weeks and increases in complexity. But given the prominence of the P100 and P200, and that the sources of these components are known, later waves are usually ignored in the post-term period, unless the early components are missing (*i.e.* in a baby that has an immature waveform). Between 32 and 40 weeks GA there is the greatest increase in the number of stellate and other association neurons and their connections with the pyramidal cells.

PATTERN STIMULI

The pattern-reversal VEP recorded in preterm infants has a different morphology and pattern of maturation in the late preterm period. The primary component is a large slow positivity seen reliably in infants 33 weeks PCA and older (Harding *et al.* 1989). The latency of this slow positivity, probably P100, is often over 300ms, but decreases rapidly with age. By term PCA the latency of the P100 is about 250ms and 200ms by 44 weeks PCA (Grose *et al.* 1989). The N300, which is the dominant wave at this age with flash VEPs, is not seen in the pattern VEP. At term age, the pattern VEPs in normal infants born preterm show a slightly accelerated maturation, in that

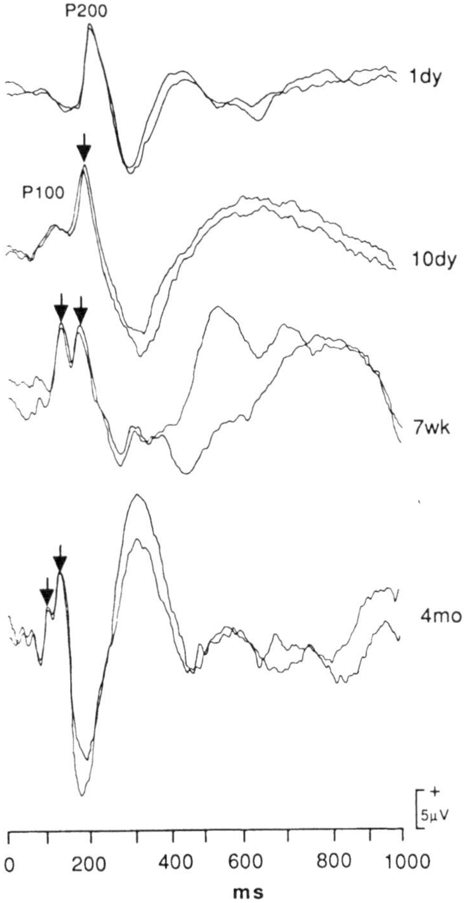

Fig. 6.3. The early postnatal maturation of the LED VEP, showing the emergence of the P100 soon after birth (in those babies in which it is not present at first recording), the clearly separated two peaks in the early months of life and rapidly decreasing latencies of the components with increasing age.

the latencies or measured acuity are better than infants born at term (Sokol and Jones 1979, Norcia *et al.* 1987).

Post-term maturation

FLASH STIMULI

After 40 weeks of age there is still rapid maturation of the recorded VEP, but the changes are primarily in latency; morphological changes are completed soon after birth. The initial single large positivity at around 200ms becomes a bifid component with an earlier positivity (P100) emerging usually before four weeks of age. The presence of both positive components at birth is not uncommon, but in our experience the presence of only P200 is more typical. With stroboscopic stimuli, Kurtzberg (1982) found the P100 present in 88 per cent of term babies. The two positive components remain quite prominent and distinct for several months despite a gradual shortening of the latency of these components (Fig. 6.3). They usually merge into a single, large positive component (P100) by six months of age, although both positive components are still seen in a percentage of young children's VEPS. The late slow waves, characteristic of the preterm VEP, are present in a fair number of post-term babies, but can be obscured with multiple smaller components.

The VEP to stroboscopic flash also shows very rapid maturation post-term, although when the waveform develops adult-like morphology appears to vary with recording parameters and laboratories. It does not appear to be affected by preterm birth (Ellingson 1986). Both morphological changes and striking latency decreases are seen over the first months of life (Ellingson *et al.* 1973, Laget *et al.* 1977); latency and amplitude changes in the primary components in later infancy are slight. There are some differences in the maturational pattern of these two types of flash VEPS, again emphasising the need for laboratory-specific norms, but the general rapid developmental progression is similar.

PATTERN STIMULI

The post-term maturational changes in pattern VEPS are dependent upon the visual angle of the patterned stimuli used to elicit the VEPS. VEPS to large and medium check sizes (*i.e.* 120′ to 60′ of arc) can be recorded from birth onwards. In the first month of life, the VEP recordings are simple waveforms with only a large, slowly rising positive component. The maturational changes to large check sizes are quite rapid with the negative components preceding and following the large positivity appearing at two months of age; latencies decrease rapidly while amplitudes increase. An adult-like VEP in terms of both morphology and latencies is recorded by six months to one year of age (Sokol 1982). For small check sizes (*i.e.* 7′ to 15′ of arc), the maturational pattern is slower, with no VEPS being recorded at birth, and only a simple, slow positive component recorded by three or four months of age, and the developmental changes continuing well into childhood (Sokol 1982, Maskowitz and Sokol 1983, McCulloch and Skarf 1991). As is seen in adults, the VEP latencies increase inversely with check size, so that normative data for the specific check sizes used must be obtained.

Several different aspects of visual system function in infants can be assessed with pattern VEPS and, though they are not widely used clinically, do deserve mention as they undergo rapid maturational changes in the early postnatal period. Contrast sensitivity can be measured by steady state VEPS to contrast gratings; although it is very immature in the neonatal period (Atkinson *et al.* 1979) it improves very rapidly until six months of life when it approaches adult values (Fiorentini *et al.* 1983). VEPS are also a reliable means of assessing the development of cortical binocularity (Braddick *et al.* 1986). Measurable VEPS to these stimuli appear between five and 20 weeks of age (Braddick *et al.* 1984; Eizenman *et al.* 1988, 1989*b*), with most infants showing binocular VEPS by nine months of age. To assess orientation specificity in infants, oblique grating patterns can be presented and orientation reversal VEPS can be recorded in normal infants from five or six weeks of age (Braddick *et al.* 1986). Finally, spatial and temporal interactions (VEPS to several check sizes, at a range of presentation rates) show that the temporal tuning function of low spatial frequencies is largely mature by three or four months of age, but that to high spatial frequencies the development is much slower (Moskowitz and Sokol 1980, Porciatti 1984).

Clinical applications

Visual system assessment

Few studies have attempted to correlate VEPS to flash stimuli with visual acuity or outcome, as the pattern VEP is so much better for the assessment of the anterior visual system function. However, two studies in which only flash VEPS could be obtained (due to preterm birth in one case and asphyxia in the other) did show an association between the neonatally obtained flash VEP and visual acuity (Placzek *et al.* 1985) and long-term visual outcome (McCulloch *et al.* 1991). Even this simple measure of the function of the visual pathway can pertain to questions of vision itself.

More typically, however, the assessment of the visual system, in terms of visual acuity, employs patterned stimuli. Visual thresholds can be determined directly from the parameters of the stimuli that elicit just detectable VEPS. A common technique is to estimate acuity by determining the smallest pattern size which elicits an identifiable VEP. With adequate testing conditions, reproducible VEPS should be obtained easily to check sizes down to 60′ of arc in newborn infants with normal vision. In those with visual impairment, VEPS are unrecordable or recordable only to much larger patterns or flash stimuli. More rigorous methods of estimating visual acuity from VEPS include: (i) extrapolation of the VEP amplitude versus pattern size function to zero or noise level (Campbell and Maffei 1970, Sokol *et al.* 1983), (ii) sweep techniques where a sequence of pattern stimuli with rapidly decreasing pattern sizes are presented (the threshold pattern size is measured where the signal-to-noise ratio of the VEP is unity—Regan 1977, Tyler *et al.* 1979, Norcia *et al.* 1987), and (iii) statistical detection of near threshold VEP signals to small stimuli (Eizenman *et al.* 1989*a*).

The accurate assessment of visual function in infants can be critical. Uncorrected visual disturbances in early life can result in permanent visual loss, since cortical development in the visual system is strongly influenced by early visual experience. Even in infants with uncorrectable visual impairment, early assessment is important for diagnosis and prompt referral to appropriate programmes to assist with the early development of the visually impaired child. It has been well demonstrated that the pattern VEP from birth onwards provides an objective measure of visual function and a quantifiable index of visual impairment. Thus it can be an extremely valuable means of assessing visual acuity in infants.

Neonatal asphyxia

Despite advances in antenatal care, fetal monitoring techniques, obstetric intervention and newborn resuscitation, the incidence of birth asphyxia among term infants remains unchanged (2.9 to 9 per 1000 livebirths) (MacDonald *et al.* 1980, Finer *et al.* 1981, Levene *et al.* 1985). It continues to be a major cause of neonatal mortality and is associated with an increased risk of chronic neurological disability in childhood (Nelson and Ellenberg 1981). Prediction of neurological sequelae is accurate only among the most mildly or severely affected infants. Difficulty in determining the prognosis of asphyxiated neonates results from an inability to determine adequately the severity of the insult by assessment of clinical status, imaging techniques, or by EEG monitoring. A number of studies have indicated that VEPS are sensitive to acute alteration in CNS function during and following asphyxia and may provide information for long-term prognosis (Hrbek *et al.* 1977, Hakamada *et al.* 1981). The generality of these earlier studies is limited by the inclusion of both term and preterm neonates, the variety of perinatal disorders affecting the infants, the lack of normal control groups and the restricted duration of follow-up.

We investigated the correlation of VEPS with long-term neurodevelopmental outcome in a uniform population of term infants asphyxiated at birth, compared to already established term controls (Whyte *et al.* 1987, Muttitt *et al.* 1991). Our infants showed a higher incidence of moderate (62 per cent) and severe asphyxia (27 per cent) and seizures (76 per cent) as compared to other studies, yet despite this predominance of more severely affected infants, our overall rates of mortality (22 per cent) and morbidity (32 per cent) are quite comparable to those reported in the current literature on asphyxiated neonates.

Our population is entirely out-born; all infants included in the study were less than 24 hours old at the time of admission. Ninety-two infants in our series have been followed for more than two years, and over a hundred have been followed for one year. Birth asphyxia was defined as an Apgar score <3 at 10 minutes, or by two of the following: (i) an Apgar score of <6 at five minutes; (ii) evidence of intrauterine asphyxia as manifested by a scalp PH<7, by late decelerations in fetal monitoring, or meconium staining of the liquor; or (iii) an abnormal neurological examination consistent with a diagnosis of birth asphyxia, including findings such as altered tone, altered consciousness or seizures. We excluded all infants with congenital anomalies, severe birth trauma or neuromuscular disease.

VEPS were performed during the first three days of life, on day seven, and weekly thereafter until death or discharge. VEPS were recorded from OZ referenced to FZ in response to binocular stimuli from LED goggles. Electroretinograms were recorded simultaneously from an infraorbital lead, also referenced to FZ. Based on detectable waveforms and latencies, VEPS were classified as normal, which included consistently normal VEPS and those with transient abnormalities of waveform, delayed latencies, or missing components of less than one week's duration; or abnormal, which included prolonged absence or abnormalities of waveform of greater than one week duration or an absent VEP recorded at any time during the first week of life. Both neurological assessments and VEPS were repeated at six weeks, three months, nine months, one year, 18 months or two years.

In infants with normal VEPs in the first three days of life, the majority (83 per cent) were neurodevelopmentally normal on follow-up. Those with normal VEPs in the first week of life, which includes those whose VEPs normalised during the week, were usually normal on follow-up (87 per cent). All of those (100 per cent) with abnormal VEPs throughout the first week or absent VEPs at any time during the first week of life, either died or were left with severe neurological sequelae. We observed a greater association between VEPs and outcome at two years than has been previously reported. Eighty-nine per cent of infants with normal VEPs in the first week of life were free of disability at follow-up. Death or severe neurological impairment could be predicted if an absent VEP was documented at any time or abnormalities of the waveform persisted beyond day four. This incidence of false positive (0.0 per cent) and negative (13 per cent) results is less than that noted by Hakamada *et al.* (1981) who found 30 per cent of infants with abnormal EPs were neurologically normal and 28.6 per cent with normal EPs were abnormal at follow-up. The prognostic reliability was highest in the moderately asphyxiated group (Muttitt *et al.* 1991), which is the most difficult group in which to prognosticate clinically. We found the VEPs to be more specific and accurate than other diagnostic tests in predicting neurological outcome. Thus we would recommend the VEPs as a relatively fast and effective means of assessing the functional integrity of the CNS following perinatal asphyxia, and as an accurate prognostic measure to aid in early management of hypoxic-ischaemic encephalopathy.

Hydrocephalus

Hydrocephalus is the pathological condition of enlarged cerebral ventricles, due to a relative imbalance between cerebrospinal fluid production and absorption. Hydrocephalus usually results in an impairment of cerebral function, but is one of the few apparently reversible insults to the CNS. In neonates, hydrocephalus can be either congenital (in isolation or in combination with brain abnormalities such as myelomeningocele) or due to perinatal events. In either case, hydrocephalus may not be clinically evident for days or months after birth. Early diagnosis and treatment are important to minimise the risk of neurological sequelae.

Several authors have studied VEPs in infants with the aim of aiding early detection, as the visual pathways have been shown to be affected by ventricular enlargement in adults (York *et al.* 1981). Ehle and Sklar (1979) found that all 15 infants they studied had abnormally delayed VEPs, which improved quickly post-shunting. Guthkelch *et al.* (1982) found that increased latencies were present only when the hydrocephalus was accompanied by increased head size (above the 98th centile); neonates who were normocephalic had normal VEPs more often than not. This effect was confirmed in a later study (Guthkelch *et al.* 1984); in addition, they found that the hydrocephalic children had slower maturation of the VEP. They also did repeat testing post-shunting in infants under four months old and found only small decreases in latency.

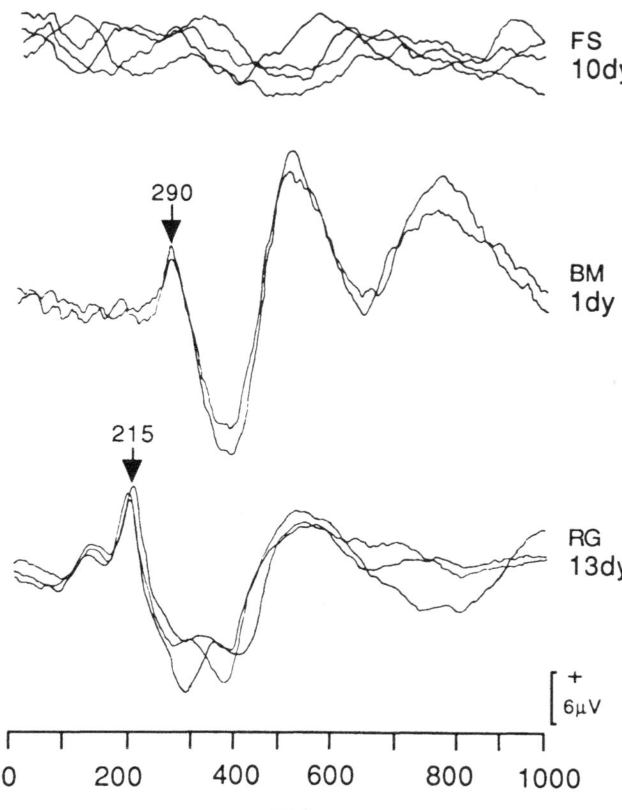

Fig. 6.4. VEPs recorded from three term hydrocephalic infants, showing examples of VEPs obtained in this population, ranging from absent responses to perfectly normal recordings. Baby FS had severely increased ventricles, a head circumference of 46cm and absent VEPs before shunting, but had VEPs within normal limits two days post-shunting. Baby BM also had severely increased ventricles, with head circumference of 38cm with delayed latency VEPs, which also recovered postoperatively. Baby RG, diagnosed prenatally, had markedly increased ventricles, a head circumference of 38cm but normal VEPs before and after shunting. All three babies went on to do well.

We have found the VEPs in young infants with hydrocephalus to be usually abnormal (83 per cent), but this did not correlate with head size or clinical status (George and Taylor 1987). In the neonates that we have now seen with hydrocephalus (>65 infants), we have found that VEPs ranged from normal to absent (Fig. 6.4), and found both normal and abnormal VEPs in babies with both enlarged head circumferences and in normocephalic infants. The abnormal VEPs did improve quickly post-shunt, however, except in infants who, due to various factors, did not improve clinically post-shunt and were left with serious neurological impairment. Thus in our experience the VEPs were most useful not in the clinical diagnosis of hydrocephalus in neonates, but in monitoring the efficacy of the shunting procedure.

Small for gestational age

Small for gestational age (SGA) infants are those who are significantly smaller at birth than one would expect for their gestational age. The term SGA infants are different from preterm neonates (although they resemble them in size and weight), as the preterms' low birthweight is due to a shorter gestational period rather than intrauterine growth retardation. Distinguishing between these groups is clinically important, as the risk factors are higher for the SGA than the preterm infants. Reliable criteria for this differentiation can be based on neurological development, an aspect of which can be assessed with VEPS. Watanabe *et al.* (1972) found that VEP latencies correlated with PCA in the SGA as well as the normal preterm infants, suggesting that neurological development in SGA infants progressed relatively normally and independently of the unfavourable intrauterine conditions which caused the slower physical growth. In contrast, Hrbek *et al.* (1982) found that although the VEPS of SGA infants generally corresponded to that of age-matched normal neonates, there was a tendency towards longer latencies in the SGA infants, as well as the presence of late slow waves, which the authors felt was a further sign of neurological immaturity. Both of these features, however, were transient. Pryds *et al.* (1989) examined eight SGA infants and found no abnormalities or unusual patterns of results.

Respiratory distress

A few studies have examined the role of VEPS in neonates suffering respiratory distress. Graziani *et al.* (1972) studied 13 preterm infants acutely during periods of severe respiratory difficulty, and found abnormal or absent VEPS in all cases, which were associated with blood gas levels. After repeated or prolonged hypoxemia, only absent VEPS were obtained, and most of these infants died. Pryds *et al.* (1989) included studies on 75 infants that required either ventilation or continuous positive airway pressure. They found no difference in the VEPS of these infants and their normal controls; the babies requiring ventilation tended to be more immature. Gambi *et al.* (1980) reported VEPS in infants with respiratory distress, graded from slight to severe. Slight respiratory distress did not affect the VEPS, while in infants with middle to severe respiratory distress the VEPS were abnormal, and in some cases the abnormalities persisted until the test at nine months. Our experience has been consistent with that of Gambi *et al.* (1980): in those who have suffered mild or transient respiratory distress, the VEPS are normal in both term and preterm neonates. In those with severe respiratory distress, the infants have usually suffered significantly hypoxic episodes, and the VEPS are more often abnormal. Rapid recovery of the VEPS following the hypoxic event, however, is usually a positive prognostic indicator. Consistently abnormal VEPS are an ominous sign, regardless of etiology.

Other applications

Hrbek *et al.* (1982) examined VEPS in a series of 10 infants born with fetal alcohol syndrome. Immature characteristics were seen in 40 per cent of the cases (which is not in itself diagnostic or uncommon), but a further 25 per cent had markedly abnormal VEPs. Multimodal EPs in this population yielded a high percentage of abnormalities, probably reflecting intrauterine damage due to substance abuse by the mother. Unfortunately, follow-up neurological data were not given to provide the necessary association with, and hence significance of, the early VEP findings.

Pryds *et al.* (1989) also examined VEPs in 23 preterm babies who went on to develop periventricular or intraventricular haemorrhage. The VEPs were not abnormal in those infants with grades 1 or 2 haemorrhage and did not predict which infants would in fact develop haemorrhage, but were abnormal in those infants with grades 3 or 4 haemorrhage. Watanabe *et al.* (1981) studied VEPs, along with electroencephalogram and auditory evoked potentials, in 16 neonates with intracranial haemorrhage. They found that the VEPs were useful in assessing the degree of brain damage, but were not useful in either diagnosis or prognosis in this population.

Ellingson (1986) found the stroboscopic VEP P2 component to have a longer latency only in the first week of life in trisomy 21 infants, with no other significant differences, despite the global cerebral dysfunction that these infants suffer.

A final application is in the assessment or quantification of delayed visual maturation. Given the marked developmental changes in the VEP in the newborn, determining an immature visual system is quite feasible. This immaturity may be secondary to other neurological disorders (*e.g.* Gambi *et al.* 1981, Guthkelch *et al.* 1984, Plazcek *et al.* 1985), or appear to be only a visual system disturbance (Fielder *et al.* 1985, Lambert *et al.* 1989). The VEPs can be used to monitor the maturation in such cases and determine when and if the baby's visual system normalises.

Summary

This chapter has reviewed the techniques most commonly used for recording flash and pattern VEPs in the newborn infant, and the developmental changes as a function of stimulus type. The very rapid maturational changes in the VEPs, including morphological changes in the preterm period and primarily latency changes post-term, provide an invaluable means for assessing and monitoring development within this aspect of the CNS. The maturational changes are such that normative values are requisite and that such norms must take into account the baby's gestational age at birth as well as the postnatal age, as maturation in the visual system is accelerated in normal preterm infants.

Given the normative base, there are many clinical applications of the VEP in the newborn period. These include assessment of various aspects of patterned vision, including acuity measures, binocularity and contrast sensitivity, quite accurate prognostic indicators of birth asphyxia, and assessment of various other disorders or conditions, such as respiratory distress, hydrocephalus or delayed intrauterine growth, which can affect the newborn infant and may lead to neurological sequelae.

Thus the VEPs are a valuable adjunct in the assessment of neonates, and their data can be useful to neurologists, neonatologists and ophthalmologists alike.

REFERENCES

Atkinson, J., Braddick, O., French, J. (1979) 'Contrast sensitivity of the human neonate measured by the VEP.' *Investigative Ophthalmology and Visual Science*, **18**, 210–213.

Braddick, O., Wattam-Bell, J., Atkinson, J. (1984) 'The onset of binocular function in human infants.' *Human Neurobiology*, **2**, 65–69.

—— Atkinson, J., Wattam-Bell, J. (1986) 'VER testing of cortical binocularity and pattern detection in infancy.' *Documenta Ophthalmologica Proceedings*, **45**, 107–115.

Campbell, F.W., Maffei, L. (1970) 'Electrophysiological evidence for the existence of orientation and size detectors in the human visual system.' *Journal of Physiology*, **207**, 635–652.

Ehle, A., Sklar, F. (1979) 'Visual evoked potentials in infants with hydrocephalus.' *Neurology*, **29**, 1541–1544.

Eizenmann, M., Skarf, B., McCulloch, D. (1988) 'Detection of early development of binocular fusion in infants.' *Investigative Ophthalmology and Visual Science*, **29**, 25.

—— McCulloch, D., Hui, R., Skarf, B. (1989*a*) 'Detection of threshold visual evoked potentials, non invasive assessment of the visual system.' *Technical Digest Series. Optical Society of America, Washington, DC*, **7**, 88–91.

—— Skarf, B., McCulloch, D. (1989*b*) 'Development of binocular vision in infants.' *Investigative Ophthalmology and Visual Science*, **30**, 313.

Ellingson, R.J. (1986) 'Development of visual evoked potentials and photic driving responses in normal full term, low risk premature, and trisomy-21 infants during the first year of life.' *Electroencephalography and Clinical Neurophysiology*, **63**, 309–316.

—— Lathrop, G.H., Danahy, T., Nelson, B. (1973) 'Variability of visual evoked potentials in human infants and adults.' *Electroencephalography and Clinical Neurophysiology*, **34**, 113–124.

Fielder, A.R., Russell-Eggitt, I.R., Dodd, K.L., Mellor, D.H. (1985) 'Delayed visual maturation.' *Transactions of the Ophthalmological Society, UK*, **104**, 653–661.

Finer, N.N., Robertson, C.M., Richards, R.T., Pinnell, L.E., Peters, K.L. (1981) 'Hypoxic-ischemic encephalopathy in term neonates: perinatal factors and outcome.' *Journal of Pediatrics*, **98**, 112–117.

Fiorentini, A., Pirchio, M., Spinelli, D. (1983) 'Development of retinal and cortical responses to pattern reversal in infants: a selective review.' *Behavioral Brain Research*, **10**, 99–106.

Gambi, D., Rossini, P.M., Albertini, G., Sollazzo, D., Torrioli, M.G., Polidori, G.C. (1980) 'Follow-up of visual evoked potential in full-term and pre-term control newborns and in subjects who suffered from perinatal respiratory distress.' *Electroencephalography and Clinical Neurophysiology*, **48**, 509–516.

George, S.R., Taylor, M.J. (1987) 'VEPs and SEPs in hydrocephalic infants before and after shunting.' *Clinical Neurology and Neurosurgery*, **89** (Suppl. I), 96.

Glaze, D.G., DeGuire, A., Frost, J.D. (1983) 'Visual evoked potentials in the newborn infant: influence of awake-asleep states.' *American Electroencephalography Society*, **56**, 31P.

Graziani, L.J., Weitzman, E.D., Pineda, G. (1972) 'Visual evoked responses during neonatal respiratory disorders in low birth weight infants.' *Pediatric Research*, **6**, 203–210.

Grose, J., Harding, G.F.A., Wilton, A.Y., Bissenden, J.G. (1989) 'The maturation of the pattern reversal VEP and flash ERG in preterm infants.' *Clinical Vision Science*, **4**, 239–246.

Groth, H., Weled, B., Batkin, S. (1970) 'A comparison of monocular visually evoked potentials in human neonates and adults.' *Electroencephalography and Clinical Neurophysiology*, **28**, 478–487.

Guthkelch, A.N., Sclabassi, R.J., Vries, J.K. (1982) 'Changes in the visual evoked potentials of hydrocephalic children.' *Neurosurgery*, **11**, 599–602.

—— —— Hirsch, R.P., Vries, J.K. (1984) 'Visual evoked potentials in hydrocephalus: relationship to head size, shunting, and mental development.' *Neurosurgery*, **14**, 283–286.

Hakamada, S., Watanabe, K., Hara, K., Miyazaki, S. (1981) 'The evolution of visual and auditory evoked potentials in infants with perinatal disorder.' *Brain and Development*, **3**, 339–344.

Harding, G.F.A., Grose, J., Wilton, A., Bissenden, J. (1989) 'The pattern reversal VEP in short-

gestation infants.' *Electroencephalography and Clinical Neurophysiology*, **74**, 76–80.
Hrbek, A., Mares, P. (1964) 'Cortical evoked responses to visual stimulation in full-term and premature newborns.' *Electroencephalography and Clinical Neurophysiology*, **16**, 575–581.
—— Hrbkova, M., Lenard, H.G. (1969) 'Somatosensory, auditory and visual evoked responses in newborn infants during sleep and wakefulness.' *Electroencephalography and Clinical Neurophysiology*, **26**, 597–603.
—— Karlberg, P., Kjellmer, I., Olsson, T., Riha, M. (1977) 'Clinical application of evoked electroencephalographic responses in newborn infants. I: Perinatal asphyxia.' *Developmental Medicine and Child Neurology*, **49**, 34–44.
—— Iversen, K., Olsson, T. (1982) 'Evaluation of cerebral function in newborn infants with fetal growth retardation.' *Advances in Neurology*, **32**, 89–95.
Kurtzberg, D. (1982) 'Event-related potentials in the evaluation of high-risk infants.' *Annals of the New York Academy of Sciences*, **388**, 557–571.
—— Vaughan, H.G. (1986) 'Preterm and post-term regional maturation of flash and pattern ERPs.' *In* Gallai, V. (Ed.) *Maturation of the CNS and Evoked Potentials.* Amsterdam: Excerpta Medica. pp. 9–15.
Laget, P., Flores-Guevara, R., D'Allest, A.M., Ostre, C., Raimbault, J., Mariani, J. (1977) 'La maturation des potentiels evoqués visuels chez l'enfant normal.' *Electroencephalography and Clinical Neurophysiology*, **43**, 732–744.
Lambert, S.R., Kriss, A., Taylor, D. (1989) 'Delayed visual maturation. A longitudinal clinical and electrophysiological assessment.' *Ophthalmology*, **96**, 524–528.
Levene, M.I., Kornberg, J., Williams, T.H.C. (1985) 'The incidence and severity of post-asphyxial encephalopathy in full-term infants.' *Early Human Development*, **11**, 21–26.
MacDonald, H.M., Mulligan, J.C., Allen, A.C., Taylor, P.M. (1980) 'Neonatal asphyxia. I. Relationship to obstetric and neonatal complications to neonatal mortality in 38,405 consecutive deliveries.' *Journal of Pediatrics*, **96**, 898–902.
McCulloch, D.L., Skarf, B. (1991) 'Development of the human visual system: monocular and binocular pattern VEP latency.' *Investigative Ophthalmology and Visual Science*, **32**, 2372–2381.
—— Taylor, M.J., Whyte, H.E. (1991) 'Visual evoked potentials and long-term visual prognosis following birth asphyxia.' *Archives of Ophthalmology*, **109**, 229–233.
Moskowitz, A., Sokol, S. (1980) 'Spatial and temporal interaction of pattern-evoked cortical potentials in human infants.' *Vision Research*, **20**, 699–707.
—— —— (1983) 'Developmental changes in the human visual system as reflected by the latency of the pattern reversal VEP.' *Electroencephalography and Clinical Neurophysiology*, **56**, 1–15.
Mushin, J., Hogg, C.R., Dubowitz, L.M.S., Skouteli, H., Arden, G.B. (1984) 'Visual evoked responses to light emitting diode (LED) photostimulation in newborn infants.' *Electroencephalography and Clinical Neurophysiology*, **58**, 317–320.
Muttitt, S.C., Taylor, M.J., Kobayashi, J.S., Whyte, H.E. (1991) 'Serial visual evoked potentials and outcome in full-term birth asphyxia.' *Pediatric Neurology*, **7**, 86–90.
Nelson, K.B., Ellenberg, J.H. (1981) 'Apgar scores as predictors of chronic neurologic disability.' *Pediatrics*, **68**, 36–44.
Norcia, A.M., Tyler, C.W. (1985) 'Spatial frequency sweep VEP: visual acuity during the first year of life.' *Vision Research*, **25**, 1399–1408.
—— —— Piecuch, R., Clyman, R., Grobstein, J. (1987) 'Visual acuity development in normal and abnormal preterm human infants.' *Journal of Pediatric Ophthalmology and Strabismus*, **24**, 70–74.
Placzek, M., Mushin, J., Dubowitz, L.M.S. (1985) 'Maturation of the visual evoked response and its correlation with visual acuity in preterm infants.' *Developmental Medicine and Child Neurology*, **27**, 448–454.
Porciatti, V. (1984) 'Temporal and spatial properties of the pattern-reversal VEPs in infants below 2 months of age.' *Human Neurobiology*, **3**, 97–102.
Pryds, O., Greisen, G., Trojaborg, W. (1988) 'Visual evoked potentials in preterm infants during the first hours of life.' *Electroencephalography and Clinical Neurophysiology*, **71**, 257–265.
—— Trojaborg, W., Carlsen, J., Jensen, J. (1989) 'Determinants of visual evoked potentials in preterm infants.' *Early Human Development*, **19**, 117–125.
Regan, D. (1977) 'Speedy assessment of visual acuity in amblyopia by the evoked potential method.' *Ophthalmologia*, **175**, 159–164.

Sokol, S. (1982) 'Infant visual development: evoked potential estimates.' *Annals of the New York Academy of Sciences*, **388**, 514–525.

—— Jones, K. (1979) 'Implicit time of pattern evoked potentials in infants an index of maturation of spatial vision.' *Vision Research*, **19**, 747–755.

—— Hansen, V., Moskowitz, A., Greenfield, P., Towle, V. (1983) 'Evoked potential and preferential looking estimates of visual acuity in paediatric patients. *Ophthalmology*, **90**, 552–564.

Stanley, O.H., Fleming, P.J., Morgan, M.H. (1986) 'Visual function in the newborn.' *Lancet*, **2**, 47–48.

—— —— —— (1987) 'Developmental wave form analysis of the neonatal flash evoked potential.' *Electroencephalography and Clinical Neurophysiology*, **68**, 149–152.

Takashima, S., Chan, F., Becker, L.E., Armstrong, D.L. (1980) 'Morphology of the developing visual cortex of the human infant.' *Journal of Neuropathology and Experimental Neurology*, **39**, 487–501.

Taylor, M.J., Farrell, E.J. (1987) 'Latency, morphological and distributional changes in VEPs with various stimuli.' *Canadian Journal of Neurological Sciences*, **14**, 244.

—— Menzies, R., MacMillan, L.J., Whyte, H.E. (1987) 'VEPs in normal full-term and premature neonates: longitudinal versus cross-sectional data.' *Electroencephalography and Clinical Neurophysiology*, **68**, 20–27.

Tyler, C.W., Apkarian, P., Levi, D.M., Nakayama, K. (1979) 'Rapid assessment of visual function: an electronic sweep technique for the pattern visual evoked potential.' *Investigation of Ophthalmology and Visual Science*, **18**, 703–713.

Umezaki, H., Morrell, F. (1970) 'Developmental study of photic evoked responses in premature infants.' *Electroencephalography and Clinical Neurophysiology*, **28**, 55–63.

Watanabe, K., Iwase, K., Hara, K. (1972) 'Maturation of visual evoked responses in low birthweight infants.' *Developmental Medicine and Child Neurology*, **14**, 425–435.

—— —— —— (1973) 'Visual evoked responses during sleep and wakefulness in pre-term infants.' *Electroencephalography and Clinical Neurophysiology*, **34**, 571–577.

—— Hara, K., Miyazaki, S., Hakamada, S., Kuroyanagi, M., Nakamura, S., Yamada, H. (1981) 'The value of EEG and cerebral evoked potentials in the assessment of neonatal intracranial hemorrhage.' *European Journal of Pediatrics*, **137**, 177–184.

Whyte, H.E., Taylor, M.J., Menzies, R., MacMillan, L.J. (1986) 'Prognostic utility of VEPs in full-term asphyxiated infants.' *Pediatric Neurology*, **2**, 220–223.

—— Pearce, J.M., Taylor, M.J. (1987) 'Changes in the VEP in preterm neonates with arousal states, as assessed by EEG monitoring.' *Electroencephalography and Clinical Neurophysiology*, **68**, 223–225.

York, D.H., Pulliam, M.W., Rosenfeld, J. G., Watts, C. (1981) 'Relationship between visual evoked potentials and intracranial pressure.' *Journal of Neurosurgery*, **55**, 909–916.

7
VISUAL ELECTROPHYSIOLOGY

G.F.A. Harding

The clinical electroretinogram (ERG) is a recording of the electrical response of the retina to a change in illumination. The ERG is a complex potential which represents an algebraic summation of all the potentials developed in a variety of retinal layers and cells to determine changes in a variety of receptors. By modifying various stimulus parameters, it is possible to reduce the response from some receptors while still stimulating others. This technique is frequently used in the clinical ERG to produce the scotopic or dark-adapted ERG (in theory coming from rod receptors), the photopic ERG (from rods and cones) and the flicker ERG (from cones alone).

The ERG consists of three waves known as a-, b- and c-waves with a further additional component called the oscillatory potentials. Granit (1933) proposed that the ERG consisted of three separate sub-systems, PI, PII and PIII. PIII was a negative potential forming the a-wave of the ERG. It is produced by the cell body of photoreceptors as two components, one from the cone response and a second one from the rod response. The PII is a positive potential produced by bipolar or Müller cells and contains two components: the first a positive peak forming the b-wave of the ERG and a later slow positive dc shift. The earlier component, *i.e.* the b-wave of the ERG, has been the subject of some contention as to its origin. Arden and Brown (1965) believed the bipolar cells to be responsible for generation of this component, though earlier Brown and Watanabe (1962) had suggested that the Müller cell was a more probable source of the b-wave. The c-wave of the ERG produced by the PI component is not the subject of much use in clinical practice.

There are some further oscillatory potentials, usually rhythmic wavelets, superimposed on the slow potential of the b-wave of the ERG. They were first described by Cobb and Morton in 1954, and although their origin is unknown, it has been suggested that they are derived from within the inner nuclear layer of the retina (Yokoyama *et al.* 1964). Some authors have suggested that the division of the a-wave into rod and cone response is actually an oscillatory potential of photopic origin which has been superimposed on the a component (Auerbach and Burian 1955, Lachapelle and Molotchnikoff 1986). However, there has been most contention over the function of the oscillatory potentials in relation to the ERG b-wave. Some authors pointed out that the oscillatory potentials are abolished in both diabetes and central retinal artery occlusion without the ERG b-wave being reduced in amplitude, and suggested that the two processes must be independent (Brunette and Desrochers 1970, Speros and Price 1981). However, other authors suggest that, since in patients with night blindness the absence of an oscillatory potential coexists with an abnormal ERG b-wave, the oscillatory potential contributes to the presence of the ERG b-wave (Lachapelle and Molotchnikoff 1986).

The level of retinal adaptation affects the ERG recording both in amplitude and latency. The ERG can be evoked by a bright light in the presence of normal background illumination, the resultant photopic response being of low amplitude and short latency. However, after 12 minutes of dark adaptation the scotopic ERG may be elicited in which the amplitude is far greater although the response is somewhat slower. Equally, by adapting the patient to a blue background and then stimulating with white or red light at 30HZ, a pure cone ERG can be obtained since the rods are unable to follow this rate of flicker.

The amplitude and latency of the a- and b-waves are also markedly affected by stimulus intensity. As the intensity of stimulation is increased, the latency of the b-wave becomes shorter and its amplitude becomes greater. With further increases in intensity the b-wave amplitude stabilises, while the a-wave reduces its latency and shows an increase in amplitude. With further increases in intensity, there are smaller oscillatory potentials whose latency remains fixed. Obviously since the pupil size will also affect the amplitude of the ERG due to the amount of illumination falling on the retina, the amplitude of the a- and b-waves will be increased if the eye is artificially dilated.

Nowadays ERG signals are almost invariably averaged except under scotopic conditions in which single sweeps are used to avoid negating the dark adaptation by the repeated flashes of light.

Neonatal ERG recording

The first neonatal ERG was recorded by Zetterström in 1951. Thirty-five term infants were recorded from birth until one year of age. No clear and consistent ERG was recordable in the first few hours of life, but after a few days a b-wave of relatively long latency was observed without any apparent a-wave being present. As the baby became older the latency of the ERG b-wave shortened and its amplitude increased. By 12 months of age the ERG was similar to that of the adult, but still the a-wave was recordable in less than 25 per cent of subjects. Zetterström concluded that the infant ERG was a scotopic phenomenon: but since the retina, apart from the macula, is fully differentiated at 40 weeks, it was presumed that the absence of the ERG at birth may have been due to the failure of normal rhodopsin response at that age. Horsten and Winkelman (1962), however, used bright flash and showed that it was possible to record ERGs from both term and preterm babies in the first day of life. The babies were dark-adapted and their pupils dilated. ERGs were demonstrated in all the newborn infants, with the a-wave clearly recognisable. The amplitude of the response was found to be small and the shape of the response was identical with that of the adults. It would therefore appear that Zetterström's failure to obtain a-waves and indeed b-waves in the initial days of life was probably due to inadequate brightness of stimulation.

Shipley and Anton (1964) studied 10 infants within the first 24 hours of life.

The pupils were dilated and the babies were dark-adapted for one hour, and a bright flash of 650,000 lux was used compared to the maximum of 160,000 lux used by Zetterström. Both a- and b-waves were clearly formed (the amplitude being equal to around 90μv) and the form of the ERG was said to be similar to that of the adult. Barnet *et al.* (1965) studied 12 infants from six hours to four days of age. The pupils were dilated and various intensities of stimulus were used. In this, the first study in which averaging of the ERG took place, both a- and b-waves were present at birth but were of relatively low amplitude (around 22μv).

Algvere and Zetterström (1967) studied 15 infants between 10 and 96 hours after birth. The pupils were dilated and all the babies were dark-adapted for five minutes. Flash rates were relatively slow, flash was dim (33,000 lux) and the authors found a delayed latency of the a-wave and reduced amplitude of the b-wave. They suggested that this was due to the stimulus threshold of the retina being markedly raised. Similar findings were obtained by Lodge *et al.* (1969), who studied babies between 13 and 38 hours of age. Algvere and Zetterström (1967) also found that oscillatory potentials were present in very young babies, being clearly observed superimposed on the b-wave of the ERG. Many of the reported ERGS, particularly those showing low amplitude and delayed responses, have used low light levels of stimulus with dark-adapted babies to produce an almost pure scotopic response. François and DeRouck (1964) showed that by modifying the intensity of the stimulus it is possible to change the ERG in infants from a small scotopic b-wave to a maximum response consisting of a large a-wave, both photopic and scotopic b-waves and a later positive-going deflection.

A carefully controlled study of the development of the scotopic ERG was carried out by Fulton and Hansen (1985). Twenty-three term infants were studied between two and 12 months of age. All the infants were dark-adapted for a period of 30 minutes prior to the investigation and the ERGS were recorded using a Dawson–Trick–Litzkow (DTL) electrode (Dawson *et al.* 1979). Blue flash stimulation was used of the whole field with relatively long interstimulus intervals of five seconds. Averaging was performed and 16 responses were averaged at each of the stimulus intensities. They found that the responses were of relatively low amplitude, but as the intensity of the stimulus increased, so the amplitude of the b-wave increased until this reached saturation. Concomitant with the increase in amplitude, of the b-wave, there was a gradual decrease in b-wave latency. It was noticeable that as the baby became older, less intense stimuli were needed to produce the ERG response and saturation was reached earlier. In terms of latency and amplitude, however, the dark-adapted ERG did not reach adult values until one year of age.

Preterm infants

A number of studies have been performed on preterm babies. Again the early studies were those of Zetterström (1952) on 30 'premature' infants between 30 and 39 weeks of post-conceptional age (PCA). Although again she found that the ERGS were not recordable during the first 24 hours, there was also evidence that the more preterm the infant the greater the delay before an ERG could be recorded. This suggested that the ERG could be used as a measure of PCA. Samson-Dollfus (1968) confirmed these findings and in 11 infants found that the ERG (consisting of both a-wave, b-wave and oscillatory potentials) was clearly recordable beyond 32 weeks PCA and appeared to show some progressive maturation. Ricci *et al.* (1983) performed serial ERG recordings on eight preterm babies from 29 to 36 weeks PCA and followed the babies at weekly intervals until four to six weeks after birth. All the infants were dark-adapted and their pupils dilated. During this period the scotopic ERG to white light was obtained. Recordings were made with a small silver chloride spiral electrode with saline-soaked cotton which was floated in the tear film. The ERG responses were averaged, usually 250 single sweeps constituting the average. Although the amplitude and latency of the a-wave were found to be constant from birth, the latency of the scotopic b-wave appeared to increase in amplitude and also show a decrease in latency with increasing PCA. Ricci *et al.* (1983) suggested that the development of the retinal circulation supplying the inner retinal layers was responsible for these changes in latency and amplitude at the b-wave, since the retinal circulation does not reach maturity until term. It is not clear, however, how the authors managed to maintain dark adaptation with five flashes per second for 250 repetitions. Using similar techniques, they investigated the photopic ERG (Ricci *et al.* 1984). They found that the a-wave was of shorter latency and higher amplitude with greater PCA, but this was only a trend between babies of different PCA. Within individuals there was no consistent variation in the amplitude of the a-wave in relation to chronological age or PCA. The b-wave was certainly related to the PCA, with clear increases in amplitude with successive weeks being 29 and 34 weeks PCA: though at this age the amplitude was equivalent to that of the response at 40 weeks. There did not appear to be a clear relationship between b-wave latency and PCA.

Grose *et al.* (1989) investigated 30 preterm babies born between 28 and 35 weeks gestational age (GA). The babies were studied longitudinally over a period of 18 weeks and all the babies appeared neurologically normal for their PCA. Each baby was investigated on at least two occasions with the first record occurring before 37 weeks PCA. ERGS were recorded using a DTL electrode (Dawson *et al.* 1979). The distal end of the electrode was secured by a blob of electrode gel on the bridge of the nose and the DTL fibre was draped across the open eye and held at the outer canthus by a pliable silver holder. All ERGS were performed under photopic conditions. Thirty sweeps were averaged to produce the ERG and the flash stimuli were presented at approximately 600ms interstimulus interval. The infants' pupils were not dilated but their eyes were held open. ERG b-waves were recorded in all the infants regardless of their PCA but in the more preterm infants it was not always possible to elicit a-waves irrespective of whether the eyes were open or closed. The b-wave consisted of a broad positive peak with a mean latency of approximately 53ms at 30 weeks PCA. As the infant grew older the latency of this wave shortened

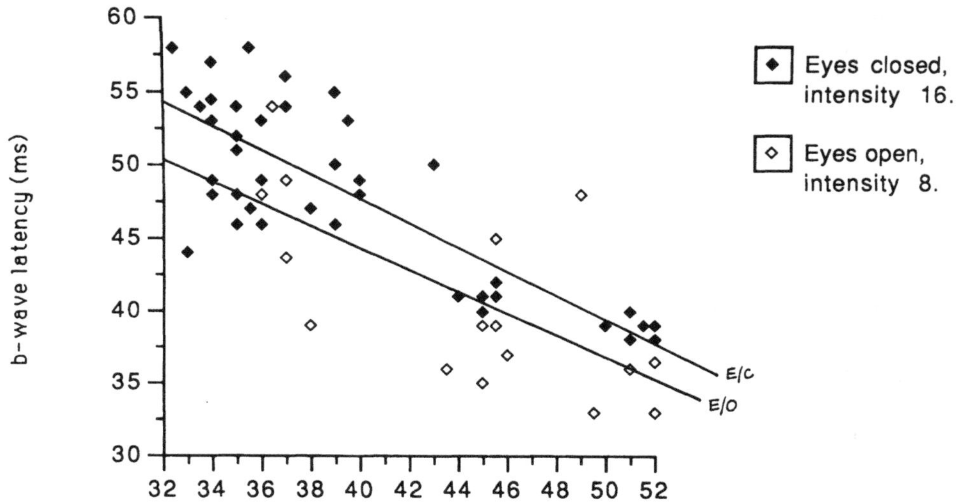

Fig. 7.1. The graph shows the latency of the ERG b-wave plotted against weeks of PCA (horizontal axis). The intensity of the stimulus was adjusted to allow for the reduced illumination with closed lids. With this adjustment there was no significant difference between the 'eyes open' and the 'eyes closed' conditions. The latency of the b-wave gradually shortens from 32 weeks to 52 weeks and is clearly negatively related to PCA.

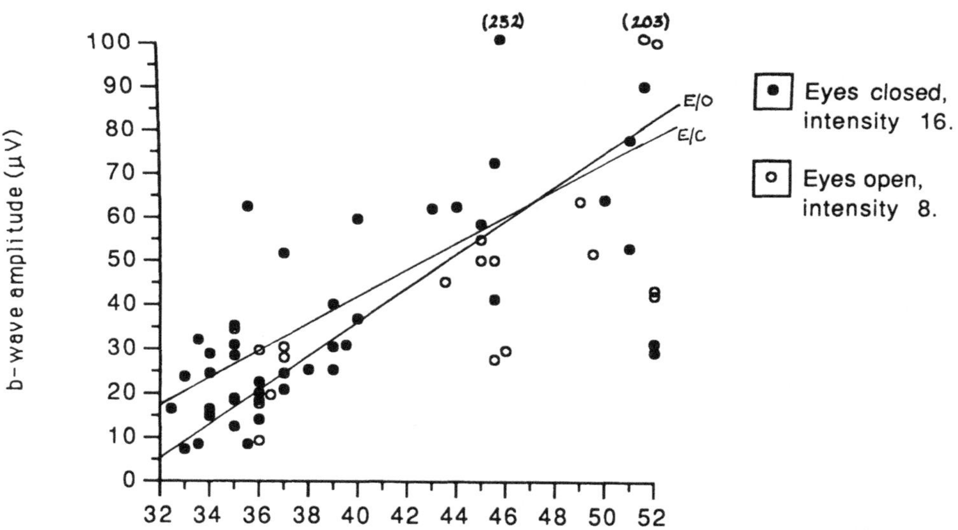

Fig. 7.2. The graph shows the b-wave amplitude in microvolts against the PCA in weeks. Although the amplitude of the b-wave was negatively correlated with PCA there is no significant difference in the amplitude under the eyes open and the eyes closed conditions allowing for the increase in intensity at the stimulus.

and there was a clear negative relationship with PCA at the time of recording (Fig. 7.1). The amplitude of the b-wave increased as the infant became older and this also showed a correlation with PCA (Fig. 7.2). The latency of the a-wave decreased slightly as the baby grew older, but this was not correlated with PCA, although a marked increase in amplitude of the a-wave was apparent from the time that it became recordable (Fig. 7.3). The authors also compared ERGs obtained with the infant's eyes closed and open. As long as there was an appropriate compensation for intensity, that is an increase in intensity from 197 to 483ms, there was no significant difference either in latency or in amplitude under the two conditions. It was felt better to record infants' ERGs with their eyes closed, since less muscle artefact was induced in babies with their eyes held open. Oscillatory potentials were only recordable in infants over 37 weeks PCA. Oscillatory potentials were recorded only when the eyes were closed—otherwise they could not be obtained even with a red stimulus.

Mactier *et al.* (1988), using similar conductive thread electrodes, were unable to find a correlation between any ERG parameter and PCA. However, 83 per cent of these infants had received phototherapy for hyperbilirubinaemia. During this period their eyes were continually patched. Mactier *et al.* (1988) did find that the amplitude and latency of the flash ERG was completely unaffected by eye closure in preterm infants ≤37 weeks PCA as long as they were Caucasian. In addition, they reported that the a-waves recorded from coloured infants were of a longer latency than those of Caucasian infants and suggested that this might be due to increased transparency of the lid in Caucasian infants.

Pattern ERGs in neonates

In recent years there has been much interest in the pattern evoked electroretinogram (PERG), which can assess retinal acuity in infants. Odom *et al.* (1983) investigated three infants around three months of age. Again a DTL electrode was used for recording, and the stimulus consisted of a reversing bar pattern at a variety of spatial frequencies between 1.25 and 4.5 cycles/degree. The black and white bars were reversed four times per second producing a steady state response which was analysed by measuring the absolute power of the second harmonic of the response. They also investigated the pattern visual evoked potential (VEP). The PERG acuity in infants was found to be considerably higher than the VEP acuity in relation to the spatial frequency of their stimuli, and they concluded that the retina is relatively more responsive to high spatial frequencies than is the visual cortex at around three months of age. Fiorentini *et al.* (1984) used skin electrodes in nine term infants aged between seven weeks and six months of age, and found similar responses in terms of visual acuity from both the VEP and the PERG. They used sine-wave gratings to a variety of spatial frequencies which were reversed 12 times/s. Again the amplitude of the second harmonic of the average response was measured. To obtain an estimate of acuity the response amplitude was extrapolated against log spatial frequency. Infant ERG acuities showed a rapid increase with age from two

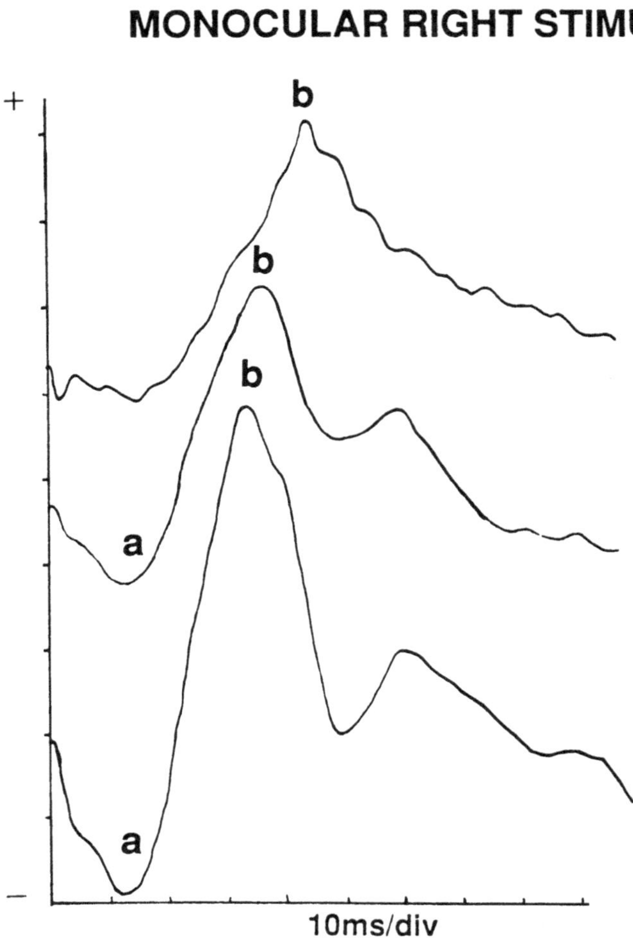

Fig. 7.3. ERG recorded on a single baby at (*top to bottom*) 33 weeks (6μv/div), 38 weeks (20μv/div) and 44 weeks (20μv/div) PCA. Initially the a-wave is not clearly present (15.32ms at 38 weeks, 15.03ms at 44 weeks), while the b-wave is apparent at 33 weeks and over successive weeks shortened in latency (44.52ms at 33 weeks, 38.89ms at 38 weeks and 34.90ms at 44 weeks).

cycles/degree at seven weeks to 12 cycles/degree at five months and the pattern VEP showed similar changes in acuity: a difference in their findings they attribute to the use of more spatial frequencies than that used by Odom *et al.* (1983).

Grose *et al.* (1989) did not report pattern ERG in preterm babies and our laboratory could not produce such a response in infants up to 53 weeks PCA.

ERG techniques

The first problem is to identify the type of electrode which should be used. Corneal electrodes were formerly used for many ERG studies, but this involved local anaesthesia. Corneal electrodes can obviously interfere with vision, removing any possibility of doing pattern ERGs; they can abrade the cornea and are generally not well tolerated (Dawson *et al.* 1979). Skin electrodes may be used and placed in close proximity to the eye, though there is a marked reduction in amplitude as soon as the electrode is placed outside the tarsal membrane (Harding and Rubinstein (1982). However, such techniques have been successfully used for ERG recording in children (Harden *et al.* 1978).

As an alternative to either corneal or skin electrodes, two similar types of electrodes have been developed. The first is known as the gold foil electrode which was developed originally by Chase *et al.* (1976). Using this technique a thin sheet of Mylar is coated with either aluminium or gold, shaped into a hook and looped over the lower lid. Later gold foil was used consistently, as this was found to make the electrode more stable (Borda *et al.* 1978, Arden *et al.* 1979). Studies were carried out of the performance of gold foil electrodes as compared with a standard contact lens electrode. In most studies a high correlation is found between a- and b-wave latency for the two electrodes. However, a- and b-wave amplitudes are found to be significantly different, the amplitude of course always being higher using the corneal electrode. Although this technique represented a novel improvement over the corneal electrode, there is no doubt that the gold foil electrode is an irritant and is not particularly well tolerated even by adults. From this point of view the gas-sterilised or DTL fibre is preferable; it is made up of filaments of spun nylon impregnated with silver. The filaments are fine enough to float on the tear film and make good contact with an attached conducting wire. Using a holder such as that described by Thompson and Drasdo (1987) the electrode is held firmly at the outer canthus, and in babies can be draped across the open eye and secured simply with a blob of electrode gel on the bridge of the nose. It should be recognised that tear production is minimal in some preterm infants, and it may be necessary to instil a drop of saline after the DTL electrode has been placed in position so that the fibre will float in the corneal tear film. Such a technique will usually lower the resistance to below 5kOhm. The reference electrode which is used for ERGs is usually a standard silver chloride disk electrode placed beyond the outer canthus.

With term infants it is frequently possible to carry out dark adaptation, which allows investigation of both rod and cone components of the ERG. In preterm infants this technique is often inappropriate. Some authors (Ricci *et al.* 1983) adapted babies to the dark using opaque eye pads, but this is frequently futile as the infant quickly light-adapts as soon as the pads are removed. Mactier *et al.* (1988) standardised retinal adaptation by using a reflective covering over the incubator in which the preterm baby was placed. However, covering the incubator makes constant monitoring impossible and therefore a video camera has to be inserted to monitor the child with infrared illumination. It is probably necessary to accept that in special care baby units it is not possible to dark-adapt the babies successfully. Frequent flash stimulation, necessary to produce an average response, completely destroys the dark adaptation.

The standard stimulus which is used for these techniques is the photostimulator or stroboscope. Certainly if infants are to be investigated with their eyes closed there is no doubt that a bright flash such as that delivered by the Grass PS22 photostimulator is necessary. Usually an intensity of around 197nitsecs is necessary (3939cd/m^2), although with closed eyes it may be necessary to deliver a stimulus of 483nitsecs (9661cd/m^2). Unfortunately this more intense stimulus sometimes produces a startle response from the babies with obvious increased electromyogram activity. The stimulus rate that has been used in studies depends on whether photopic or scotopic stimulation is attempted. For scotopic stimulation it is best to use single trials separated by around 10s as long as no more than four repetitions are carried out. For photopic ERGs the situation is much easier and stimulation rates as high as 1.75Hz may be used (Grose *et al.* 1989). Under these circumstances, and with the use of averaging, clear evoked responses are obtained after only 30 sweeps of averaging. There are a variety of commercial averagers available, all of which can be used either in the laboratory or as portable units.

Since the ERG a- and b-waves contain components between 21 and 50Hz (Orpin and McCulloch 1972), the band pass used has to exceed this range. The high pass cut-off is usually set at less than 3Hz and the upper (low-pass) cut-off around 70 to 100Hz except where it is necessary to record oscillatory potentials. In these circumstances the low pass filter should be set at 250Hz or more due to the higher frequency of these potentials.

Clinical value of the ERG infants

Electrophysiological assessment of the visual system in infants is usually only carried out in those suspected of a visual impairment. Although this chapter considers the use of the ERG in isolation, such an isolated investigation should not be performed in infants. The combination of flash ERG and flash VEP is essential in the assessment of the infant as the two techniques are entirely complementary. While the ERG will give an assessment of retinal function, and the amplitude of the ERG is directly proportional to the area of active retina stimulated, the VEP reflects the neural representation of visual space. It is therefore a much better reflector of macular problems in the retina itself and of any problems that occur along the optic nerves, the optic tracts or in the visual cortex. Nowadays many investigators also include the use of the pattern ERG (Odom *et al.* 1983) or alternatively the pattern VEP even in preterm babies down to 30 weeks (Harding *et al.* 1989*a*, Grose *et al.* 1989). All of these techniques are entirely non-invasive and therefore represent an effective measure of physiological function which may be correlated with the results of anatomical investigations. Although responses show inter-individual variability, this variability is not greater than that seen in normal adults (Fulton *et al.* 1989). It is, however, standard ERG technique to compare the responses between the two eyes since, like all evoked activity, intra-subject variability is much less than inter-subject variability. It has been suggested that to increase the sensitivity of the ERG technique, there should be a comparison between the b-wave amplitude at the point at which it saturates to high-intensity stimulation, and the intensity necessary to evoke half that amplitude (Fulton and Hansen 1982). Using this technique it was shown that at 12 months of age the ERG b-wave sensitivity matched that of the adult. These types of measures provide more normative values against which any patient can be tested. In later follow-up studies Fulton *et al.* (1989) presented normative data on infants from two to 12 months of age with the amplitude of the b-wave expressed as a percentage of the amplitude in the adult. Similar findings for photopic ERGs were published by Barnet *et al.* (1965). Norms for the flash preterm ERG have been given by Grose *et al.* (1989).

The variability of the ERG both within a subject and between subjects is in fact no greater with infants than with normal adults (Fulton *et al.* 1989) and neither is the intraocular range any greater. There is little doubt, therefore, that the ERG can be as clinically useful in newborn infants as it is in adults. However, there are very few reported studies of direct application of the ERG to neonatal visual problems.

There have been several studies of the ERG in retinopathy of prematurity. Negata (1977) reported that the amplitude of the ERG is markedly subnormal even in the very early stages, and that the ERG is extinguished in later evolved stages of the disease. François and De Rouck (1983) used the classification of Patz and Payne (1976) and classified their cases between stage I and stage V. Spontaneous regression occurred in any active stage: 80 per cent of patients in stage I showed such an effect, whereas stages IV and V always left significant residue. They examined 196 eyes of patients with retinopathy of prematurity and reported that an extinguished ERG is always seen in stages IV and V. It is subnormal in stages II and III but may well be normal in stage I. Their conclusion was that the more preserved the ERG, the milder the retinopathy, and if the ERG is within normal limits the degree of retinopathy could not be greater than stage II. Cases with an extinguished ERG always gave a poor prognosis.

Taurine deficiency in children has been reported to produce an increase in the latency of the scotopic ERG (Geggel *et al.* 1982). However, in a study of preterm babies who might be expected to show some signs of taurine deficiency, there was no difference in ERGs or VEPs in babies fed on taurine or taurine-free diets (Harding *et al.* 1989*b*).

Microphthalmos is sometimes associated with ERG abnormalities (Panagakis *et al.* 1982). In their study eight of 18 eyes produced normal ERGs: two showed a slight reduction of the ERG amplitude, three eyes showed a markedly reduced ERG and no ERG was recordable in five of the eyes. However, in many of the cases there were other abnormalities such as cataracts, retinal degeneration, or coloboma of the iris or the optic nerve. Although three of the cases with normal ERGs had a coexisting cataract, ophthalmoscopy performed after extraction revealed no pathological findings from the eye fundus, indicating the prognostic value of the ERG when the fundus is unobservable.

Algvere, P., Zetterström, B. (1967) 'Size and shape of the electroretinogram in newborn infants.' *Acta Ophthalmologica*, **45**, 399–410.

Arden, G.B., Brown, K.T. (1965) 'Some properties of the cat electroretinogram revealed by local recording under oil.' *Journal of Physiology (London)*, **176**, 429–461.

Arden, G.B., Carter, R.M., Hogg, C., Siegel, I.M., Margolis, S. (1979) 'A gold foil electrode: extending the horizons for clinical electroretinography.' *Investigative Ophthalmology*, **18**, 421–426.

Auerbach, E., Burian, H.M. (1955) 'Studies on the photopic-scotopic relationship in the human electroretinogram.' *American Journal of Ophthalmology*, **40**, 42–60.

Barnet, A.B., Lodge, A., Armington, J.C. (1965) 'Electroretinogram in newborn human infants.' *Science*, **148**, 651–654.

Borda, R.P., Gilliam, R.M., Coats, A.C. (1978) 'Gold-coated Mylar (GCM) electrode for electroretinography.' *Documenta Ophthalmologica Proceedings Series*, **15**, 339–354.

Brown, K.T., Watanabe, K. (1962) 'Isolation and identification of a receptor potential from the pure cone fovea of the monkey retina.' *Nature*, **193**, 958–960.

Brunette, J.R., Desrochers, R. (1970) 'Oscillatory potentials: a clinical study in diabetics.' *Canadian Journal of Ophthalmology*, **5**, 373–380.

Chase, W.W., Fradkin, N.E., Tsuda, S. (1976) 'A new electrode for electroretinography.' *American Journal of Optometry and Physiological Optics*, **53**, 668–671.

Cobb, W.A., Morton, H.B. (1954) 'A new component of the human electroretinogram.' *Journal of Physiology*, **123**, 36P–37P.

Dawson, W.W., Trick, G.L., Litzkow, C.A. (1979) 'Improved electrode for electroretinography.' *Investigative Ophthalmology and Visual Science*, **18**, 988–991.

Fiorentini, A., Pirchio, M., Sandini, G. (1984) 'Development of retinal acuity in infants evaluated with pattern electroretinogram.' *Human Neurobiology*, **3**, 93–95.

François, J., De Rouck, A. (1964) 'The electroretinogram in young children (single stimulus, twin flashes, and intermittent stimulation).' *Documenta Ophthalmologica*, **18**, 330–343.

—— —— (1983) 'Retrolental fibroplasia and ERG.' *Documenta Ophthalmologica Proceedings Series*, **37**, 278–291.

Fulton, A.B., Hansen, R.M. (1982) 'Background adaptation in human infants: analysis of b-wave responses.' *Documenta Ophthalmologica Proceedings Series*, **31**, 191–197.

—— —— (1985) 'Electroretinography: application to clinical studies of infants.' *Journal of Pediatric Ophthalmology and Strabismus*, **22**, 251–255.

—— Hartmann, E.E., Hansen, R.M. (1989) 'Electrophysiologic testing techniques for children.' *Documenta Ophthalmologica*, **71**, 341–354.

Geggel, H.S., Heckenlively, J.R., Martin, D.A., Ament, M.E., Kopple, J.D. (1982) 'Human retinal dysfunction and taurine deficiency.' *Documenta Ophthalmologica Proceedings Series*, **31**, 199–207.

Granit, R. (1933) 'The components of the retinal action potential in mammals and their relation to the discharge of the optic nerve.' *Journal of Physiology*, **77**, 207–239.

Grose, J., Harding, G.F.A., Wilton, A.Y., Bissenden, J.G. (1989) 'The maturation of the pattern reversal VEP and flash ERG in pre-term infants.' *Clinical Vision Sciences*, **4**, 239–246.

Harden, A., Picton-Robinson, N., Bradshaw, K., Pampiglione, G. (1978) *In* Barber, C. (Ed.) *Evoked Potentials: Proceedings of International Evoked Potentials Symposium, Nottingham.* Lancaster: MTP Press.

Harding, G.F.A., Grose, J., Wilton, A., Bissenden, J.G. (1989*a*) 'The pattern reversal VEP in short gestation infants.' *Electroencephalography and Clinical Neurophysiology*, **74**, 76–80.

—— Grose, J., Wilton, A.Y., Bissenden, J.G. (1989*b*) 'The pattern reversal VEP in short-gestation infants on taurine or taurine-free diet.' *Documenta Ophthalmologica*, **73**, 103–109.

—— Rubinstein, M.P. (1982) 'The visually evoked subcortical potential to flash stimulation in normal subjects and patients with lesions of the visual pathway.' *Advances in Neurology*, **32**, 31–39.

Horsten, G.P.M., Winkelman, J.E. (1962) 'Electrical activity of the retina in relation to histological differentiation in infants born prematurely and at full-term.' *Vision Research*, **12**, 269–276.

Lachapelle, P., Molotchnikoff, S. (1986) 'Components of the electroretinogram: a reappraisal.' *Documenta Ophthalmologica*, **63**, 337–348.

Lodge, A., Armington, J.C., Barnet, A., Shanks, B.L., Newcomb, C.N. (1969) 'Newborn infants'

electroretinograms and evoked electroencephalographic responses to orange and white light.' *Child Development*, **40**, 267–293.
Mactier, H., Dexter, J.D., Hewett, J.E., Latham, C.B., Woodruff, C.W. (1988) 'The electroretinogram in pre-term infants.' *Journal of Pediatrics*, **113**, 607–612.
Negata, M. (1977) 'Treatment of acute proliferative retrolental fibroplasia with xenon-arc photocoagulation.' *Japanese Journal of Ophthalmology*, **21**, 436–459.
Odom, J.V., Maida, T.M., Dawson, W.W., Romano, P.E. (1983) 'Retinal and cortical pattern responses: a comparison of infants and adults.' *American Journal of Optometry and Physiological Optics*, **60**, 369–375.
Orpin, J.A., McCulloch, C. (1972) 'Power analysis of the electroretinogram.' *Canadian Journal of Ophthalmology*, **7**, 454–461.
Panagakis, E., Moschos, M., Angelopoulos, A., Palimeris, G., Velissaropoulos, P. (1982) 'ERG findings in children with microphthalmos.' *Documenta Ophthalmologica Proceedings Series*, **31**, 217–227.
Patz, A., Payne, J.W. (1976) 'Retrolental fibroplasia.' *In* Duane, T.D. (Ed.) *Clinical Ophthalmology, Vol. 3.* New York: Harper & Row. Chapter 20.
Ricci, B., Falsini, B., Valentini, P., Molle, F., Rufi, L. (1983) 'Development of the main electroretinographic components in premature infants during the first week of life.' *Arch. Soc. Oftal. Optom.*, **17**, 159.
—— —— —— —— —— (1984) 'L'elettroretinaogramma fotopica nei prematura.' *Annali Ottalmologica e Clinica Occulista*, **110**, 771–780.
Samson-Dollfus, D. (1968) 'Développement normal de l'ERG dupuis l'âge foetal de seizieme et demi: jusqu'à l'âge de quatre mois après la naissance à terme.' *Bulletin Société d'Ophthalmologie de France*, 423–431.
Shipley, T., Anton, M.T. (1964) 'The human electroretinogram in the first day of life.' *Journal of Pediatrics*, **65**, 733–739.
Speros, P., Price, J. (1981) 'Oscillatory potentials. History, techniques and potential use in the evaluation of disturbances of retinal circulation.' *Survey of Ophthalmology*, **251**, 237–252.
Thompson, D.A., Drasdo, N. (1987) 'An improved method for using the DTL fibre in electroretinography.' *Ophthalmic and Physologio Optics*, **7**, 315–319.
Yokoyama, M., Kaneko, K., Nakai, Y.T. (1964) 'The oscillatory potential in the retina and optic nerve of the rabbit.' *Mie Medical Journal*, **13**, 109–122.
Zetterström, B. (1952) 'The electroretinogram in premature children.' *Acta Ophthalmologica*, **30**, 405–408.

8

ASSESSMENT OF MOTOR PATHWAYS

J.A. Eyre and S. Miller

Sensorimotor integration plays an important role in the acquisition of motor skills in animals (Sakamoto *et al.* 1989) and in man (Bernstein 1967, Stelmach 1976, Hildreth and Hollerbach 1987, Neilson *et al.* 1988). Such integration not only involves peripheral reflex pathways, but also occurs at many levels within the central nervous system (CNS) (Lundberg 1982, Sakamoto *et al.* 1989). The process is complex and detailed and forms the basis of internal computations within the CNS, as has been demonstrated in animals (Miller and Oscarsson 1969; Oscarsson 1973; Lundberg 1975, 1979, 1982). To study the development of the central nervous control of movement, therefore, requires investigation of both motor and sensory systems. Somatosensory pathways are discussed in Chapter 4, and this chapter describes the development of the corticospinal pathway and sensorimotor reflex integration at the spinal level.

In the perinatal period, there is rapid maturation of neurons in the central and peripheral nervous system. Broadly, as discussed in Chapter 1, there is maturation of the cell body with increasing size of the soma and extension of the dendritic tree (Marin-Padilla 1988, Miller 1988). In parallel, the axon enlarges in length and diameter. However the most striking changes, and perhaps the most significant for movement control, concern synaptic projections within the CNS. Axonal projections become more focused with withdrawal of collateral branches (Innocenti 1981, Ivy *et al.* 1984). At the same time there is a redistribution of synapses over the soma-dendritic surface. The overall density of synaptic terminals initially rises and then falls (Rakic *et al.* 1986), but the relative proportion of synapses on dendrites to soma increases (Conradi 1976). The morphological types of synaptic terminals also change with age, with an increasing density of terminals ascribed to inhibitory function, particularly on the soma (Bodian 1966, Conradi 1976). These remarkable organisational changes are reflected in developing motor control and in neurophysiological measurements. The process continues into adulthood, but is most rapid during the perinatal period and first two postnatal years. In neurophysiological terms, the 'snapshot' of the perinatal period must be considered as part of this overall continuum of development.

Noninvasive stimulation of the corticospinal pathway

Neurophysiological investigation of the corticospinal pathway in man depends on the ability to stimulate the neurons of the motor cortex through the intact skull. Gualterotti and Patterson (1954) first reported stimulation of the unexposed motor cortex in baboons and humans using repetitive electrical shocks. However, owing

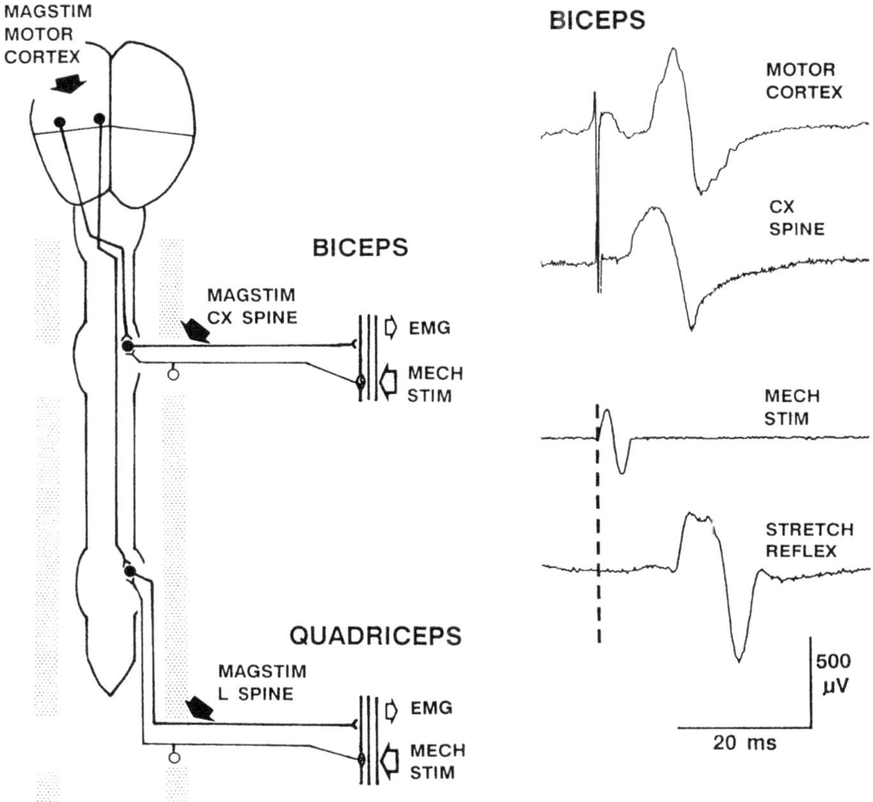

Fig. 8.1. Motor evoked potentials from biceps brachii obtained from a newborn baby. *Left*: experimental protocol, and *right*: sample records. The upper two traces show motor action potentials evoked following electromagnetic stimulation of the motor cortex and cervical motor nerve respectively. The third trace represents the mechanical stimulus applied to biceps brachii tendon and the lowest trace the evoked phasic stretch reflex in biceps brachii. Shaded area represents the vertebral column. Magstim, electromagnetic stimulation; Cx, cervical; L, lumbar; mech stim, mechanical stimulation.

to the large electrical resistance of the skull bones, a high and intensely painful voltage of stimulation was required. Merton and Morton (1980) succeeded in activating muscles in the hand and upper limb by applying a single short (50μs) high-voltage electrical pulse to the scalp above the contralateral motor cortex. It was later found that the same technique could also be used for activating peripheral motor nerves at their point of exit from the vertebral foramina (Merton *et al.* 1982, Plassman and Gandevia 1989). By subtracting the latency of the motor nerve responses from those following cortical stimulation, estimates could be made of the central conduction delays of the fastest conducting fibres within the corticospinal pathway (Fig. 8.1) (Merton *et al.* 1982). This technique has since been successfully applied to the study of corticospinal tract transmission in normal adult subjects and those with central motor disorders (Rossini *et al.* 1987, Rothwell *et al.* 1987*b*).

Despite a very brief stimulus, however, the technique is too painful to be used in unanaesthetised children.

Painless excitation of the motor cortex was first achieved by Barker *et al.* (1985, 1987) using electromagnetic induction, the magnetic field being generated with a coil placed above the scalp. The ability to stimulate biological structures with currents induced by time varying magnetic fields had been appreciated for many years. Indeed the flashes of light (known as magnetophosphenes), stimulated by electromagnetically induced currents in the retina, have been studied since the late 19th century (d'Arsonval 1896, Thompson 1910). Other nervous structures have higher thresholds for activation, however, and it proved a technical challenge to induce a magnetic field of sufficient magnitude and rate of change. In 1965 Bickford and Fremming first reported stimulating unexposed human peripheral nerves using a 500Hz sinusoidal magnetic field of 4 Tesla peak amplitude lasting 20ms. Although clear muscular contractions were observed, the duration of the magnetic field precluded the recording of peripheral nerve or muscle activity because of the artefacts induced in the recording equipment by the large changes of magnetic flux. Bickford and Fremming suggested the possible use of magnetic fields to stimulate the brain, but were unable to demonstrate this. Polson *et al.* (1982) achieved activation of peripheral nerves using a *single* magnetic pulse of short duration, so that motor action potentials could be recorded from a nearby muscle. It was the further development of this technique which first enabled the painless stimulation of the motor cortex in humans. Since then, electromagnetic stimulation of the human motor cortex to evoke muscle action potentials in skeletal muscle has developed into a widely used, noninvasive technique for evaluating descending motor pathway function in humans (Berardelli *et al.* 1987, Mills *et al.* 1987, Rossini *et al.* 1987, Rothwell *et al.* 1987*a*, Ingram *et al.* 1988, Koh and Eyre 1988, Eyre *et al.* 1991*a*).

Evidence for activation of corticospinal neurons following electromagnetic stimulation of the motor cortex

It is now several years since Barker and his colleagues first described the technique of electromagnetic stimulation of the brain. Since then several investigators have confirmed their original observations and have provided indirect evidence that the responses involve activation of the corticospinal pathway.

1. There is preferential activation of the distal muscles of the hand (Rothwell *et al.* 1987*b*).

2. Very short central motor conduction delays have been found from cortex to spinal motor nerve, between 5 and 7ms in children and adults (Rothwell *et al.* 1987*a*, Eyre *et al.* 1991*a*).

3. Patients with documented lesions of the corticospinal pathway have delayed or absent responses in the contralateral muscles following motor cortex stimulation (Mills *et al.* 1987, Rossini *et al.* 1987, Rothwell *et al.* 1987*a*).

The conclusion that the electromagnetic stimulus excites corticospinal neurons is supported by neurophysiological studies in the Macaque monkey where short latency responses have been recorded in the corticospinal pathway (Amassian *et al.* 1987; Edgley *et al.* 1989, 1990*a*,*b*). These observations have been further confirmed in the Macaque monkey in recordings from single axons in the corticospinal projection (Edgley *et al.* 1991). In fact electromagnetic stimulation powerfully excites the majority of myelinated fibres in the corticospinal pathway, with responses recorded in axons over the conduction velocity range of 15 to 100m/s.

Observations in human subjects that the latencies of muscle action potentials following electrical stimulation of the motor cortex were 2 to 3ms shorter than those following magnetic stimulation (Hess *et al.* 1987) have provoked considerable debate. Hess *et al.* (1987) originally proposed that electrical stimulation activated the axons of corticospinal neurons at a site distal to the cortex, while electromagnetic stimulation activated the neurons within the cortex itself. Day *et al.* (1989) questioned this proposal because, given a conduction velocity in the fastest conducting fibres of 70m/s, the delay of 2 to 3ms would mean activation at a site 14cm below the cortex. They suggested that electrical stimulation activated corticospinal neurons directly while electromagnetic stimulation activated other cortical neurons which excited corticospinal neurons transsynaptically. Indirect support was obtained from studies in human subjects.

The pendulum has now swung back to the original proposal of Hess *et al.* (1987). Neurophysiological studies in the monkey have established that both electrical and electromagnetic stimulation can activate corticospinal neurons directly. At threshold intensities both stimuli excite the axon within the cortex (Edgley *et al.* 1989, 1990*a*,*b*, 1992), but at higher stimulus intensities the electrical stimulus excites the axon at progressively more distal sites down to at least the level of the medullary pyramid. Excitation by electromagnetic stimulation is restricted to within the cortex at all stimulus intensities. Distal axonal excitation with increasing electrical stimulus intensities has subsequently been confirmed in humans with extradural recordings of the corticospinal volley at upper cervical spinal levels (Burke *et al.* 1990). The previous studies in human subjects comparing the latencies following electrical and electromagnetic stimulation (*e.g.* Day *et al.* 1989) were made at suprathreshold intensities. It is likely that the differences in the response characteristics are due to more distal excitation of the axon by electrical compared with electromagnetic stimulation.

Safety of electromagnetic stimulation of the brain

The safety record of electromagnetic stimulation of the brain in children and adults is very high indeed. Since the first report of the technique (Barker *et al.* 1985), tens of thousands of adults—and about a thousand babies and children in our laboratory alone—have been studied with no adverse consequences. There is one report of a generalised epileptic seizure occurring during electromagnetic brain stimulation in a 57-year-old man with a very large right hemispheric infarct; a previous electroencephalogram (EEG) had shown a right-sided abnormality (Hömberg and

Netz 1989). The incidence of seizure following stroke has been reported to be up to 40 per cent. Many thousands of subjects have now been studied after stroke and this is the only report of a seizure occurring during stimulation. It is therefore likely to be a chance occurrence.

The maximal currents and the charge induced in the brain during magnetic stimulation have been calculated by Barker *et al.* (1987), who stated that the maximal charge of approximately 50μc/pulse induced by magnetic stimulation is 0.05 to 0.005 per cent of the charge used in electroconvulsive therapy. Furthermore, the amount of thermal energy deposited in tissue with electromagnetic stimulation is very small, representing less than 0.01 per cent of the heat generated by normal cerebral basal metabolism. The peak magnetic field applied is similar to the static fields used in whole body and head magnetic imaging scanners. No hazards due to these fields have yet been reported, despite prolonged periods of continuous exposure.

The safety of the technique has also been explored in studies in the cat (Eyre *et al.* 1990). The experiments were designed to test whether prolonged runs of maximal electromagnetic stimulation at 12 per minute might evoke changes in cerebral bloodflow, heart rate and blood pressure, as well as EEG, somatosensory evoked potentials and motor evoked potentials. No stimulus-related changes were observed, even when the brain had been subjected to severe anoxic episodes in which cerebral autoregulation had been lost. No evidence of kindling was observed even during or following anoxia, although it should be noted from studies in the rat and cat that electrical stimuli applied at 3Hz or less, irrespective of the number of stimuli applied, could not cause kindling (Goddard *et al.* 1969).

Electromagnetic stimulation of motor pathways

When an electromagnetic stimulus is applied to the brain, activity is evoked in the corticospinal pathway (Edgley *et al.* 1989, 1990*a,b*, 1992) which in turn activates spinal motor neurons to excite action potentials in muscle (Barker *et al.* 1987, Koh and Eyre 1988, Eyre *et al.* 1991*a*). The electromagnetic stimulus can also be used to excite the spinal motor nerves as they emerge from the vertebral column, which enables the peripheral motor conduction delay to be estimated in the upper limb (Plassman and Gandevia 1989, Ugawa *et al.* 1989, Eyre *et al.* 1991*a*). This method cannot be used for estimating peripheral motor conduction delay in the lower limb, since the stimulus appears not to excite the spinal motor nerves in their prolonged descent through the vertebral canal, but only at their exit from the vertebral foramina. Estimates of peripheral motor conduction delay in the lower limb can, however, be derived directly from the F response (Kimura 1974), although the method may be painful, or indirectly from the timing of stretch reflexes. Subtraction of the peripheral from the overall motor conduction delay provides an estimate of central motor conduction delay (Fig. 8.1) (Eyre *et al.* 1991*a*).

In our studies, a MagStim 200 (MagStim Co. Ltd) electromagnetic stimulator

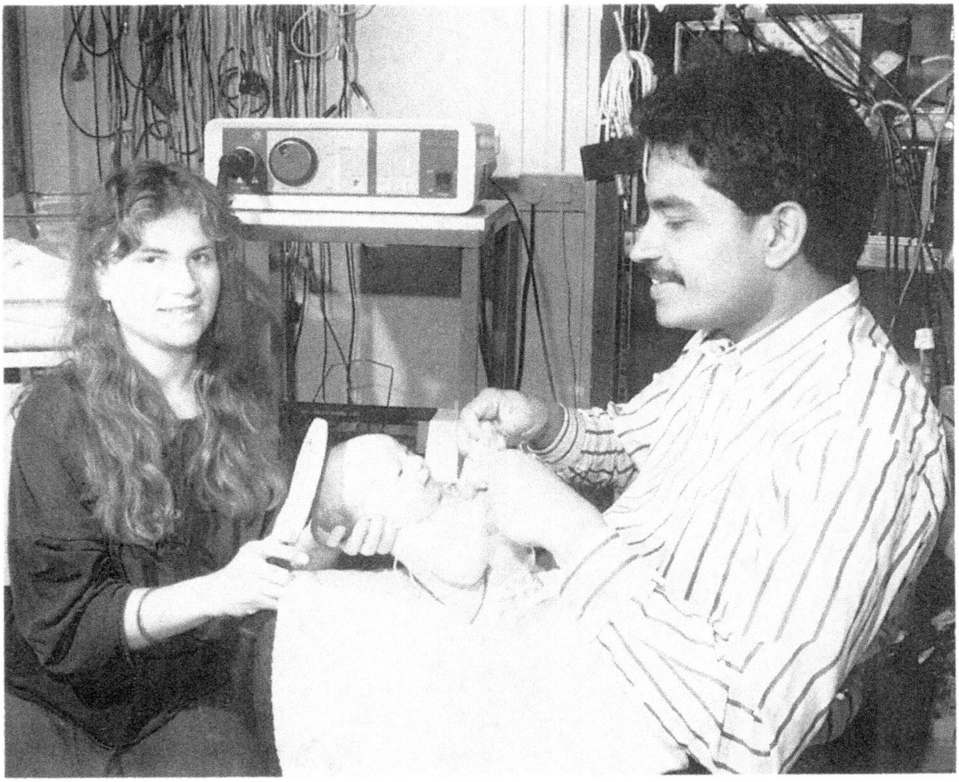

Fig. 8.2. Electromagnetic stimulation of the motor cortex in a newborn infant using a 9cm coil. Background muscle activity in biceps brachii is being evoked using the traction reflex. Motor action potentials in biceps brachii are being recorded using surface-mounted electrodes.

has been used to make estimates of conduction delays from the motor cortex to biceps brachii and hypothenar muscles in the upper limb and quadriceps in the lower limb. The MagStim 9cm circular coil was placed in the tangential plane above the vertex of the head, to stimulate the motor cortex (Fig. 8.2). The stimulus intensity was gradually increased until the threshold level was reached, when a response in the muscle being studied could be obtained in 50 per cent of trials. It is important to note the threshold level because this varies with age and with central motor pathology (see below). The stimulus intensity was then set so that responses could be obtained in all trials. The *shortest* latency in any trial between cortical stimulation and the muscle response was noted, since this has been shown to provide the basis for the best estimate of central motor conduction delay (Hess *et al.* 1987, Eyre *et al.* 1991*a*).

To stimulate the cervical motor roots a MagStim 6cm circular coil was placed in the coronal plane overlying the fifth to eighth cervical spines (Fig. 8.3). As described above, the stimulus intensity was increased until the threshold level was

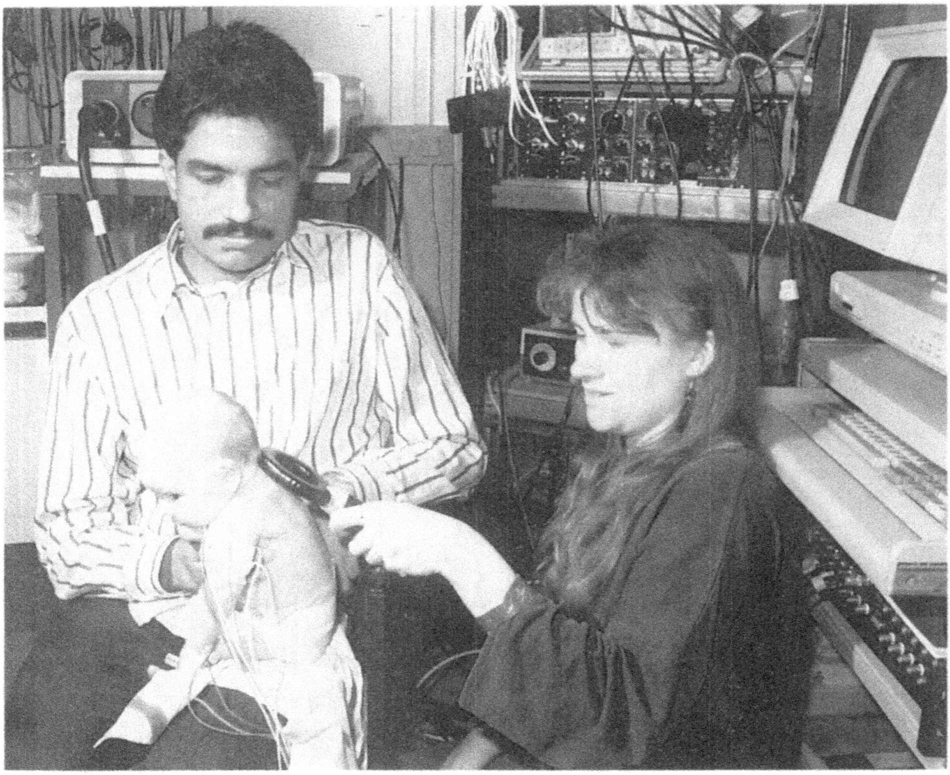

Fig. 8.3. Electromagnetic stimulation of the spinal motor nerve in a newborn baby by placing the 6cm coil over the cervical spine.

achieved. With this stimulus intensity the coil was then moved in small steps laterally to obtain the *longest* latency for evoking muscle action potentials. The longest latency response to percutaneous electrical stimulation applied at threshold to the cervical spine has been shown to arise from excitation of the motor roots close to their exit from the intervertebral foramina (Plassman and Gandevia 1989), and it is reasonable to assume that the same would apply in the case of electromagnetic stimulation. Identification of the longest onset latency following electromagnetic stimulation over the cervical spines was not made in the study of Ugawa *et al.* (1989), who only reported average latencies of the responses.

Electromyograms (EMGS) were recorded from either the left or right biceps brachii, hypothenar muscles and quadriceps femoris during *contraction*, since electromagnetic stimulation of the cortex does not evoke responses in relaxed muscles in children under six years of age (Koh and Eyre 1988). In subjects older than two years, contraction in the muscles being studied was achieved by asking the subject to hold a 200g weight or to extend the knee from a flexed position. In subjects of two years and under, the responses were measured during periods of spontaneous EMG activity.

The EMG was recorded with skin-mounted Ag/AgCl EEG cup electrodes (standard 5mm diameter) filled with saline jelly. The skin was cleaned with surgical spirit and prepared by gently rubbing with Omniprep. Pairs of electrodes were placed 15mm apart over the belly of biceps, over the hypothenar eminence, and for quadriceps femoris over the anterior aspect of the thigh midway between the knee and hip. The impedance of the electrodes was maintained in the 1 to 5kOhm range throughout the recordings. The EMG signals were amplified, filtered with a −3dB bandpass of 5 to 1500Hz and recorded onto magnetic tape using a Racal Store 4 recorder. The latencies of the responses were analysed off-line by computer (1401 Interface and Signal Averager Program: Cambridge Electronic Design Ltd). For the upper limb, the central motor conduction delay was estimated by subtracting the *longest* latency of onset of the muscle action potential evoked following cervical root stimulation from the *shortest* latency of onset of the muscle action potential evoked following cortical stimulation (Fig. 8.1). For the lower limb the stretch reflex was used to estimate the peripheral motor conduction delay (see p. 128). To allow for synaptic delay, 1ms was subtracted from the total latency of the stretch reflex. The remaining latency was apportioned according to the relative mean maximum conduction velocities for age in motor and sensory components of muscle nerves (Vecchierini-Blineau and Guiheneuc 1979). The stimulus intensity was expressed as the percentage of the maximum power output of the stimulator, calculated as a function of the square of the voltage fed to the coil from the stimulator output.

Results in normal subjects

For investigation of motor pathways to the upper limb, measurements were made in 444 healthy normal subjects ranging in age from 31 weeks gestation to 55 years; 150 were preterm or term infants and 270 of the subjects were aged two years or under. Fifty subjects have been studied so far to characterise the development of motor pathways to quadriceps muscle. Healthy preterm and term infants were defined as having Apgar scores of eight or more at one and five minutes after birth, with no significant neurological complications and normal ultrasound scans.

In all subjects, EMG responses in the muscles studied were obtained following electromagnetic stimulation over the cortex and cervical spines. The total and central motor conduction delays in the preterm and term baby were relatively high, compared with adult values (Fig. 8.4). The central motor conduction delays shorten slightly in the first year and then decrease rapidly to achieve adult values by 2½ years (Fig. 8.4). The rapid reduction in the delays observed reflects the process of myelination and the more than sevenfold increase in axon diameter in the corticospinal pathway which occurs over this period (Nathan and Smith 1955, Yakovlev and Lecours 1967). It is also possible that the linkage from corticospinal

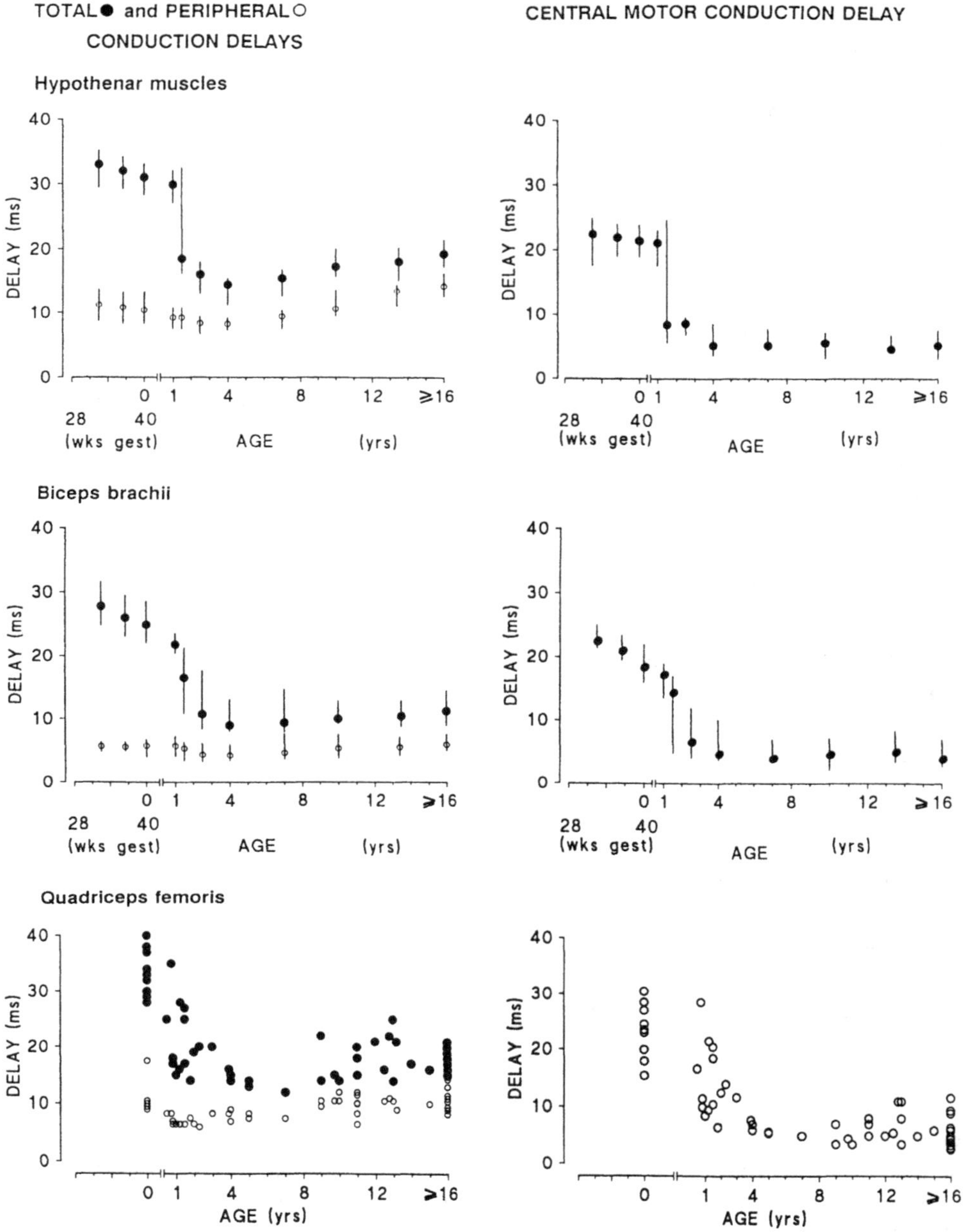

Fig. 8.4. The latency of motor evoked potentials in relation to subject age in the hypothenar muscles, biceps brachii and quadriceps femoris. The symbols in the graphs for biceps brachii and hypothenar muscles represent the median values and the bars the 10th to 90th centile range. The graphs on the left represent the total and peripheral conduction delays; those on the right represent the estimated central motor conduction delays.

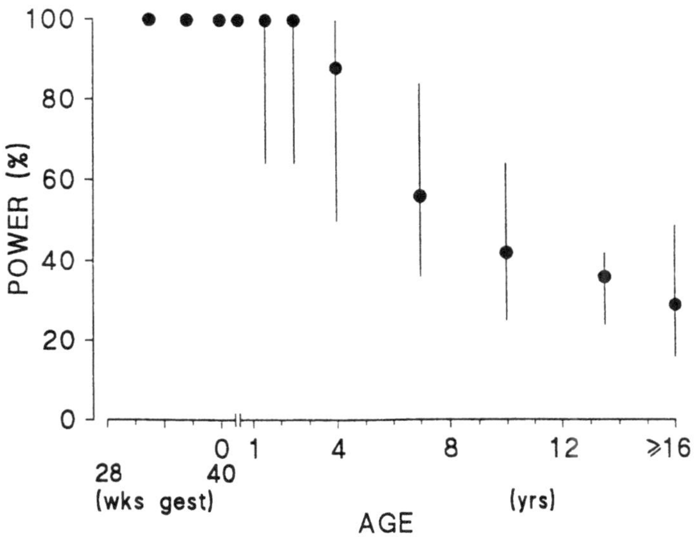

Fig. 8.5. The threshold stimulus intensity for evoking motor action potentials in biceps brachii in relation to age. The symbols represent the median value and the bars the 10th to 90th centile range. The stimulus intensity is expressed as power and is calculated as a percentage of the maximum power output of the stimulator. A similar pattern of change in threshold with age was found for the hypothenar muscles and quadriceps.

axons to motor neurons changes from polysynaptic to monosynaptic over this period (Lawrence and Hopkins 1976).

The peripheral motor delay remains relatively constant in the first 1½ years and then decreases slightly around the age of four years (Fig. 8.4). This pattern of delays reflects the combination of increasing arm length during growth and the increase in conduction velocities in motor nerves (Thomas and Lambert 1960, Vecchierini-Blineau and Guiheneuc 1979).

There is a progressive increase in the total motor conduction delay from the age of four years. This is entirely attributable to the increase in peripheral motor conduction delay, which is in proportion to increasing arm length (Eyre *et al.* 1991*a*). In contrast, adult values for central motor conduction delay are achieved from the age of two to four years, and these remain constant throughout childhood and adolescence despite a more than twofold increase in stature. The constancy of central motor conduction delays can only be achieved by increasing conduction velocities in the corticospinal pathway throughout childhood. The implication of these observations is that, within the corticospinal pathway, axons have progressively increasing diameters in proportion to stature, in contrast to peripheral nerves where there is no further increase in axon diameter after three to five years of age (Rexed 1944, Nathan and Smith 1955, Gutrecht and Dyck 1970).

The threshold stimulus intensity required to excite responses through the corticospinal pathway remains high for the first two years after birth. It then falls exponentially with age to reach adult values by 16 years (Fig. 8.5).

Electromagnetic stimulation of the brain in children with cerebral palsy

Electromagnetic stimulation of the brain has been studied in two groups of cerebral-palsied children: those with spastic hemiplegia (15 children aged four to 16 years) and those with spastic quadriplegia (15 children aged five to 16 years). Children with spastic hemiplegia demonstrated abnormalities of corticospinal transmission to the hemiplegic side with absent responses or prolonged central motor conduction delays and/or high thresholds for activation (Eyre *et al.* 1989). The degree of abnormality in corticospinal transmission was found to be in proportion to the impairment of hand function. In one child with spastic hemiplegia and mirror movements of the hands, Farmer *et al* (1990) also demonstrated abnormal corticospinal projections from the normal motor cortex to homologous muscles on both the contralateral and ipsilateral sides.

Surprisingly, studies of the 15 children with severe spasticity involving all four limbs revealed no abnormality of cortocospinal transmission (Eyre *et al.* 1989). Furthermore, in a longitudinal study of 63 children born prematurely, the 14 children with signs of spastic quadriplegia at 18 months had displayed normal development of corticospinal transmission (Eyre *et al.* 1991*b*).

Therefore, it appears that while unilateral abnormalities in corticospinal transmission may be predictive of spastic hemiplegia, early studies of corticospinal function are not of prognostic significance for spastic quadriparesis.

Further studies are currently being conducted to determine if more subtle abnormalities of corticospinal function can be demonstrated in those with spastic quadriparesis.

Development of spinal reflex pathways

In studies in the cat, descending motor pathways modulate the activity of both excitatory and inhibitory interneurons of spinal reflex pathways, as well as acting directly on the alpha motor neuron. Normal movement control may therefore be reinforced by the selection by descending pathways of spinal reflex patterns most appropriate to achieve the desired movement (Lundberg and Voorhoeve 1962; Lundberg 1975, 1979, 1982). Changes in spinal reflex patterns occurring during development, therefore, are likely to be of fundamental importance in the overall development of motor control. The development of two spinal reflex patterns has been studied in the newborn and young infant: the phasic stretch reflex (Myklebust *et al.* 1986, O'Sullivan *et al.* 1991) and the cutaneous reflex (Issler and Stephens 1983, Rowlandson and Stephens 1985*a*), which are described in detail below.

Phasic stretch reflex

Primary muscle spindle afferents predominantly excite alpha motor neurons of the homonymous muscle (forming the basis of the phasic stretch reflex) and to a lesser degree motor neurons of synergistic muscles, in the cat (Eccles *et al.* 1957*a, b*) and baboon (Hongo *et al.* 1984). In the limbs, activation of primary spindle afferents also evokes reciprocal inhibition of alpha motor neurons of antagonistic muscles through Group I_A inhibitory interneurons (see Hultborn's 1972 study in the cat). Comparable reflex patterns of excitation and inhibition have been observed in adult human subjects between muscles of the limbs (Tanaka 1974, Day *et al.* 1984, Plant and Miller 1990, O'Sullivan *et al.* 1991).

In the newborn animal and the human neonate, the patterns of stretch reflexes and reciprocal inhibition are less well defined, but it is notable that the mature patterns are not yet established. Excitatory reflex actions from muscle afferents predominate (Skoglund 1960, Saito 1979, Myklebust 1990). The kitten has been shown to have excitatory monosynaptic projections between primary afferents and alpha motor neurons of non-homonymous and non-synergistic muscles, which become greatly reduced in comparison to the adult cat (Eccles *et al.* 1963). Indeed, many excitatory intersegmental projections from primary afferents to motor neurons disappear during development (as shown by Saito's 1979 study in the rat). In the human neonate, Myklebust *et al.* (1986) and Myklebust (1990) observed that a tendon tap to triceps surae evoked excitatory reflex activity, not only in triceps surae but also in its antagonist, tibialis anterior, and to more distant muscles of the lower limb, quadriceps femoris and the hamstring muscles. They termed the radiation of the reflex to tibialis anterior 'reciprocal excitation', and that to quadriceps and the hamstrings 'reflex irradiation'. Using indirect evidence, Myklebust *et al.* (1986) concluded that the radiated responses resulted from monosynaptic or oligosynaptic excitatory projections from primary muscle afferents of triceps surae to alpha motor neurons of the other muscles, projections which later become masked or eliminated during normal development. Continuing these studies, Myklebust (1990) presented preliminary evidence in 15 children that reflex radiation in the lower limb becomes restricted over the first six years of life.

To characterise further the development of the phasic stretch reflex, a large cross-sectional study was conducted in which the stretch reflex in biceps brachii and the degree of radiation of the reflex among muscles of the upper limb at different ages were examined (O'Sullivan *et al.* 1991). The study was performed on 444 subjects, ranging from preterm babies of 31 weeks gestation to adults of 55 years. The subjects were all healthy and had no past history or clinical signs of neurological disorder. The 149 preterm and term infants studied all had Apgar scores of greater than eight at one and five minutes after birth and normal cerebral ultrasound scans.

Methods

Subjects of less than six months were studied in a supine position with the head in a midline anatomical position (Fig. 8.6). Subjects aged more than six months were seated either on a parent's knee or on a chair, and the reflexes were studied with the head in the midline position. In all subjects the left elbow was positioned in approximately 45° of flexion from full extension; in those subjects where the responses to contralateral stimulation were recorded by applying the stimulus to the right biceps tendon, the right elbow was similarly positioned in approximately 45° of flexion from full extension.

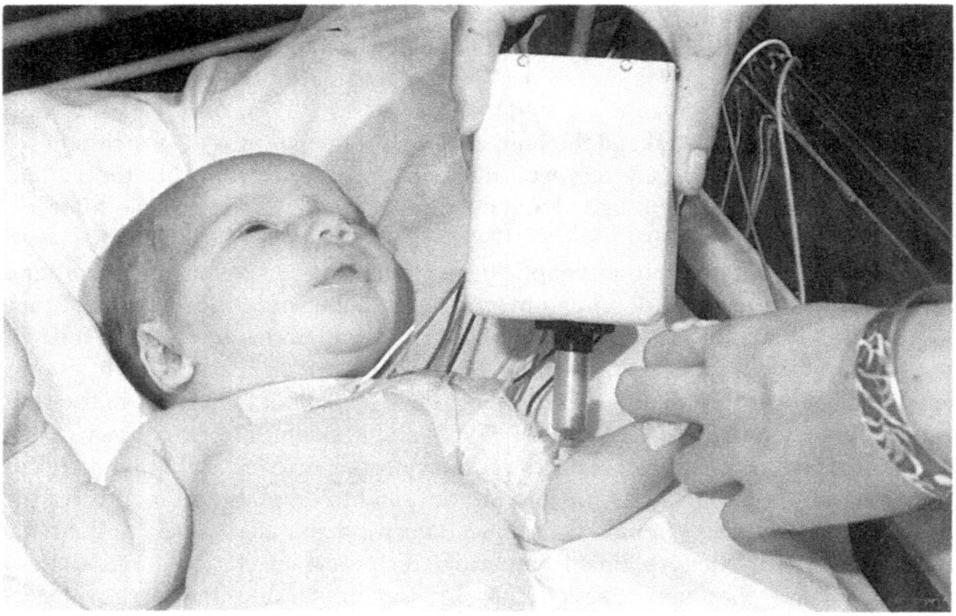

Fig. 8.6. Newborn infant having a phasic stretch reflex evoked in biceps brachii with a hand-held electromagnetic vibrator.

Subjects under one month were studied while quietly awake or asleep, and their state of sleep was determined either by observation (N 138) or by polygraphic recording (N 11) using the method of Anders *et al.* (1971). Subjects over one month were studied while awake.

The phasic stretch reflex was elicited in biceps brachii with a hand-held electromechanical vibrator (Ling Altec 200) delivering a single cycle of 150Hz sine wave over a peak to peak amplitude range of 0.2 to 3.1mm (O'Sullivan *et al.* 1991). Each stimulus began from the zero crossing point of the sine wave giving an initial outward deflection. The stylus of the vibrator, a circular plastic disc of 1cm diameter, was applied to the skin overlying the tendon of biceps brachii within the cubital fossa (Fig. 8.6). The peak-to-peak amplitude of the stimulus was increased until a reflex response could be elicited in biceps brachii in 50 per cent of the trials, and this was defined as the threshold. The amplitude was then set to be 1.2 times the threshold so that a reflex response could be obtained in biceps brachii in all trials. In each subject an attempt was first made to elicit the reflex and define the threshold in *relaxed* muscle. If no reflex response was obtained even at maximum peak-to-peak amplitude of the stimulus, the reflex was then elicited in the presence of background muscle activity in biceps brachii and the threshold defined in *contracting* muscle. Subjects older than two years were given a 200g weight to hold in the left hand; in subjects aged two years and under, the reflexes were measured during periods of spontaneous EMG activity.

EMGs were recorded using standard Ag/AgCl skin-mounted EEG electrodes, (5mm in diameter with centres separated by 15mm) from the following muscles of the left upper limb: biceps brachii, triceps brachii, deltoid, pectoralis major and those of the hypothenar eminence. In each case the recording electrodes were placed in the vertical anatomical plane over the belly of biceps brachii, the lateral head of triceps brachii and the hypothenar eminence, and in the horizontal plane over the clavicular fibres of pectoralis major and over the lateral aspect of deltoid. The EMGs were amplified and filtered using a −3dB bandpass of 5 to 1500Hz. The impedance of the recording electrodes was measured and maintained between 1 and 5kOhms.

In each subject, controls were carried out to determine if responses in muscles other than biceps brachii could be attributed to their direct response to mechanical spread of the stimulus through the tissues of the limb. The same stimulus magnitude used to evoke reflex responses (*i.e.* 1.2 times the threshold for evoking a reflex in biceps brachii) was also applied to the skin on either side of the biceps tendon in the cubital fossa and to the medial and lateral epicondyles of the humerus. If these stimuli evoked a reflex response in any of the muscles, including biceps brachii, direct excitation of the muscles by mechanical spread was assumed and the data from the subject were excluded from further analysis.

Results in normal subjects

In all 444 subjects tested, a phasic stretch reflex in either relaxed or contracting biceps brachii was evoked by the vibratory stimulus applied to the skin overlying the tendon. Figure 8.7A shows representative recordings of the biceps stretch reflex in subjects ranging in age from 31 weeks gestation to 25 years. It should be noted that in nearly all subjects under the age of two years the reflex could be elicited in relaxed muscle, whereas background muscle activity in biceps brachii was required in the large majority of subjects older than two years. Figure 8.7B shows the percentage of subjects with age in whom it was not possible to elicit the phasic stretch reflex in relaxed biceps brachii and in whom facilitatory background muscle contraction was required. The peak-to-peak amplitude of the vibratory stimulus at threshold for eliciting the reflex in relaxed and contracted muscle is shown in relation to the subjects' ages in Figure 8.7C. The data in the three parts of Figure 8.7 support the conclusion that in the first 12 to 24 months after birth there is a rapid increase in threshold for eliciting the phasic stretch reflex, and that this process continues to the age of six years.

The shortest onset latency was determined from examination of at least 20 trials and is shown in relation to age in Figure 8.8A. The latency initially falls over the first year after birth and then progressively increases to adult values, which are reached between 13 and 15 years of age.

To investigate whether the stretch reflex might have monosynaptic linkage at birth, estimates of the central transmission delay were made in 175 subjects. The peripheral conduction delay in the motor nerve to biceps brachii was measured by

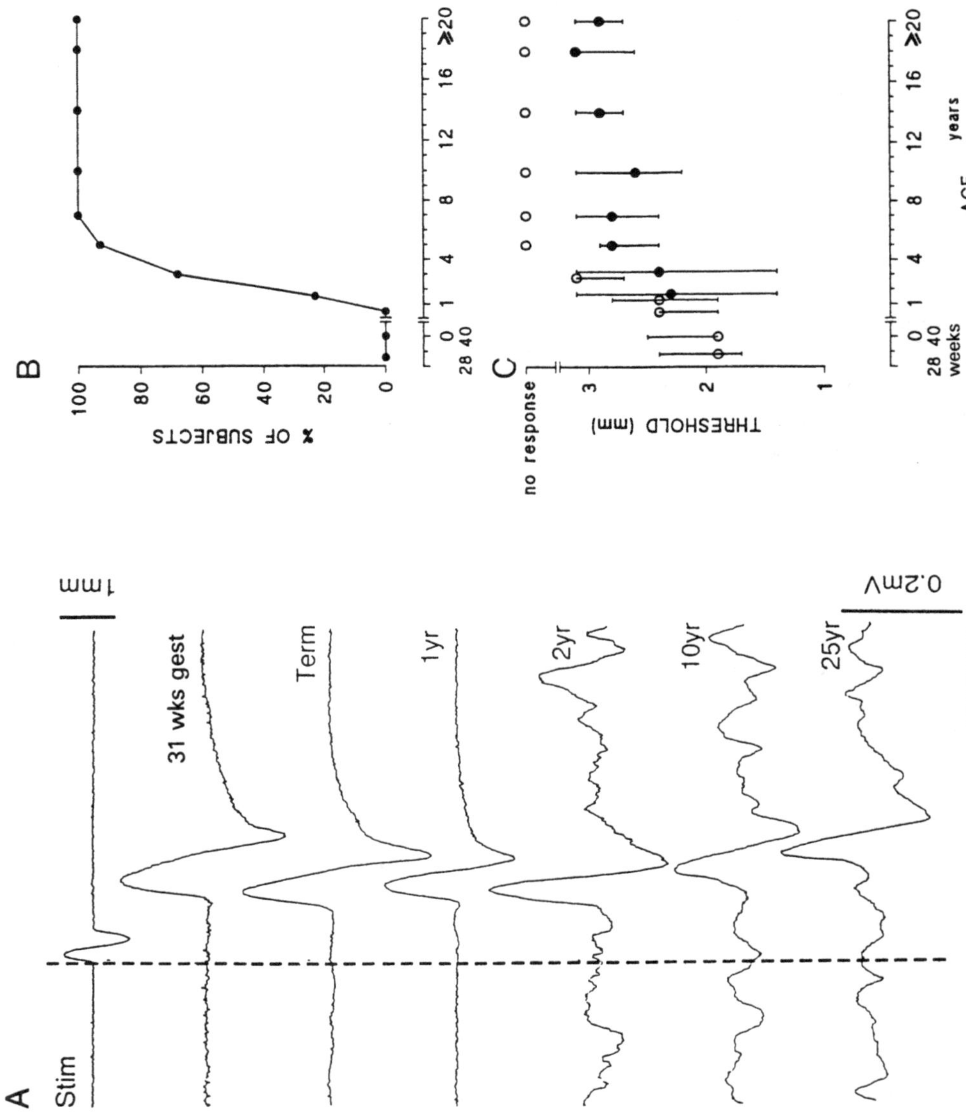

Fig. 8.7. *A*: phasic stretch reflexes in subjects of different ages: weeks gest, weeks of gestation; term, 40 weeks gestation. Dashed line indicates the onset of stimulation. *B*: percentage of subjects in which it was not possible to elicit the phasic stretch reflex in relaxed muscle. *C*: threshold of the phasic stretch reflex in biceps brachii with age. The threshold is expressed as the peak-to-peak amplitude of the vibratory stimulus (mm). The symbols represent the median values and the bars the 10th to 90th centile range. The open circles are recordings made in relaxed muscles and the filled circles in contracting muscle.

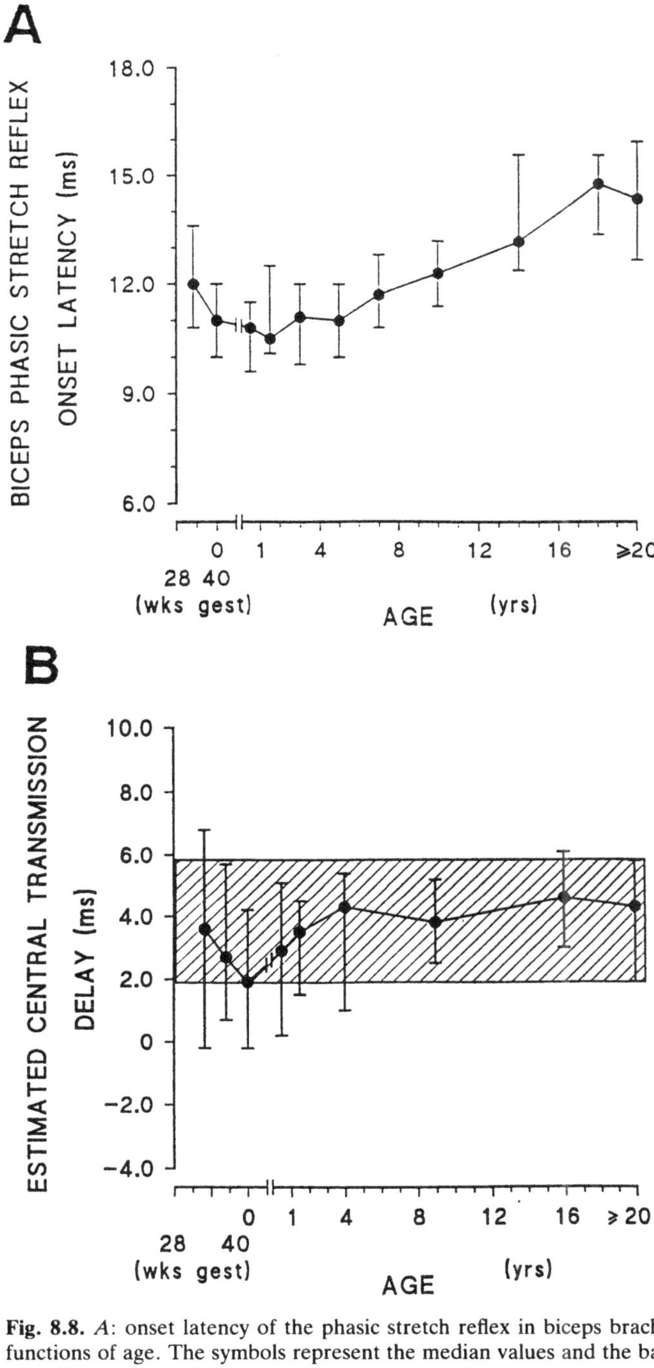

Fig. 8.8. *A*: onset latency of the phasic stretch reflex in biceps brachii. *B*: estimated central delay as functions of age. The symbols represent the median values and the bars the 10th to 90th centile range. The hatched area indicates the 10th to 90th centile range for adults.

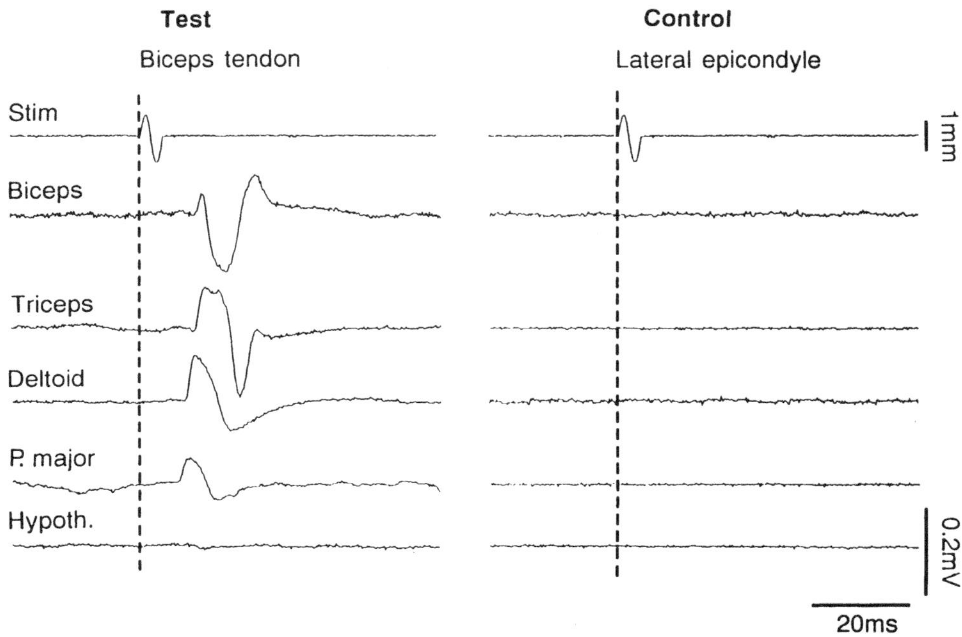

Fig. 8.9. Phasic stretch reflex in biceps brachii and radiated responses in other muscles in a neonate of 40 weeks gestation, evoked with the vibrator placed on the tendon of ipsilateral biceps brachii (left-hand panel). No muscle responses occurred in these muscles in the control when the same stimulus was applied to the lateral epicondyle at the elbow (right-hand panel). Dotted line indicates the onset of stimulation.

electromagnetic stimulation applied over the cervical spines. The delay in the afferent reflex arc to the intervertebral foramina was taken to be equal to the measured efferent delay, scaled according to the relative mean maximum conduction velocities for age in motor and sensory components of muscle nerves (Vecchierini-Blineau and Guiheneuc 1979).

The central transmission delay was estimated by subtracting the sum of the conduction delays in the efferent and afferent arcs, as defined above, from the minimum onset latency of the phasic stretch reflex. This delay will also include a period for conduction in motor and sensory roots within the vertebral canal, the synaptic delay and the period for the rising phase of the composite excitatory postsynaptic potential in the motor neurons. Figure 8.8B shows these estimated central transmission delays in relation to age. The delays at all ages, including the perinatal period, are similar to or shorter than those in adults, with the implication that the early component of the phasic stretch reflex is monosynaptic at all ages.

When a vibratory stimulus was applied to the tendon of biceps, a stretch reflex was recorded (as described above). In some subjects excitatory responses were also recorded in the EMGs of the ipsilateral triceps, deltoid, pectoralis major and hypothenar muscles, and these are referred to as radiated responses (Fig. 8.9). Figure 8.10 shows the percentage of subjects in whom such radiated responses were

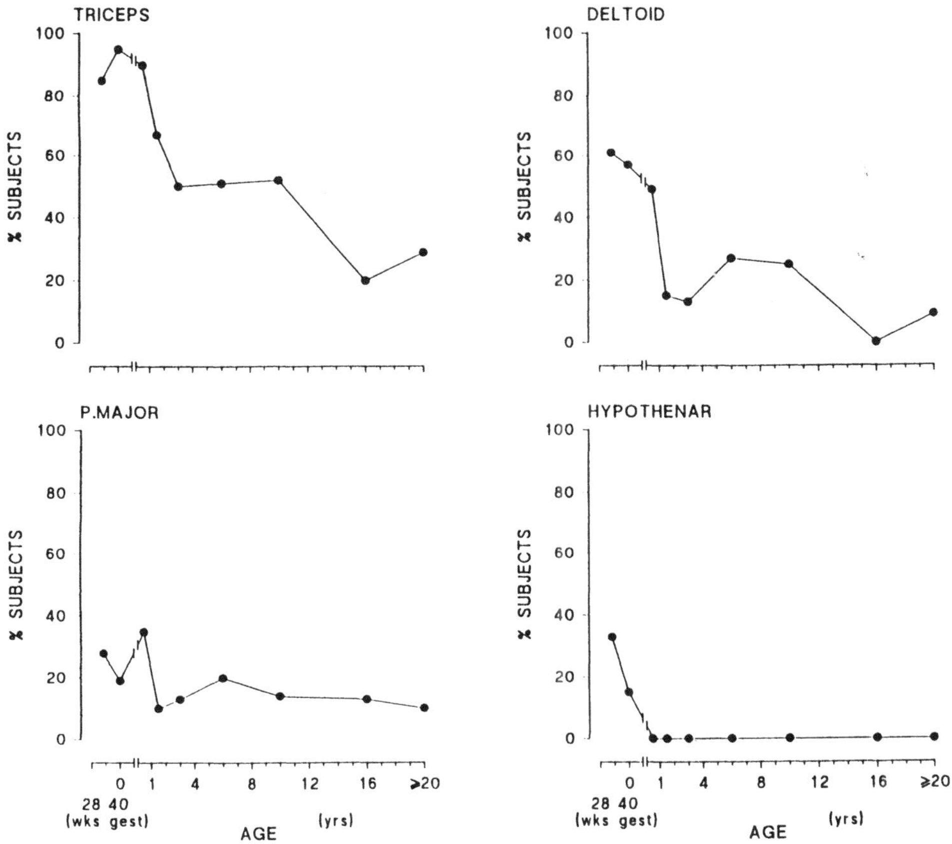

Fig. 8.10. Percentage of subjects showing radiated responses in relation to age. Radiated responses were considered to be present if the reflex ratio (see text) was equal to or greater than 0.1, since those of lesser magnitude were not significantly greater than background muscle activity. The numbers indicate the subjects in each age group. P.MAJOR = pectoralis major.

observed for each muscle studied. No contralateral radiated responses were observed in the muscles studied in the left limb when the same vibratory stimulus was applied to evoke a stretch reflex in the right biceps brachii.

In order to obtain estimates of the magnitudes of the ipsilateral radiated responses, the ratio was calculated of the area of the average of 20 radiated responses to the area of the average of 20 responses in biceps brachii. The relative magnitudes of the radiated responses in the muscles studied in relation to age are shown in Figure 8.11. Values of reflex ratio greater than 1 occurred in 41 subjects, all below the age of one year, indicating radiated responses which were larger than the stretch reflex in biceps brachii, with the standardised stimulus strengths used.

At all ages the probability and magnitude of a radiated response were highest in triceps brachii, followed by deltoid and pectoralis major. In the hypothenar muscles a small radiated response was recorded in only three subjects, all neonates.

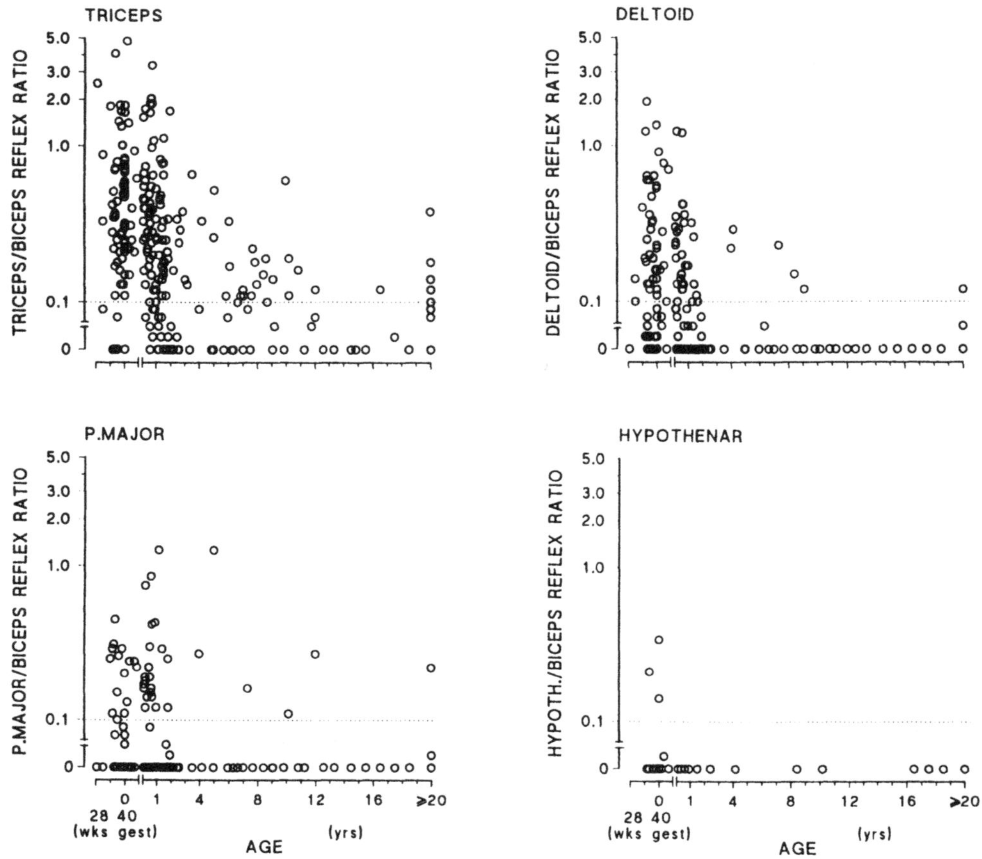

Fig. 8.11. Reflex ratios of radiated responses in different muscles in relation to the subjects' ages. The reflex ratio is given by the area of the average of 20 radiated responses divided by the area of the average of 20 phasic stretch reflexes in biceps brachii. The reflex ratio is plotted on a log scale. Reflex ratios of less than 0.1 indicate radiated responses not significantly greater than the background muscle activity. P.MAJOR = pectoralis major.

The probability and magnitude of a radiated response was greatest in the preterm and term neonates and decreased with age. For all the muscles, restriction of radiated responses was most marked within the first two postnatal years. In adults a small radiated response was observed in only five subjects in triceps, in one subject in deltoid and in one subject in pectoralis major (Figs 8.10, 11).

Where a radiated response occurred, the onset latency of the biceps stretch reflex was subtracted from the onset latency of the radiated response in each of the muscles. Figure 8.12 shows these differences in relation to age. In the newborn infant and up until the age of two years the differences for triceps brachii have a median of 0ms and an interquartile range of −0.4ms to +0.5ms, after which they increase to a median value of approximately 4ms in adults. For deltoid, in newborn babies and infants up to two years, the differences have a median of −0.3ms with

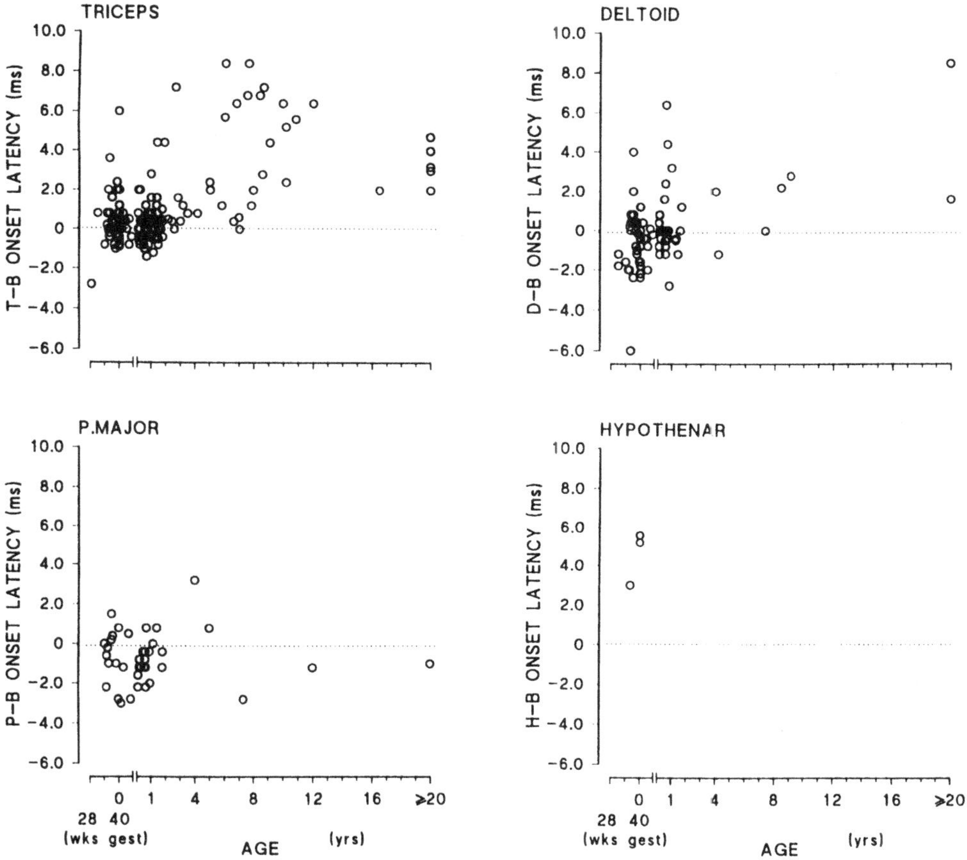

Fig. 8.12. Onset latencies of radiated responses in different muscles in relation to age. The onset latency of the phasic stretch reflex in each subject has been subtracted from the onset latency of each radiated response. P.MAJOR = pectoralis major.

an interquartile range of −1.2ms to +0.4ms. For pectoralis major up to two years of age, the median value is −1ms with an interquartile range of −1.2ms to −0.2ms. For both deltoid and pectoralis major there is no evident change in the relative latencies with age. In the three newborn babies in whom radiated responses were obtained in hypothenar muscles, differences of 3.0, 5.1 and 5.7ms were obtained.

Of the 149 subjects aged less than one month, 25 were studied awake, 58 in active sleep and 66 in quiet sleep. No significant differences were observed in the onset latency, amplitude and threshold of the biceps stretch reflex with the various states of arousal. There was no significant difference in the probability of radiated responses with the exception of that in deltoid, which occurred less frequently in the awake state than would be expected; nor were there significant differences in the amplitudes of the radiated responses with the different states of arousal.

Conclusion

This study has revealed a clear pattern for the development of the stretch reflex. In the newborn there is a low activation threshold, which increases rapidly in the postnatal period. In addition there is a high probability of radiation of excitation from biceps brachii afferents to the motor neurons of its antagonist, triceps brachii, and other muscles of the upper limb in early postnatal life, but this radiation becomes restricted with age.

Developmental studies in children using H-reflexes describe a similar pattern of development. Thomas and Lambert (1960) and Mayer and Mosser (1969) demonstrated H-reflexes to small muscles of the hand and foot in the neonate which cannot be evoked after the age of 12 months. However, attempts to quantify the change of threshold during development using H:M ratios (Mayer and Mosser, 1969, Vecchierini-Blineau and Guiheneuc 1981) have led to inconclusive results. The difficulties in these studies are likely to be due to the complex nature of the H-reflex stimulus (Burke *et al.* 1983) and to be compounded by the small numbers of subjects studied.

Postnatal changes in the responsiveness of primary muscle afferents are unlikely to be responsible for the increase in threshold of the phasic stretch reflex. Muscle spindles in cat and man are innervated at an early stage of fetal development and rapidly differentiate (Gregory and Proske 1988). In the cat, Skoglund (1960) demonstrated rapidly adapting responses to stretch at birth. Gregory and Proske (1988) noted increased sensitivity and firing rate of muscle spindle afferents to standard muscle stretch with increasing age, which would suggest the reverse of an increase of threshold. The increase in threshold of the phasic stretch reflex in human development is likely to reflect changes within the spinal cord of the size, input resistance and membrane properties of the alpha motor neurons and of the distribution, density and efficacy of the synapses they receive: processes which, on the basis of the present results, are most marked in the neonatal period but which are likely to continue to the age of six years.

In the neonate the magnitude of the radiated responses often exceeded those of the phasic stretch in biceps brachii (Fig. 8.11), which may indicate a powerful synaptic input to these non-homonymous and non-synergistic motor neurons early in development. On the evidence of timing in the present study it is likely that at least the initial component of the radiated responses in other muscles of the upper limb results from direct projections of muscle afferents from biceps brachii, which activate the relevant motor neurons monosynaptically. This conclusion is drawn from the observations that the radiated response in triceps brachii shares the same onset latency as biceps (Fig. 8.10), where the efferent arc is of approximately the same length, and that the radiated responses in deltoid and pectoralis major both occur earlier than that of biceps, corresponding to the shorter efferent arcs to these muscles relative to that of biceps.

A wide range of non-homonymous, monosynaptic muscle afferent projections have been reported in fetal, newborn and adult animals. In the kitten, Eccles *et al.*

(1963) reported monosynaptic connections between primary afferents and alpha motor neurons of non-homonymous or non-synergistic muscles, a small proportion of which persisted in the adult cat (Eccles *et al.* 1957*a*, *b*). In the fetal rat, Saito (1979) demonstrated monosynaptic projections from afferents in L_1 to L_6 dorsal roots to motor neurons of L_3 segment; while in the fetal sheep, Anggard *et al.* (1961) observed radiation of stretch reflexes from gastrocnemius to other muscles of the lower limb including direct antagonists. These observations also support the conclusion that the radiated responses arise from direct projections of biceps muscle afferents.

Reduction of radiation of primary afferents to non-homonymous or non-synergistic motor neurons has been observed in animal studies. The intersegmental radiation in the fetal rat (Saito 1979) became restricted so that at birth only the L_3 dorsal root could evoke responses in L_3 ventral root. Administration of strychnine restored the radiated responses in the postnatal period but failed to do so at later ages. Saito concluded that the early restriction of radiation arose in part from spinal inhibitory neuronal mechanisms, but that later the intersegmental projections providing the radiated responses had been eliminated. The observation that fewer monosynaptic projections to motor neurons from non-homonymous muscles are present in the adult can than in the kitten (Eccles *et al.* 1957*a*,*b*, 1963) supports the suggestion that monosynaptic non-homonymous afferent projections are eliminated during development.

Development of the phasic stretch reflex in children with cerebral palsy

To determine if there is an abnormal pattern of development of the stretch reflex in children with spastic cerebral palsy, a longitudinal study is currently being conducted in 63 children who were born preterm and are at risk of developing cerebral palsy (Eyre *et al.* 1991*b*). Fourteen children at 18 months have signs of developmental delay and spasticity involving all four limbs. These children all displayed an abnormal pattern of development of the stretch reflex, with a persisting low threshold for activation and a failure to show the normal pattern of progressive restriction in the radiation of the phasic stretch reflex to other muscles of the upper limb. The remaining 42 children, who were clinically normal at 18 months, have so far shown a normal pattern of development of the stretch reflex. The conclusion that there is an abnormal pattern of development of the phasic stretch reflex in children with spastic cerebral palsy is supported by the low threshold for activation of the stretch reflex and an increased probability for radiated responses observed in children and adults with spastic cerebral palsy (Myklebust *et al.* 1982, O'Sullivan 1991). While subjects with spasticity after brain damage sustained in adulthood show a decreased threshold for the stretch reflex, they do not have an increased probability of a radiated response (Myklebust *et al.* 1982). These observations support the conclusion that direct projections to homonymous motor neurons are withdrawn during the process of normal development, a process which may fail to take place in children with perinatal brain damage.

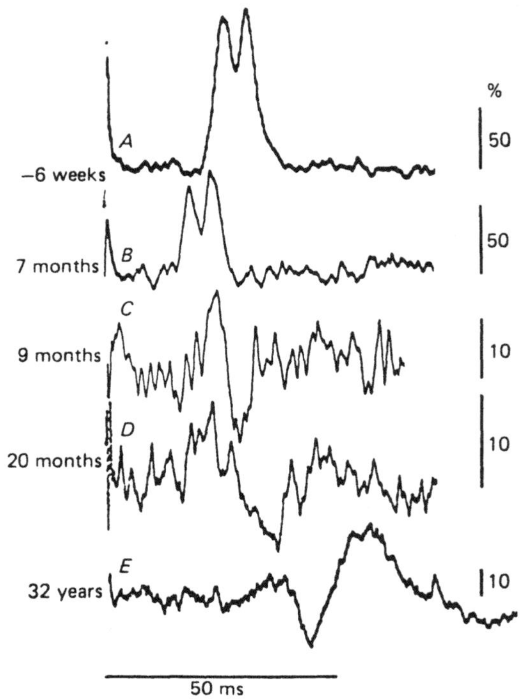

Fig. 8.13. Changes in cutaneous reflex EMG responses with age. *A* to *E*: average rectified reflex EMG recorded from forearm extensor muscles following single electrical stimuli delivered to the fingers. Vertical calibration: *A*, *B*: 50 per cent increase in amplitude of averaged rectified EMG signal; *C* to *E*: 10 per cent increase in amplitude. (Reproduced from Issler and Stephens 1983, by permission.)

Cutaneous reflexes

In adult human subjects, cutaneous reflexes can be evoked in muscles of the upper and lower limbs by electrical and mechanical stimuli (Meinck *et al.* 1983). Muscle contraction of 5 to 10 per cent of maximum voluntary contraction is required to provide a background level of activity in the EMG upon which the reflexes can be observed. The typical pattern of response is triphasic (Caccia *et al.* 1973, Garnett and Stephens 1980, Jenner and Stephens 1982, Issler and Stephens 1983, Meinck *et al.* 1983). An initial period of excitation, designated E_1, is followed by inhibition, I_1, and a further period of excitation, E_2 (Fig. 8.13, lowest trace). From recordings of the compound action potential evoked by electrical stimulation it has been established that fast conducting Group II cutaneous fibres are responsible for the reflexes (Caccia *et al.* 1973, Garnett and Stephens 1980). For the E_1 and I_1 components of the response, the central latencies have been estimated to be about 2 to 4ms, indicating oligosynaptic pathways in the spinal cord (Jenner and Stephens 1982). This synaptic linkage is comparable to short-latency excitation and inhibition of spinal motor neurons in the cat, evoked by stimulation of cutaneous nerves (Baldissera *et al.* 1981).

The local sign of these cutaneous reflexes differs in the upper and lower limbs. In the muscles of the forearm and hand, the triphasic response to light cutaneous stimulation is generally observed in flexors and extensors irrespective of functional agonist/antagonist muscle relationships (Meinck *et al.* 1983). In muscles of the lower limb the triphasic response (E_1, I_1, E_2) is observed in functional flexors (*e.g.* tibialis anterior), but the responses in physiological extensors (*e.g.* triceps surae) have a different pattern with initial short-latency inhibition followed by a later variable excitatory component. These differences probably underlie the greater reflex complexity involved in manipulatory movements of the hand and fingers.

The peak of the longer excitatory reflex component (E_2) occurs in adult human subjects approximately 40ms after the peak of the early excitatory response (E_1) (Jenner and Stephens 1982). Some authors have hypothesised that the E_2 component represents a fast reflex involving a pathway to and from the sensorimotor cortex. Jenner and Stephens (1982) and Evans *et al.* (1989) demonstrated that the latency of the E_2 component is compatible with the sum of the conduction delays in the dorsal column pathway to the cortex and in the corticospinal pathway to the spinal cord. Furthermore, the E_2 component of the reflex disappears and the E_1 component is exaggerated in subjects with lesions of the dorsal columns or of the corticospinal pathway (Choa and Stephens 1982, Jenner and Stephens 1982). The hypothesis is attractive, particularly as the E_2 component is prominent when relatively independent finger movements are attempted (Evans *et al.* 1989).

Cutaneous reflexes recorded in babies and children

Electrical stimulation can evoke cutaneous reflexes in the upper and lower limbs of babies and children, and the methods described below are taken from their papers (Issler and Stephens 1983, Rowlandson and Stephens 1985*a*).

Methods

The surface EMG was recorded in the upper limb using pairs of disk electrodes (Type 650466, Beckman RIIC Ltd) with 15mm centre to centre spacing. One electrode pair was placed over the superficial extensor group of muscles of forearm just distal to the lateral epicondyle of the humerus. Another electrode pair was placed over the superficial flexor muscles just proximal to the wrist. In the lower limb the surface EMG of tibialis anterior was recorded using bipolar electrodes consisting of two Ag/AgCl strips (7 × 20mm), 20mm apart, making skin contact through felt pads soaked in saline (Type EL2210M, Medelec Ltd). The electrodes were strapped to the skin adjacent to the tibial crest and over the belly of the muscle at the junction of its proximal third and distal two thirds. Issler and Stephens (1983) commented that the reflex responses are best visualised by rectification of the EMG and signal averaging.

Ring electrodes (Type E/D S-K, Medelec Ltd) were attached to fingers or toes for digital nerve stimulation. For the fingers, one electrode was placed around the

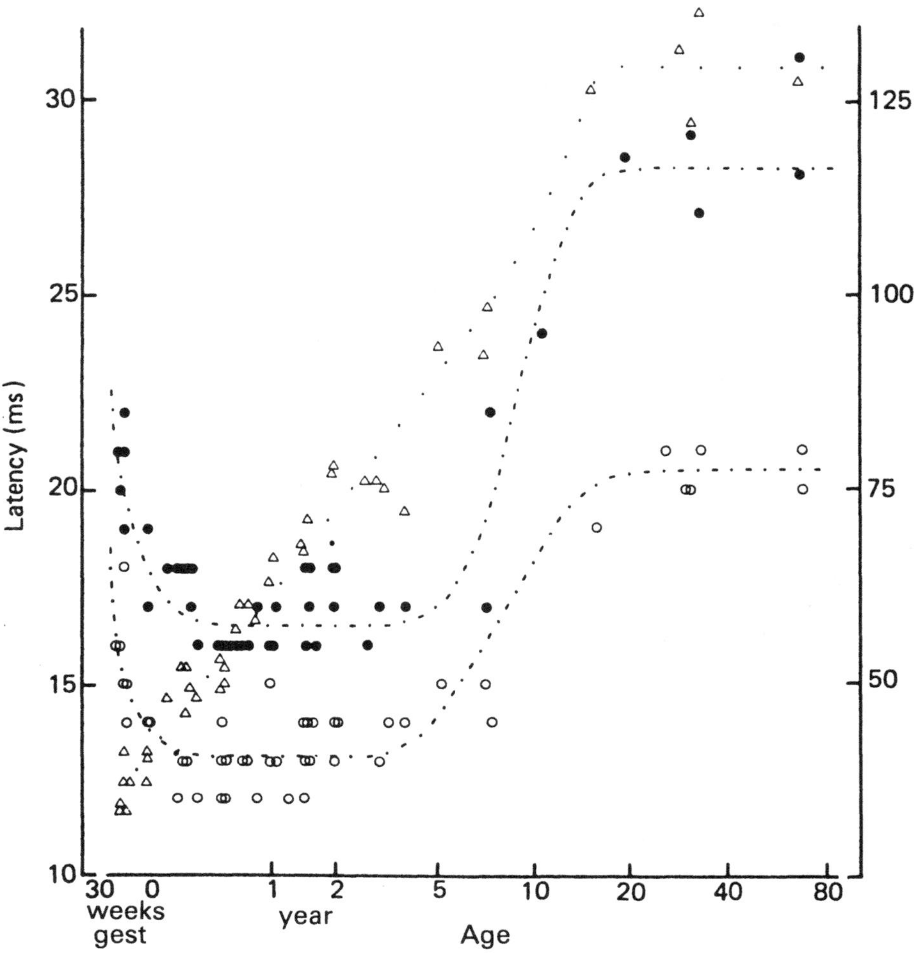

Fig. 8.14. Changes in latency of reflex responses with age. Filled circles, latency of first component of cutaneous reflex in forearm muscles following stimulation of the fingers; open circles, latency of tendon jerk; open triangles, axonal conduction distance for cutaneous reflex measuring from fingers to spinous process C7 and from C7 to middle of forearm. (Reproduced from Issler and Stephens 1983, by permission.)

base of the index finger and the other around the base of the ring finger, the electrode on the ring finger acting as cathode. For the toes, one electrode was placed around the second toe and the other around the fourth toe. A constant current stimulator provided pulses of 100μs duration at 3 pulses/s. For the fingers the current was set at 10mA and for the toes at 10 to 15mA. In adult subjects these stimulus intensities correspond to approximately twice the perceptual threshold and they are not painful. In babies these stimuli generally pass unnoticed.

Muscle contraction was required as a background for recording the reflexes.

Muscle activity in the forearm was obtained by manipulative tasks such as building a tower or holding a biscuit, as appropriate for the age of the child. Muscle activity in tibialis anterior was obtained by manipulation of the foot and in getting the subject to stand.

In infants aged six weeks or under, recordings were made within one hour of the next feed and when the subject was awake (behavioural states 3 and 4 of Prechtl and Beintema 1964).

Development of cutaneous reflexes

The cutaneous reflex can be readily excited in the normal neonate and consists entirely of a single brief wave of increased muscle activity (Fig. 8.13) (Issler and Stephens 1983, Rowlandson and Stephens 1985*a*). The latencies of the responses were high in the preterm infant and followed a plateau to approximately five years when they increased to reach adult values at 10 to 20 years (Fig. 8.14). The central latency of this neonatal reflex is about 3ms and corresponds to the latency of E_1 of the adult cutaneous reflex (Issler and Stephens 1983). This single excitatory component of the neonatal reflex has also been designated E_1. Between 18 months and two years of postnatal life a second excitatory wave (E_2) appears in the reflex, separated from E_1 by a variable inhibitory phase. During subsequent development the E_2 component gradually increases, becoming equal in amplitude to E_1 at four to eight years. The E_1 component progressively diminishes in amplitude, leaving at the age of 12 to 16 years the larger and dominant E_2 component (Issler and Stephens 1983, Rowlandson and Stephens 1985*a*, Evans *et al.* 1990).

In adults the E_2 component of the cutaneous reflex was particularly marked when elicited during the performance of tasks involving relatively independent finger movements. The question was then whether the appearance of the E_2 component, involving a postulated cortical reflex loop, might be associated with the development of manipulative skills. Evans *et al.* (1990) studied the cutaneous reflex in the first dorsal interosseous muscle in 127 children aged between three and 18 years. At all ages the E_2 component was significantly smaller in reflexes elicited during a power grip of the hand than during the relatively independent finger movement of abduction of the index finger. Despite these observations, however, no clear relationship was noted between the magnitude of the E_2 component and the ability to produce rapid finger movements.

Cutaneous reflexes in children with central nervous disorders

Cutaneous reflexes in the first dorsal interosseous muscle were recorded in 21 children with cerebral palsy, aged four to 17 years (Evans *et al.* 1991). The E_1 response was not abnormally large, as had been observed in adults with signs of corticospinal damage, and did not become exaggerated in the whole hand grip (Choa and Stephens 1982, Jenner and Stephens 1982). In some children the E_2 component was comparable in its occurrence and magnitude to that of normal children of an appropriate age. These were unexpected findings, and Evans *et al.*

(1991) argued that even though manual dexterity is impaired in these subjects with cerebral palsy, some plasticity in descending pathways may have taken place during motor development which does not occur in subjects suffering brain damage in adulthood. The authors advanced some evidence for this idea from animal experiments and from other human studies (Farmer *et al.* 1990). We need further neurophysiological and behavioural studies of motor development in cerebral-palsied children, particularly in the period from birth to two years, when the neural substrate for sensorimotor control is undergoing marked reorganisation and development (see above and Chapter 1).

Cutaneous reflexes have also been examined in a small sample of children aged five to 15 years with various neurological disorders (N 8) or learning difficulties (N 15) (Rowlandson and Stephens 1985*b*). In cases with involvement of the motor cortex the E_1 response tends to be exaggerated. Where severe disease of the spinal cord occurs, the reflex responses were observed at abnormally prolonged latency. In some cases with minimal cerebral dysfunction the normal E_2 response may be absent or replaced by a longer-latency excitatory response. Finally, the authors suggest that an abnormally absent or delayed E_2 response in the group with learning difficulties would be consistent with the hypothesis that the cortical control of spinal cutaneous reflexes is impaired. Further prospective longitudinal studies are required.

Conclusion

Cutaneous reflexes to muscles of the upper and lower limbs undergo marked maturation in the neonatal period. Like corticospinal transmission and the stretch reflex, this maturation continues into adolescence. Assessment of cutaneous reflexes during the first two postnatal years may provide measures of the development of normal or abnormal sensorimotor control at the spinal level and in the cerebral cortex.

ACKNOWLEDGEMENTS

We acknowledge with gratitude our collaborators whose work contributed to parts of this review: K. Anderson, S.A. Edgley, M. Gibson, T.H.H.G. Koh, M.C. O'Sullivan, R.N. Lemon, R.D. Plant, V. Ramesh and C. Watts. The studies on the corticospinal pathway and the phasic stretch reflex were supported by the Medical Research Council, Wellcome Trust and Spastics Society.

REFERENCES

Amassian, V.E., Quirk, G.J., Stewart, M. (1987) 'Magnetic coil versus electrical stimulation of monkey motor cortex.' *Journal of Physiology*, **394**, 119P.

Anders, T.F., Emde, R., Parmelee, A.H. (1971) *A Manual of Standardised Terminology Techniques and Criteria for Scoring of States of Sleep and Wakefulness in Newborn Infants.* UCLA Brain Information Service BRI Publications Office: LA California NNDS Neurological Information Network.

Anggard, L., Bergstrom, R., Bernhard, C.G. (1961) 'Analysis of prenatal spinal reflex activity in sheep.' *Acta Physiologica Scandinavica*, **53**, 128–136.

d'Arsonval, A. (1896) 'Dispositifs pour la mesure des courants alternatifs de toutes fréquences.' *Communications of the Royal Society of Biology*, **3**, 450–457.

Baldissera, F., Hultborn, H, Illert, M. (1981) 'Integration in spinal neuronal systems.' *In* Brookhart, J.M., Mountcastle, V.B., Brooks, V.B., Geiger, S.R. (Eds) *Hand Book of Physiology VII, Section 1: The Nervous System Motor Control. Part 1.* Maryland: American Physiological Society.

Barker, A.T., Jalinous, R, Freeston, I.L. (1985) 'Non invasive magnetic stimulation of the human motor cortex,' *Lancet*, **1**, 1106–1107.

—— Freeston, I.L., Jalinous, R., Jarratt, J.A. (1987) 'Magnetic stimulation of the human brain and peripheral nervous system: an introduction and the results of an initial clinical evaluation.' *Neurosurgery*, **20**, 100–109.

Berardelli, A., Inghilleri, M., Manfredi, M., Zamponi, A., Cecconi, V., Dolce, G. (1987) 'Cortical and cervical stimulation after hemisphere infarction.' *Journal of Neurology, Neurosurgery and Psychiatry*, **49**, 251–257.

Bernstein, N. (1967) *The Co-ordination and Regulation of Movements.* Oxford: Pergamon.

Bickford, R.G., Fremming, B.D. (1965) 'Neuronal stimulation by pulsed magnetic fields in animals and man.' *Digest of the 6th International Conference of Medical Electronics and Biological Engineering.* p. 112.

Bodian, D. (1966) 'Development of fine structure of spinal cord in monkey fetuses.' *Bulletin of the Johns Hopkins Hospital*, **119**, 129–149.

Burke, D., Gandevia, S.C., McKeon, B. (1983) 'The afferent volleys responsible for spinal proprioceptive reflexes in man.' *Journal of Physiology*, **339**, 535–552.

—— Hicks, R.G., Stephen, J.P.H. (1990) 'Corticospinal volleys evoked by anodal and cathodal stimulation of the human motor cortex.' *Journal of Physiology*, **425**, 283–300.

Caccia, M.R., McComas, A.J., Upton, A.R.M., Blogg, T. (1973) 'Cutaneous reflexes in small muscles of the hand.' *Journal of Neurology, Neurosurgery and Psychiatry*, **36**, 960–977.

Choa, B.H.G., Stephens, J.A. (1982) 'Cutaneous reflex responses and central nervous lesions studied in the lower limb in man.' *Journal of Physiology*, **328**, 23–24P.

Conradi, S. (1976) 'Functional anatomy of the anterior horn motor neuron.' *In* Landon, D.N. (Ed.) *The Peripheral Nerve.* London: Chapman & Hall. pp. 279–329.

Day, B.L., Marsden, C.D., Obeso, J.A., Rothwell, J.C. (1984) 'Reciprocal inhibition between the muscles of the human forearm.' *Journal of Physiology*, **349**, 519–534.

—— Dressler, D., Maertens de Noordhout, A., Marsden, C.D., Nakashima, K., Rothwell, J.C., Thompson, P.D. (1989) 'Electrical and magnetic stimulation of human motor cortex: surface EMG and single motor unit responses.' *Journal of Physiology*, **412**, 449–473.

Eccles, J.C., Eccles, R.M., Lundberg, A. (1957*a*) 'Synaptic actions on motoneurones in relation to the two components of the group 1 muscle afferent volley.' *Journal of Physiology*, **136**, 527–546.

—— —— —— (1957*b*) 'The convergence of monosynaptic excitatory afferents onto many different species of alpha motoneurones.' *Journal of Physiology*, **137**, 22–50.

—— Shealy, C.N., Willis, W.D. (1963) 'Patterns of innervation of kitten motoneurones.' *Journal of Physiology*, **165**, 392–402.

Edgley, S.A., Eyre, J.A., Lemon, R.N., Miller, S. (1989) 'Direct activation of corticospinal neurones by electromagnetic stimulation in anaesthetised and conscious monkeys.' *Journal of Physiology*, **414**, 8P.

—— —— —— —— (1990*a*) 'At what level is the corticospinal pathway excited by electromagnetic and percutaneous stimulation of the brain? Evidence from the anaesthetised Macaque monkey.' *Journal of Physiology*, **420**, 47P.

—— —— —— —— (1990*b*) 'Excitation of the corticospinal tract by electromagnetic and electrical stimulation of the scalp in the Macaque monkey.' *Journal of Physiology*, **425**, 301–320.

—— —— —— —— (1992) 'Direct and indirect activation of corticospinal neurones by electrical and magnetic stimulation in anaesthetised Macaque monkey.' *Journal of Physiology, in press.*

Evans, A.L., Harrison, L.M., Stephens, J.A. (1989) 'Task dependent changes in cutaneous reflexes recorded from various muscles controlling finger movement in man.' *Journal of Physiology*, **418**, 1–12.

—— —— —— (1990) 'Maturation of the cutaneomuscular reflex recorded from the first dorsal interosseous muscle in man.' *Journal of Physiology*, **428**, 425–440.

——— ——— ——— (1991) 'Cutaneomuscular reflexes recorded from the first dorsal interosseous muscle of children with cerebral palsy.' *Developmental Medicine and Child Neurology*, **33**, 541–551.

Eyre, J.A., Gibson, M., Koh, T.H.H.G., Miller, S., O'Sullivan, M.C., Ramesh, V. (1989) 'Corticospinal transmission excited by electromagnetic stimulation of the brain is impaired in children with spastic hemiparesis but not in those with quadriparesis.' *Journal of Physiology*, **414**, 9P.

—— Flecknell, P.A., Kenyon, B.R., Koh, T.H.H.G., Miller, S. (1990) 'Effects of electromagnetic stimulation of the brain on cortical activity, cortical blood flow, blood pressure and heart rate in the cat: an evaluation of safety.' *Journal of Neurology, Neurosurgery and Psychiatry*, **53**, 507–514.

—— Miller, S., Ramesh, V. (1991*a*) 'Constancy of central conduction delays during development in man: investigation of motor and somatosensory pathways.' *Journal of Physiology*, **434**, 441–452.

—— —— O'Sullivan, M.C., Ramesh, V., Watts, C. (1991*b*) 'The development of corticospinal tract function in normal children and its pathophysiology in those with cerebral palsy.' *Journal of Physiology*, **438**, 32P.

Farmer, S.F., Harrison, L.M., Ingram, D.A., Stephens, J.A. (1990) 'Evidence for plasticity of central motor pathways in children with hemiplegic cerebral palsy.' *Journal of Physiology*, **429**, 40P.

Garnett, R., Stephens, J.A. (1980) 'The reflex responses of single motor units in human first dorsal interosseous muscles following cutaneous afferent stimulation.' *Journal of Physiology*, **303**, 351–364.

Goddard, G.V., McIntyre, D.C., Leech, C.K. (1969) 'A permanent change in brain function resulting from daily electrical stimulation.' *Experimental Neurology*, **25**, 295–330.

Gregory, J.E., Proske, U. (1988) 'Development of proprioception.' *In* Meisami, E., Timiras, P.S. (Eds) *Handbook of Human Growth and Developmental Biology, Vol. 1, Part B.* Florida: CRC Press. pp. 95–101.

Gualterotti, T., Patterson, A.S. (1954) 'Electrical stimulation of the unexposed cerebral cortex.' *Neurosurgery*, **20**, 195–197.

Gutrecht, J.A., Dyck, P.J. (1970) 'Quantitative teased fibre and histological studies of human sural nerve during postnatal development.' *Journal of Comparative Neurology*, **138**, 117–130.

Hess, C.W., Mills, K.R., Murray, N.M.F. (1987) 'Responses in small hand muscles from magnetic stimulation of the human brain.' *Journal of Physiology*, **388**, 397–419.

Hildreth, E.C., Hollerbach, J.M. (1987) 'Artificial intelligence: computational approach to vision and motor control.' *In* Mountcastle, V.B., Plum, F., Geiger, S.R. (Eds) *Handbook of Physiology, Vol. 5.* Bethesda: American Physiological Society. pp. 605–643.

Homberg, V., Netz, J. (1989) 'Generalised seizures induced by transcranial magnetic stimulation of motor cortex.' *Lancet*, **2**, 1223.

Hongo, T., Lundberg, A., Phillips, C.G., Thompson, R.F. (1984) 'The pattern of monosynaptic 1a-connections to hindlimb motor nuclei in the baboon: a comparison with the cat.' *Proceedings of the Royal Society of London*, **221**, 261–289.

Hultborn, H. (1972) 'Convergence on interneurones in the reciprocal 1a inhibitory pathway to motoneurones.' *Acta Physiologica Scandinavica* (Suppl. 375), 1–42.

Ingram, D.A., Thompson, A.J., Swash, M. (1988) 'Central motor conduction in multiple sclerosis: evaluation of abnormalities revealed by transcutaneous magnetic stimulation of the brain.' *Journal of Neurology, Neurosurgery and Psychiatry*, **51**, 487–494.

Innocenti, G.M. (1981) 'Growth and reshaping of axons in establishment of visual callosal connections.' *Science*, **212**, 824–831.

Issler, H., Stephens, J.A. (1983) 'The maturation of cutaneous reflexes studied in the upper limb in man.' *Journal of Physiology*, **335**, 643–654.

Ivy, G.O., Yould, H.J., Killackery, H.P. (1984) 'Variability in the distribution of callosal projections in adult parietal cortex.' *Brain Research*, **306**, 53–61.

Jenner, J.R., Stephens, J.A. (1982) 'Cutaneous reflex responses and their central pathways studied in man.' *Journal of Physiology*, **333**, 405–419.

Kimura, J. (1974) 'F-wave velocity in the central segment of the median and ulnar nerves: a study in normal subjects and in patients with Charcot-Marie-Tooth disease.' *Neurology*, **24**, 539–546.

Koh, T.H.H.G., Eyre, J.A. (1988) 'Maturation of the corticospinal tract from birth to adulthood measured by electromagnetic stimulation of the motor cortex.' *Archives of Disease in Childhood*,

63, 1347–1352.

Lawrence, D.G., Hopkins, D.A. (1976) 'The development of motor control in the Rhesus monkey: evidence concerning the role of cortico-motoneuronal connections.' *Brain*, **99**, 235–254.

Lundberg, A. (1975) 'The control of spinal mechanisms from the brain.' *In* Tower, D.B. (Ed.) *The Nervous System, Vol. 1.* New York: Raven Press. pp. 253–265.

—— (1979) 'Multisensory control of spinal reflex pathways.' *Progress in Brain Research*, **50**, 11–28.

—— (1982) 'Inhibitory control from the brain stem of transmission from primary afferents to motoneurons, primary afferent terminals and ascending pathways.' *In* Sjolund, B., Bjorklund, A. (Eds) *Brain Stem Control of Spinal Mechanisms.* Amsterdam: Elsevier Biomedical. pp. 179–224.

—— Voorhoeve, P. (1962) 'Effects from the pyramidal tract on spinal reflex arcs.' *Acta Physiologica Scandinavica*, **56**, 201–219.

Marin-Padilla, M. (1988) 'Early ontogenesis of the human cerebral cortex.' *In* Peters, A., Jones, E.G. (Eds) *Cerebral Cortex, Vol. 7. Development and Maturation of Cerebral Cortex.* New York: Plenum Press. pp. 1–30.

Mayer, R.F., Mosser, R.S. (1969) 'Excitability of motoneurones in infants.' *Neurology*, **19**, 932–945.

Meinck, H.M., Benecke, R., Kuster, S., Conrad, B. (1983) 'Cutaneomuscular (flexor) reflex organisation in normal man and in patients with motor disorders.' *In* Desmedt, J.E. (Ed.) *Motor Control Mechanisms in Health and Disease.* New York: Raven Press. pp. 787–796.

Merton, P.A., Morton, H.B. (1980) 'Stimulation of the cerebral cortex in the intact subject.' *Nature*, **285**, 227.

—— —— Hill, D.K., Marsden, C.D. (1982) 'Scope of a technique for electrical stimulation of human brain, spinal cord and muscle.' *Lancet*, **2**, 596–600.

Miller, M.W. (1988) 'Development of projection and local circuit neurons in neocortex.' *In* Peters, A., Jones, E.G. (Eds) *Cerebral Cortex, Vol. 7. Development and Maturation of Cerebral Cortex.* New York: Plenum Press. pp. 133–166.

Miller, S., Oscarsson, O. (1969) 'Termination and functional organization of spino-olivocerebellar paths.' *In* Fields, W.S., Willis, W.D. (Eds) *The Cerebellum in Health and Disease.* St Louis: W.H. Green. pp. 172–200.

Mills, K.R., Murray, N.M.F., Hess, C.W. (1987) 'Magnetic and electrical transcranial brain stimulation: physiological mechanisms and clinical applications.' *Neurosurgery*, **20**, 164–168.

Myklebust, B.M. (1990) 'A review of myotatic reflexes and the development of motor control and gait in infants and children: a special communication.' *Physical Therapy*, **70**, 188–203.

—— Gottlieb, G.L., Penn, R.D., Agarwal, G.C. (1982) 'Reciprocal excitation of antagonist muscles as a differentiating feature in spasticity.' *Annals of Neurology*, **12**, 367–374.

—— —— Agarwal, G.C. (1986) 'Stretch reflexes of the normal infant.' *Developmental Medicine and Child Neurology*, **28**, 440–449.

Nathan, P.W., Smith, M.C. (1955) 'Long descending tracts in man. 1. Review of present knowledge.' *Brain*, **78**, 249–303.

Neilson, P.D., Neilson, M.D., O'Dwyer, N.J. (1988) 'Internal models and intermittency: a theoretical account of human tracking behaviour.' *Biological Cybernetics*, **58**, 101–112.

Oscarsson, O. (1973) 'Functional organization of spino-cerebellar paths.' *In* Iggo, A. (Ed.) *Handbook of Sensory Physiology. Vol. 2.* Berlin: Springer. pp. 339–380.

O'Sullivan, M.C. (1991) 'The development of the phasic stretch reflex in man and its pathophysiology in central motor disorders.' University of Newcastle upon Tyne: PhD Thesis.

—— Eyre, J.A., Miller, S. (1991) 'Radiation of phasic stretch reflex in biceps brachii to muscles of the arm in man and its restriction during development.' *Journal of Physiology*, **439**, 529–543.

Plant, R.D., Miller, S. (1990) 'Short latency inhibitory reflexes in shoulder and trunk muscles in spastic hemiplegia following stroke.' *In* Beradelli, A., Benecke, R., Manfredi, M., Marsden, C.D. (Eds) *Motor Disturbances II.* London: Academic Press. pp. 367–377.

Plassman, B.L., Gandevia, S.C. (1989) 'High voltage stimulation over the spinal cord: sources of latency variation.' *Journal of Neurology, Neurosurgery and Psychiatry*, **52**, 213–217.

Polson, M.J.R., Barker, A.T., Freeston, L. (1982) 'Stimulation of nerve trunks with time varying magnetic fields.' *Medical and Biological Engineering and Computing*, **20**, 243–244.

Prechtl, N.R.F., Beintema, D. (1964) *The Neurological Examination of the Full Term Newborn Infant. Clinics in Developmental Medicine, No. 12.* London: SIMP with Heinemann Medical.

Rakic, P., Bourgeois, J.P., Eckenhoff, M.F., Zecevic, N., Goldman Rakic, P. (1986) 'Concurrent over-

production of synapses in diverse regions of the primate cerebral cortex.' *Science*, **232**, 232–235.
Rexed, B. (1944) 'Contributions to the knowledge of the postnatal development of the peripheral nervous system in man.' *Acta Psychiatrica et Neurologica* (Suppl. 33), 1–205.
Rossini, P.M., Caramia, M.D., Zarola, F. (1987) 'Mechanisms of nervous propagation along central motor pathways: non-invasive evaluation in healthy subjects and in patients with neurological disease.' *Neurosurgery*, **20**, 183–191.
Rothwell, J.C., Day, B.L., Thompson, P.D., Dick, J.P.R., Marsden, C.D. (1987*a*) 'Some experiences of techniques for stimulation of the human cerebral motor cortex through the scalp.' *Neurosurgery*, **20**, 156–163.
—— Thompson, P.D., Day, B.L., Dick, J.P.R., Kachi, T., Cowan, J.M.A., Marsden, C.D. (1987*b*) 'Motor cortex stimulation in intact man. I. General characteristics of EMG responses in different muscles.' *Brain*, **110**, 1173–1190.
Rowlandson, P.H., Stephens, J.A. (1985*a*) 'Maturation of cutaneous reflex responses recorded in the lower limb in man.' *Developmental Medicine and Child Neurology*, **27**, 425–433.
—— —— (1985*b*) 'Cutaneous reflex responses recorded in children with various neurological disorders.' *Developmental Medicine and Child Neurology*, **27**, 434–447.
Sakamoto, T., Arissian, K., Asanuma, H. (1989) 'Functional role of the sensory cortex in learning skills in the cat.' *Brain Research*, **503**, 258–264.
Saito, K. (1979) 'Development of spinal reflexes in the rat fetus studied in vitro.' *Journal of Physiology*, **294**, 581–594.
Skoglund, S. (1960) 'The activity of muscle receptors in the kitten.' *Acta Physiologica Scandinavia*, **50**, 203–221.
Stelmach, G.E. (1976) *Motor Control Issues and Trends*. New York: Academic Press.
Tanaka, R. (1974) 'Reciprocal inhibition during voluntary movements in man.' *Experimental Brain Research*, **21**, 529–540.
Thomas, J.E., Lambert, E.H. (1960) 'Ulnar nerve conduction velocity and H-reflex in infants and children.' *Journal of Applied Physiology*, **15**, 1–9.
Thompson, S.P. (1910) 'A physiological effect of an alternating magnetic field.' *Proceedings of the Royal Society*, **82**, 396–398.
Ugawa, Y., Rothwell, J.C., Day, B.L., Thompson, P.D., Marsden, C.D. (1989) 'Magnetic stimulation over the spinal enlargements.' *Journal of Neurology, Neurosurgery and Psychiatry*, **52**, 1025–1032.
Vecchierini-Blineau, M.F., Guiheneuc, P. (1979) 'Electrophysiological study of the peripheral nervous system in children. Changes in proximal and distal conduction velocities from birth to age five years.' *Journal of Neurology, Neurosurgery and Psychiatry*, **42**, 753–759.
—— —— (1981) 'Excitability of the monosynaptic reflex pathway in the child from birth to four years of age.' *Journal of Neurology, Neurosurgery and Psychiatry*, **44**, 309–314.
Yakovlev, P.I., Lecours, A.R. (1967) 'Myelogenetic cycles of regional maturation of the brain.' *In* Minkowski, A. (Ed.) *Regional Development of the Brain in Early Life*. Oxford: Blackwell. pp. 3–70.

9
NERVE CONDUCTION

Josette Khater-Boidin and Bernard Duron

Measurement of nerve fibre conduction velocities is fundamental to the assessment of postnatal maturation of the peripheral nervous system. Moreover, motor and sensory conduction velocities provide an objective method of diagnosing neuromuscular diseases in the early stages of life. It is therefore essential to know the range of normal values for each age-range, not only for the various categories of nerve fibres but also for each nerve. Following the initial study by Thomas and Lambert (1960), many further studies of the motor fibres of preterm and term newborn babies have been published (Cerra and Johnson 1962, Gamstorp 1963, Raimbault and Laget 1963, Dunn *et al.* 1964, Ruppert *et al.* 1967, Blom and Finnström 1968, Dubowitz *et al.* 1968, Radtke 1969, Wagner and Buchthal 1972, Cruz-Martinez *et al.* 1977, Duron *et al.* 1977, Vecchierini-Blineau and Guiheneuc 1979). Nevertheless, except for the report of Wagner and Buchthal, which collated the results of several authors, generally these studies are concerned with only one or two nerves. There is little information in the literature on 1_A proprioceptive and non-nociceptive cutaneous fibres.

The aim of this chapter is to review data concerning conduction velocities in motor, 1_A proprioceptive and non-nociceptive cutaneous fibres of both upper and lower limbs between 28 and 42 weeks post-conceptional age (PCA). Most of these data derive from our own studies of 145 term and 77 preterm infants with no apparent disease of the nervous system (Khater-Boidin *et al.* 1988, Khater-Boidin and Duron 1989). The conduction velocities of the motor fibres and afferent 1_A fibres of the ulnar, median, tibial and peroneal nerves were studied, as well as those of the non-nociceptive cutaneous fibres of the ulnar, median and sural nerves.

Methods to determine nerve conduction

The conventional method for measuring motor fibre conduction velocities involves stimulating the motor nerve successively at two points along its course and recording an evoked potential from the muscle it supplies. Subtraction of the shorter from the longer latency gives the conduction time along a segment of the nerve. If the length of the nerve between the two points of stimulation is measured, the conduction velocity can be calculated by dividing it by the conduction time. The main difficulty in infants is determining the exact distance between the two points of stimulation: an error of a few millimetres in this measurement can lead to significant variation in the calculation of conduction velocity.

Proprioceptive 1_A fibre conduction velocity is measured using the monosynaptic Hoffmann reflex. As previously described by Thomas and Lambert (1960), in term and preterm newborn infants weak stimuli are able to excite sensory but not motor fibres to elicit an 'H' reflex response in small hand or foot muscles. Thus if one stimulates the nerve with appropriate intensity successively at two different points (the same points as in the motor fibre conduction velocity study), the conduction velocity of 1_A fibres can be calculated by dividing the distance between the two points of stimulation by the latency difference between the two 'H' reflex responses.

For non-nociceptive fibre conduction, the digital nerves may be stimulated in the upper limbs by means of rings taped to the fingers in order to record orthodromic sensory potentials from two proximal sites on the course of the nerve. In lower limbs, nerve sensory potentials are recorded after stimulating cutaneous nerve branches by means of bipolar electrodes taped to the skin.

Stimulation

Stimulation of the motor nerve fibres and of the proprioceptive 1_A fibres is conducted using bipolar surface electrodes (*e.g.* DISA 13 L25), the poles set about 1cm apart. The electrodes are held on the stimulation points by the investigator during the short time necessary for the examination. To study motor fibres the cathode must be distal in comparison with the anode, whereas for 1_A fibres the opposite applies. The cathode position is marked by a small stroke made on the skin with a dermal pencil to enable measurement of the distance between the two stimulation points. Activation of the motor fibres needs single square pulses of current (duration 0.1 to 0.2ms at 1HZ), the supramaximal intensity—generally about 30mA—being progressively determined by following the recruitment of the muscle response on the screen. For 1_A fibre study it is preferable to stimulate with single shocks of longer duration (0.5 to 1ms) with low progressive intensity and low frequency ($<$0.5HZ). In these conditions maximal 'H' reflex response can be elicited without direct muscle response. In babies, as in adults, the nerves which are most easily accessible to stimulation are the median and ulnar nerves for the upper limb, the tibial and peroneal nerves for the lower limb. The common points of stimulation are the wrist, elbow and axilla for upper limb nerves and the ankle and knee for lower limb nerves. However, in babies sometimes the medial epicondyle and the fibular head are not very prominent and so the nerve course can be difficult to localise.

Cutaneous nerve distal branches are stimulated by means of two small bands (2mm wide), cut from silver self-sticking surface electrodes used in electrocardiography (*e.g.* Dorvit DVTE). These electrodes are wrapped around the first or the fifth finger in order, respectively, to stimulate the median or ulnar nerve's cutaneous fibres. To stimulate the sural nerve they are applied on the skin of the external side of the foot. In all cases, since stimulation is at the cathode, the stimulating electrodes are placed with the cathode nearest the recording electrodes. The output impulse is constituted by a square wave (duration 0.1 to 0.2ms, intensity 5 to 8mA), delivered at a frequency of 2 or 3HZ.

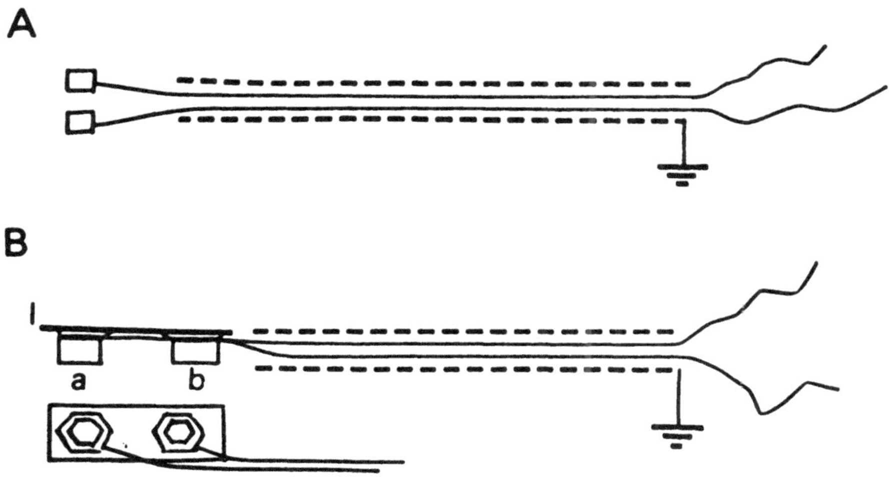

Fig. 9.1. Recording electrodes. *A*: bipolar surface electrodes for muscle potentials. *B*: bipolar surface electrodes for cutaneous fibres action potentials. *a,b*: silver cupolae filled with conductive gel. I: insulating strip.

Recording

Muscle potentials are recorded by means of bipolar surface electrodes taped to the skin over the muscle being activated, either directly over the motor fibres or indirectly by activation of 1_A afferent fibres. In our experience the handiest electrodes are two small silver plates, 3 to 4mm in diameter, spaced at 0.5 to 1cm apart, depending on the muscle (Fig. 9.1A). To record the cutaneous fibre action potentials, we use bipolar surface electrodes consisting of two small silver cupolae filled with conductive gel (Fig. 9.1B), attached above the nerve course by means of adhesive tape.

The ground electrode (a small silver band, 0.5cm wide and 5cm long) is fastened between the stimulating and recording electrodes by means of a small bracelet. A little band of sponge soaked with conductive gel is intercalated between the skin and the ground electrode. It should be noted that the adhesive tape and bracelet are very convenient but care must be taken to ensure that they are not too tight.

After amplification (A.C., filter setting 20 to 2000HZ), nerve and muscle potentials are displayed on a screen and simultaneously recorded on paper. Cutaneous nerve activity must first be averaged electronically; generally the summation of 200 responses is sufficient. Figure 9.2 shows examples of electrode positioning and recordings obtained.

Calculation of conduction velocities

As mentioned above, the conduction velocity is obtained by dividing the conduction distance by the latency difference between the two responses. If the

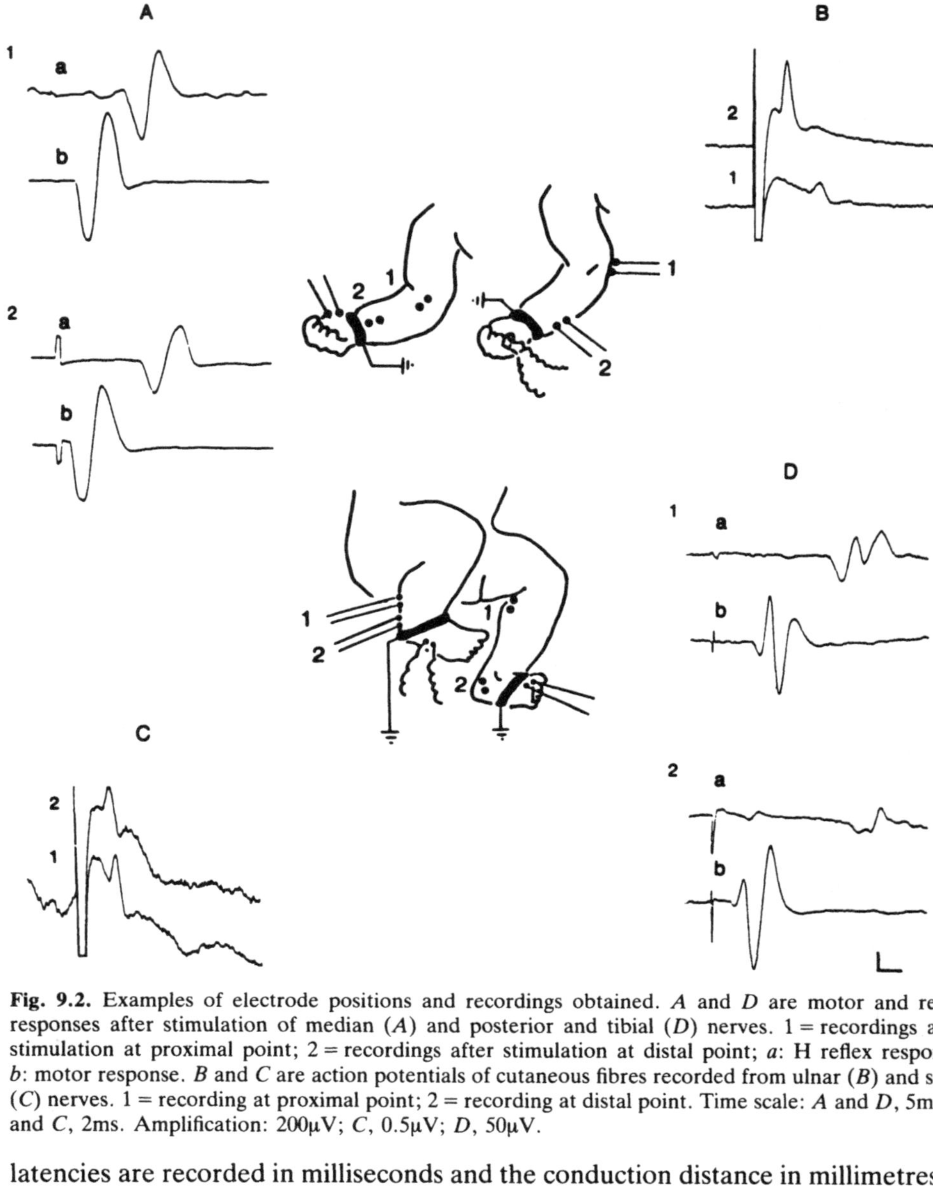

Fig. 9.2. Examples of electrode positions and recordings obtained. *A* and *D* are motor and reflex responses after stimulation of median (*A*) and posterior and tibial (*D*) nerves. 1 = recordings after stimulation at proximal point; 2 = recordings after stimulation at distal point; *a*: H reflex response; *b*: motor response. *B* and *C* are action potentials of cutaneous fibres recorded from ulnar (*B*) and sural (*C*) nerves. 1 = recording at proximal point; 2 = recording at distal point. Time scale: *A* and *D*, 5ms; *B* and *C*, 2ms. Amplification: 200μV; *C*, 0.5μV; *D*, 50μV.

latencies are recorded in milliseconds and the conduction distance in millimetres, it is easy to calculate the conduction velocity in metres per second. The latency of a response corresponds to the delay between artefact stimulation and the start of the potential. The conduction distance corresponds to the length of nerve between the two stimulation points for motor and 1_A fibres and to the distance between the two reception electrodes for cutaneous fibres. In adults this length is generally estimated by measuring directly on the skin surface the distance between the points

TABLE 9.I

Mean values of conduction times and conduction velocities for term newborn infants

Conduction times (ms)	*Mean*	*SD*	*Conduction velocities (m/s)*	*Mean*	*SD*	*N**
Ulnar nerve						
Motor fibres						
wrist	2.8	0.3	elbow-wrist	29.2	3.4	57
elbow	4.8	0.5	axilla-elbow	28.8	3.8	43
axilla	6.8	0.7				
I_A fibres						
wrist	17.7	2.0	elbow-wrist	35.0	4.4	25
elbow	16.2	1.3				
Cutaneous fibres						
wrist	2.0	0.3	wrist-elbow	25.8	4.4	24
elbow	4.7	0.7				
Median nerve						
Motor fibres						
wrist	3.2	0.4	elbow-wrist	26.4	2.8	44
elbow	5.3	0.6	axilla-elbow	26.9	3.9	20
axilla	7.5	0.8				
I_A fibres						
wrist	18.7	1.6	elbow-wrist	30.1	3.0	20
elbow	17.1	2.1				
Cutaneous fibres						
wrist	2.1	0.3	wrist-elbow	26.8	4.0	23
elbow	4.3	0.4				
Tibial nerve						
Motor fibres						
ankle	4.2	1.0	knee-ankle	21.7	3.5	27
knee	8.4	1.3				
I_A fibres						
ankle	28.4	2.1	ankle-knee	25.2	4.4	17
knee	24.9	1.7				
Peroneal nerve						
Motor fibres						
ankle	4.0	1.1	fibular head-ankle	25.4	2.5	27
fibular head	6.5	1.1				
I_A fibres						
ankle	26.4	2.1	ankle-fibular head	26.7	3.2	10
fibular head	24.0	2.1				
Sural nerve						
Cutaneous fibres						
malleolus	2.1	0.4	malleolus-foreleg	25.2	3.2	18
foreleg	2.7	0.4				

* Number of values for each series

of stimulation or reception. In babies, because the length of the nerve is particularly short and because limbs are generally plump, it is better to estimate this distance with a divider.

Normal data

Our data are presented in terms of the mean (±SD) values, calculated for each series of results. Linear correlations were determined by the method of least squares. Statistical significance ($p<0.05$) was assessed according to the number of values recorded: the Student t test was used for numbers greater than 20 and the non-parametric Mann–Whitney U test for lesser numbers.

Term infants

Numerous studies have been conducted since 1960. These studies are generally concerned with one or two nerves and a relatively small population of subjects. The results we report here, taken from tests conducted in our laboratory, concern 145 term infants, examined within six days after birth. The PCA of the population was 40.3 ± 1.3 weeks. This large population allowed us, for each nerve and for each group of nerve fibres, to obtain series of 10 to 57 values. The conduction times and conduction velocities obtained for the ulnar and median nerves (motor fibres, 1_A fibres, non-nociceptive cutaneous fibres), for the tibial and peroneal nerves (motor fibres, 1_A fibres) and for the sural nerve (non-nociceptive cutaneous fibres) are given in Table 9.I. As is well known, nerve conduction velocities in fullterm infants are roughly half those in adults. In our technical conditions the amplitudes of muscle action potentials (recorded with surface electrodes) were never below 2mv. They ranged between 4 and 8mv on the small muscle of the hand and between 2 and 6mv on the small muscles of the foot.

For motor fibres, in the different nerves studied, the averaged conduction velocities are significantly different except between the median and peroneal nerves. The conduction velocities of 1_A fibres are in all instances significantly greater than those of motor fibres. For 1_A fibres the averaged conduction velocities are significantly different in the different nerves except between the peroneal and tibial nerves. The values obtained for the non-nociceptive cutaneous fibres are not statistically different for the three nerves studied. Interestingly, the conduction velocities of the non-nociceptive cutaneous fibres are the same in the upper and lower limbs. Moreover, in contrast to the results found in cats by Skoglund and Romero (1965), our findings do not support the idea that in humans there may be a difference in maturation between motor and cutaneous fibres. Indeed, our average values in the median nerve for the motor and cutaneous fibres are identical. For the ulnar nerve there is a difference between the two types of fibres, and consistent with the findings of Skoglund and Romero in cats, the conduction velocity of the motor fibres is greater than that of the cutaneous fibres.

The values we obtained for motor fibre conduction velocities are quite similar to those of other authors (Thomas and Lambert 1960, Gamstorp 1963, Dunn *et al.* 1964, Blom and Finnström 1968, Dubowitz *et al.* 1968, Wagner and Buchthal 1972, Cruz-Martinez *et al.* 1977, Vecchierini-Blineau and Guiheneuc 1979), as shown in Figure 9.3. We also found, as did Blom and Finnström (1968), that in term newborn infants the motor fibre conduction velocities in the upper limbs generally are faster than those in the lower limbs. For 1_A fibre conduction velocities also, the values we found are similar to those reported previously (Cruz-Martinez *et al.* 1977,

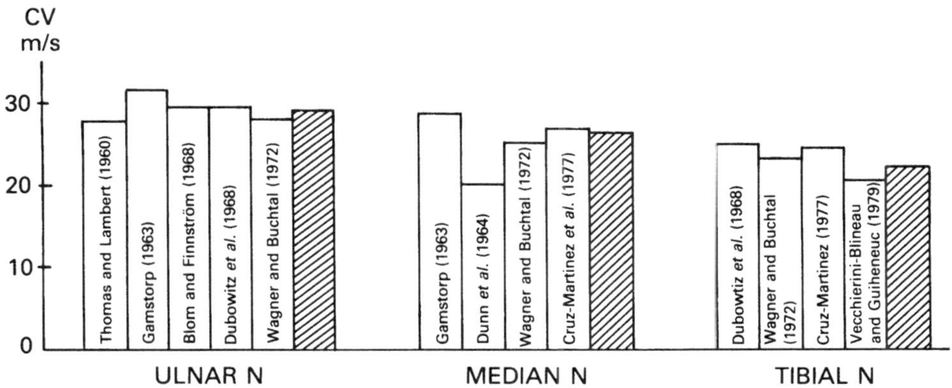

Fig. 9.3. Motor fibres (term infants). Averaged values of conduction velocity (CV) obtained by various authors for ulnar, median and tibial nerves. Hatched columns are our averaged values.

Duron *et al.* 1977, Vecchierini-Blineau and Guiheneuc 1979). In accord with Raimbault and Laget (1963), we obtained significantly greater velocities for 1_A than for motor fibres. In general, the conduction velocities of non-nociceptive cutaneous fibres have been measured in infants over one month old (Gamstorp and Shelburne 1965, Minejima *et al.* 1971, Audry-Chaboud *et al.* 1984, Brunon *et al.* 1984). Therefore our results for non-nociceptive cutaneous fibres can be compared with those of other authors only for the ulnar and median nerves. For the ulnar nerve, our averaged value is virtually the same as the value calculated from the regression line of Wagner and Buchthal (1972) at 40 weeks PCA (26 m/s) and as the averaged value of Cruz-Martinez *et al.* (1978) (25.2 ± 3.6 m/s). For the median nerve, our values are similar to those given by Desmedt *et al.* (1973) (20 to 34 m/s), but less than those of Cruz-Martinez *et al.* (1978) (30.6 ± 2.9 m/s).

Preterm infants

As with term infants, the most widely studied fibres in preterm infants have been the motor fibres (Thomas and Lambert 1960, Cerra and Johnson 1962, Ruppert *et al.* 1967, Blom and Finnström 1968, Dubowitz *et al.* 1968, Schulte *et al.* 1968, Moosa and Dubowitz 1971, Wagner and Buchthal 1972, Cruz-Martinez *et al.* 1977, Cruz-Martinez *et al.* 1983, Kesson *et al.* 1985). To our knowledge, in preterm infants 1_A fibre conduction velocity has been studied by Bougle *et al.* (1990) and cutaneous conduction velocity by Wagner and Buchthal (1972) only.

Our study was conducted on 77 preterm infants (44 male, 33 female), examined between one and 50 days after birth, at PCAs between 28 and 39 weeks. In this work we measured the conduction velocities of the motor fibres and afferent 1_A fibres of the ulnar, median and tibial nerves as well as those of non-nociceptive cutaneous fibres of the ulnar and median nerves. The peroneal and sural nerves

TABLE 9.II

Mean values of conduction velocities (m/s) for preterm infants at different PCAs and equations of regression lines calculated from individual values of both the preterm and term newborn infants

PCA (wks)	*29–31*			*31–33*			*33–35*			*35–37*			*29–42*		
	Mean	*SD*	*N**	*Mean*	*SD*	*N**	*Mean*	*SD*	*N**	*Mean*	*SD*	*N**	*Regression lines*	*r†*	*N**
Ulnar nerve															
Motor fibres	17.2	1.9	7	21.5	3.4	13	23.6	2.0	20	24.8	3.3	22	1.1 × −14.5	0.79	119
IA fibres	18.9	3.3	4	22.5	5.6	8	26.7	5.8	10	28.2	4.8	10	1.5 × −25.9	0.77	57
Cutaneous fibres				19.6	3.2	7	19.4	2.3	13	23.1	1.7	7	0.9 × −11.7	0.62	52
Median nerve															
Motor fibres				18.2	2.9	8	20.7	2.0	10	23.2	3.4	10	0.9 × −12.0	0.78	75
IA fibres				19.7	2.2	8	24.6	2.4	10	27.4	4.6	9	1.1 × −15.6	0.78	48
Cutaneous fibres				19.3	3.2	6	19.9	1.9	6	23.3	2.2	6	1.0 × −13.2	0.70	44
Tibial nerve															
Motor fibres				16.0	2.7	10	17.1	2.5	14	19.1	1.7	11	0.8 × − 9.3	0.71	69
IA fibres				18.4	3.6	5	20.0	4.1	6	22.9	3.0	7	1.0 × −14.7	0.68	36

* Number of values for each series
† Correlation coefficients

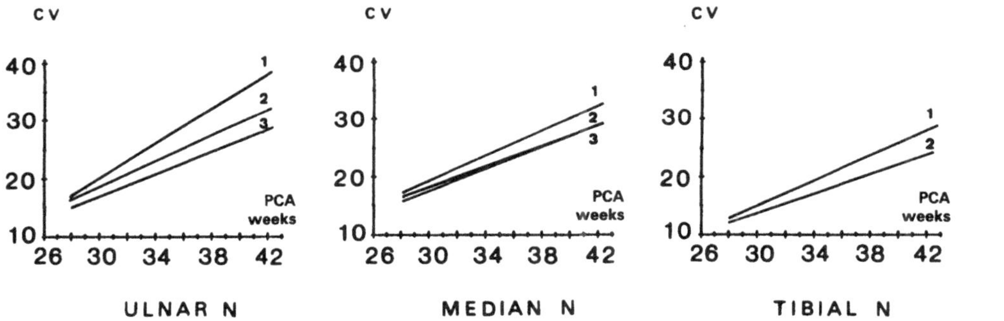

Fig. 9.4. Regression lines (preterm and term infants) obtained for each nerve studies. 1 = I_A fibres; 2 = motor fibres; 3 = cutaneous fibres. CV = conduction velocity, in m/s.

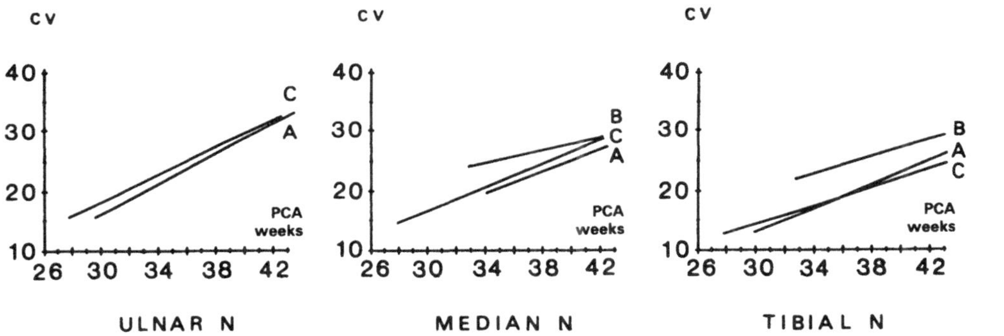

Fig. 9.5. Motor fibres (preterm and term infants). Regression lines obtained for ulnar, median and tibial nerves by: *A*, Wagner and Buchthal (1972); *B*, Cruz-Martinez *et al.* (1983); *C*, Khater-Boidin and Duron (1989). CV = conduction velocity, in m/s.

were not studied because it was difficult to set the electrodes in good position on the very small limbs of these infants.

Whatever the age of the preterm infant, as in term newborn infants, the conduction velocities of 1_A fibres are greater than those of both motor and cutaneous fibres for a given nerve (Table 9.II). Moreover, for the muscular nerve fibres (motor and 1_A), conduction velocities in the upper limbs are greater than those in the lower limbs. An interesting point is that, contrary to the results of Hakamada *et al.* (1988), monosynaptic reflexes can easily be elicited in preterm infants, of whatever age, in both upper and lower limbs. The segmental monosynaptic circuits involved in 'H' reflexes are functional from as early as 28 weeks PCA. The regression lines calculated from individual values for both the preterm and term infants are shown in Figure 9.4. The increase in conduction velocity per week of PCA ranged from 0.8 to 1.5 m/s (see Table 9.II). For each nerve the slope of regression line for 1_A fibres is more pronounced than those for motor and cutaneous fibres.

Wagner and Buchthal (1972), taking into account their own results and data from Thomas and Lambert (1960), Gamstorp (1963), Ruppert *et al.* (1967), Blom and Finnström (1968), Dubowitz *et al.* (1968) and Schulte *et al.* (1968), correlated motor fibre conduction velocities in ulnar, median and tibial posterior nerves with PCA (from 30 to 42 weeks). Cruz-Martinez *et al.* (1983) established the same correlation in median and tibial posterior nerves at PCAS of 33 to 45 weeks. The regression lines we obtained for the ulnar, median and tibial posterior nerves can be virtually superimposed on those of Wagner and Buchthal (Fig. 9.5). The differences between our results and those of Cruz-Martinez *et al* (1983) may be due to the fact that those authors' regression line was established from values obtained from slightly older children: the lack of very young preterm infants and the presence of some one-month-old babies may modify the slope of the regression line.

For the 1_A fibres, our results are in agreement with those obtained by Cruz-Martinez and Ferrer (1978) after percutaneous nerve stimulation (median and ulnar nerves) at the wrist. Indeed, in this type of stimulation all the fibres (motor, cutaneous and 1_A) of mixed nerves are activated, and therefore the conduction velocity measured in these conditions is that of the fastest nerve fibres. In a recent study Bougle *et al.* (1990) measured the motor and 1_A nerve conduction velocities in three groups of infants—a group of normal term newborn infants and two groups of preterm babies tested at the expected date of term. In these conditions, which differ from ours, the authors found no difference in the motor nerve conduction velocities between the three groups of infants at the same PCA. This is in agreement with the results of Cruz-Martinez *et al.* (1977), which correlated motor conduction velocity only with gestational age. Proprioceptive 1_A nerve conduction, however, was significantly lower at the time of term in preterm compared to term newborn infants. Nevertheless, although the mean motor conduction velocity for the group of term newborn infants (25.74 ± 3.95 m/s) is in accord with our results and those of other authors, the mean 1_A conduction velocity for the lower limb (31.96 ± 7.38 m/s) seems high in comparison with values reported for the upper limb (Cruz-Martinez *et al.* 1977, Duron *et al.* 1977, Vecchierini-Blineau and Guiheneuc 1979). Also, the distribution of the individual values seems widely dispersed, as indicated by the standard deviation. Thus the hypothesis of Bougle *et al.* (1990), suggesting that the maturation of proprioceptive nerve fibres in preterm infants is slowed during the weeks before the expected term date, must be confirmed.

No extensive study such as our own has been reported for cutaneous fibres between the wrist and elbow of preterm neonates. Nevertheless, our mean values for the ulnar nerve are similar to those given by Wagner and Buchthal (1972) for the ulnar and median nerves between the digits and wrist. This confirms what Wagner and Buchthal demonstrated, that the increase in conduction velocity with age is the same in the proximal segment of the nerve as in the distal. The differences between absolute values of conduction velocities measured in the distal and proximal segments of nerve can be due to variations in temperature. In order to avoid such fluctuations, it seems preferable to measure cutaneous sensory conduction velocities on the proximal segments of nerves.

Pattern of abnormality

The measurement of conduction velocity is an objective test, and a painless and reliable method of investigation of the peripheral nervous system. In babies and children it can be used to study progressive changes in nerve conduction during growth and disease. Nevertheless, for an initial test it is essential to know the normal ranges at different ages with statistical validity. It was the aim of our preliminary study to determine the normal ranges in preterm and term newborn infants. In routine neonatal testing of preterm babies without sign of neurological disease the measurement of nerve conduction velocities appears useful in determining PCA, as suggested by Dubowitz *et al.* (1968) and Miller *et al.* (1983). Moreover, study of different categories of nerve fibres is able to bring greater precision to this determination.

Except for obstetrical injuries of the brachial plexus, pathology of the peripheral nervous system is relatively rare at birth, in contrast to pathology of the central nervous system. Nevertheless, electrophysiological study (nerve fibre conduction velocity and electromyography) of the peripheral nervous system appears helpful in two circumstances at least. The first is when, in the absence of any clinical sign, a probability of hereditary neuropathy exists. In this case, even in the absence of electrophysiological abnormalities, the first examination can constitute a helpful reference for eventual follow-up.

The second circumstance is represented by the complex group of the neonatal hypotonias in which proximal hereditary motor neuropathy (HMN) is included. As underlined by Harding (1984), in the type I of proximal HMN (Werdnig–Hoffmann disease) sensory nerve conduction velocity is normal; motor nerve conduction velocity, generally normal, may be slightly reduced; and electromyography usually demonstrates typical neurogenic activities. In our experience it appears that one of the most important signs in Werdnig–Hoffmann disease is the very small amplitude of the evoked compound muscle potential (<2mv) recorded on the small hand or foot muscles after the corresponding nerve stimulation. Nevertheless, absence of short circuits due to perspiration at the recording sites must be confirmed before any interpretation concerning variations in amplitudes of the potentials. In some cases, results need to be checked using needle electrodes. A typical example is a two-month-old baby in whom only motor fibre conduction velocity was reduced (21 and 16m/s in the ulnar and median nerves respectively)—the amplitudes of muscle action potentials were 0.26 and 0.54mv on the hypothenar and thenar eminences respectively. A second interesting example is a term infant examined two weeks after birth. In this baby the motor fibre conduction velocities were strictly normal (32 and 30m/s on the hypothenar and thenar eminences respectively). Both these two babies died before six months of age, and the diagnosis of Werdnig–Hoffmann disease was confirmed histologically.

REFERENCES

Audry-Chaboud, D., Soichot, P., Giroud, M., Nivelon, J.L. (1984) 'Intérêt de l'étude des vitesses de conduction nerveuse sensitive à l'aiguille chez l'enfant au dessous de 3 ans.' *Revue d'Electroencéphalographie et de Neurophysiologie Clinique*, **13**, 336–339.

Blom, S., Finnström, O. (1968) 'Motor conduction velocities in newborn infants of various gestational ages.' *Acta Paediatrica Scandinavica*, **57**, 377–384.

Bougle, D., Denise, P., Yaseen, K., Tranier, S., Voirin, J., Pottier, M., Venezia, R. (1990) 'Maturation of peripheral nerves in preterm infants. Motor and proprioceptive nerve conduction.' *Electroencephalography and Clinical Neurophysiology*, **75**, 118–121.

Brunon, A.M., Chauplannaz, G., Berard, C., Bady, B. (1984) 'Vitesses de conduction sensitive normales des nerfs médian et cubital chez l'enfant de la naissance à quinze ans.' *Revue d'Electroencéphalographie et de Neurophysiologie Clinique*, **14**, 69–73.

Cerra, D., Johnson, E.W. (1962) 'Motor nerve conduction velocity in premature infants.' *Archives of Physical Medicine and Rehabilitation*, **43**, 160–164.

Cruz-Martinez, A., Pérez-Conde, M.C., Ferrer, M.T. (1977) 'Motor conduction velocity and H-reflexes in infancy and childhood. I. Study in newborns, twins and small-for-dates.' *Electromyography and Clinical Neurophysiology*, **17**, 493–505.

—— Del Campo, F., Barrio, M., Gutierrez, A.M., Lopez, E. (1978) 'Sensory and mixed conduction velocity in infancy and childhood. I. Normal parameters in median, ulnar and sural nerves.' *Electromyography and Clinical Neurophysiology*, **18**, 487–504.

—— Ferrer, M.T. (1978) 'Sensory and mixed conduction velocity in infancy and childhood. II. Ratio between the amplitude of sensory evoked potentials at the wrist, stimulating the different fingers in both hands.' *Electromyography and Clinical Neurophysiology*, **18**, 505–515.

—— —— Martin, J.M. (1983) 'Motor conduction velocity and H-reflex in prematures with very short gestational age.' *Electromyography and Clinical Neurophysiology*, **23**, 13–19.

Desmedt, J.E., Noel, P., Debecker, J., Nameche, J. (1973) 'Maturation of afferent conduction velocity as studied by sensory nerve potentials and by cerebral evoked potentials.' *In* Desmedt, J.E. (Ed.) *New Developments in Electromyography and Clinical Neurophysiology*. Basel: Karger.

Dubowitz, V., Whittaker, G.F., Brown, B.H., Robinson, A. (1968) 'Nerve conduction velocity. An index of neurological maturity of the newborn infant.' *Developmental Medicine and Child Neurology*, **10**, 741–749.

Dunn, H.G., Buckler, W.St.J., Morrison, G.C.E., Emery, A.W. (1964) 'Conduction velocity of motor nerves in infants and children.' *Pediatrics*, **34**, 708–727.

Duron, B., Marlot, D., De Marles, O. (1977) 'Réflexes d'Hoffmann chez le nouveau-né normal. Evolution postnatale des vitesses de conduction des fibres alpha motrices et des fibres sensitives IA du nerf cubital.' *Revue d'Electroencéphalographie et de Neurophysiologie Clinique*, **7**, 509–521.

Gamstorp, I. (1963) 'Normal conduction velocity of ulnar, median and peroneal nerves in infancy, childhood and adolescence.' *Acta Paediatrica Scandinavica* (Suppl. 146), 68–76.

—— Shelburn, S.A. (1965) 'Peripheral sensory conduction in ulnar and median nerves of normal infants, children and adolescents.' *Acta Paediatrica Scandinavica*, **54**, 309–313.

Harding, A.E. (1984) 'Inherited neuronal atrophy and degeneration predominantly of lower motor neurons.' *In* Dyck, P.J., Thomas, P.K., Lambert, E.H., Bunge, R. (Eds) *Peripheral Neuropathies, Vol. II*. Philadelphia: W.B. Saunders.

Hakamada, S., Hayakawa, F., Kuno, K., Tanaka, R. (1988) 'Development of the monosynaptic reflex pathway in the human spinal cord.' *Developmental Brain Research*, **42**, 239–246.

Kesson, A.M., Henderson-Smart, D.J., Pettigrew, A.G., Edwards, D.A. (1985) 'Peripheral nerve conduction velocity and brainstem evoked responses in small for gestational age preterm infants.' *Early Human Development*, **11**, 213–219.

Khater-Boidin, J., Marlot, D., Duron, B. (1988) 'Vitesses de conduction des fibres motrices, sensitives cutanées et proprioceptives I_A chez le nouveau-né normal à terme.' *Neurophysiologie Clinique*, **18**, 59–72.

—— Duron, B. (1989) 'Evolution of motor, IA and cutaneous nerve-fibre conduction velocities in premature and fullterm newborns.' *Developmental Medicine and Child Neurology*, **31**, 47–55.

Miller, G.A., Heckmatt, J.Z., Dubowitz, L.M., Dubowitz, V. (1983) 'Use of nerve conduction velocity to determine gestational age in infants at risk and in very-low-birth-weight infants.' *Journal of

Pediatrics, **103**, 109–112.
Minejima, T.F., Sato, K., Sugiyama, S. (1971) 'Sensory nerve action potentials in infants and children.' *In Abstracts of the IVth International Electromyography Congress. Brussels.* pp. 100–101.
Moosa, A., Dubowitz, V. (1971) 'Postnatal maturation of peripheral nerves in preterm and full-term infants.' *Journal of Pediatrics*, **79**, 915–922.
Radtke, H.W. (1969) 'Motorische Nervenleitgeschwindigkeit bei normalen Säuglingen und Kindern.' *Helvetica Paediatrica Acta*, **24**, 390–398.
Raimbault, J., Laget, P. (1963) 'Etude de la vitesse de conduction des fibres nerveuses chez le jeune enfant.' *Revue Neurologique*, **108**, 204–209.
Ruppert, E.S., Robertson, A.F., Johnson, E.W. (1967) 'Motor nerve conduction velocities in infants of low birth weight (LBW).' *Journal of Pediatrics*, **70**, 693–694.
Schulte, F.J., Michaelis, R., Linke, I., Nolte, R. (1968) 'Motor nerve conduction velocity in term, preterm and small-for-dates newborn infants.' *Pediatrics*, **42**, 17–26.
Skoglund, S., Romero, C. (1965) 'Postnatal growth of spinal nerves and roots. A morphological study in the cat with physiological correlations.' *Acta Physiologica Scandinavica* (Suppl. 260).
Thomas, J.E., Lambert, E.H. (1960) 'Ulnar nerve conduction velocity and H reflex in infants and children.' *Journal of Applied Physiology*, **15**, 1–9.
Vecchierini-Blineau, M.F., Guiheneuc, P. (1979) 'Electrophysiological study of the peripheral nervous system in children.' *Journal of Neurology, Neurosurgery and Psychiatry*, **42**, 753–759.
Wagner, A.L., Buchthal, F. (1972) 'Motor and sensory conduction in infancy and childhood: reappraisal.' *Developmental Medicine and Child Neurology*, **14**, 189–216.

10
THE ASSESSMENT OF THE AUTONOMIC NERVOUS SYSTEM

Phyllis M. Gootman and Norman Gootman

The autonomic nervous system

The autonomic nervous system (ANS) is concerned with regulation of every visceral organ in the body. For years it was thought to be simpler anatomically than the central nervous system (CNS), since ANS function is largely involuntary or 'automatic', but now its anatomy is known to be as complex as in the rest of the neuraxis. More recent and current anatomical studies have clarified the localisation of preganglionic and postganglionic cell bodies as well as the connections within the CNS with the preganglionic motor neurons. In addition, recent investigations using new immunocytochemical and/or histochemical techniques have shown that there are more than 20 putative chemical messengers within the ANS (Potter 1988), if one includes the neuropeptides located within the enteric system as well as within the CNS or functioning as co-transmitters with the classical neurotransmitters, norepinephrine (NE) and acetylcholine (ACh). It has been suggested that urinary levels of neuropeptide Y might be a clinically useful marker for diagnosis of paediatric neuroblastoma (Kogner *et al.* 1990), while vasoactive intestinal polypeptide has been reported absent from Auerbach's plexus in children with Hirschsprung's disease (Tsuto *et al.* 1989).

Although there have been attempts to include afferents within the ANS (Freire-Maia and Azevedo 1990, Prechtl and Powley 1990), Langley's seminal work (1921) describing the system as motor (or efferent) is still the most logical. It cannot be said that afferent inputs are just somatic or just visceral, *i.e.* autonomic. Afferents cause alterations in both somatic and autonomic efferents, leading to alterations in effector functions.

Figure 10.1 summarises the autonomic innervation of visceral organs. The preganglionic neurons of both the sympathetic (thoracolumbar) and parasympathetic (craniosacral) divisions are located in the brain and spinal cord. The *afferent* limbs of autonomic reflexes may be in any afferent nerve. Preganglionic sympathetic soma are primarily located in the intermediolateral cell column of the thoracolumbar spinal cord. The preganglionic sympathetic fibres are usually myelinated and leave the spinal roots as white rami communicantes synapsing in ganglia making up the sympathetic chain (paravertebral). Unmyelinated postganglionic fibres rejoin the anterior spinal roots. Some preganglionic sympathetic fibres traverse the sympathetic chain and synapse in the more peripheral prevertebral ganglia (*e.g.* coeliac). The urogenital system is innervated by sympathetic fibres

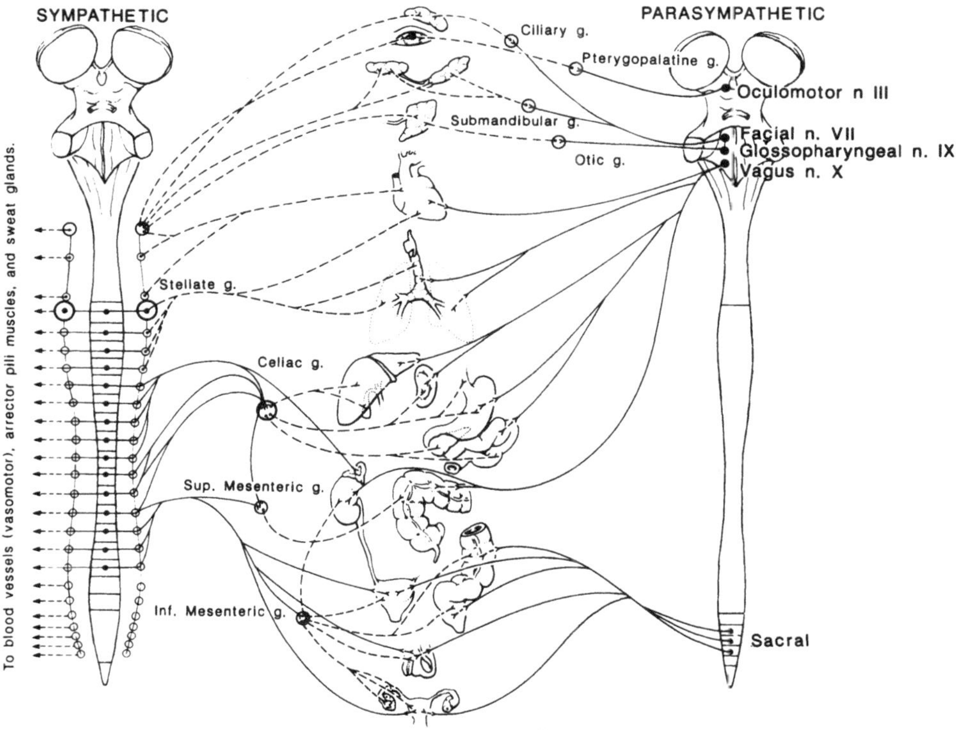

Fig. 10.1. Schematic representation of ANS innervation of visceral organs. *Left:* sympathetic outflow. *Right:* parasympathetic outflow. Preganglionic fibres indicated by solid lines; postganglionic fibres by dashed lines.

that follow the arrangement of parasympathetic fibres and synapse in the most peripheral (terminal) ganglia.

Parasympathetic preganglionic neurons are located in the brainstem (cranial nerves III, VII, IX, X) and the intermediolateral cell column of the sacral spinal cord. The preganglionic neurons synapse with postganglionic soma in ganglia located close to or within the effector (terminal ganglia).

The excitatory transmitter at all preganglionic terminals is ACh. The receptor type is not blocked by atropine and is classified as a (ganglionic) nicotinic receptor. Ganglionic transmission has been shown to involve other cholinergic receptors which are blocked by atropine, *i.e.* muscarinic receptors, as well as other neurotransmitters such as dopaminergic and serotonergic (Greengard and Kebabian 1974, Eränkö *et al.* 1986). While the complexity of ganglionic transmission was first shown for sympathetic ganglia with the presence of interneurons, *i.e.* small intensely fluorescent (SIF) cells (Eränkö 1976, Chiba 1978), such complexity has also been verified for parasympathetic ganglia (de Groat and Booth 1980, Bornstein *et al.* 1988). The latter also receive an inhibitory innervation from postganglionic sympathetic fibres (Surprenant 1986). The pelvic ganglia have also been reported to contain SIF cells (Kanerva and Hervonen 1976; de Groat and Booth 1980, 1984).

ANS development

Embryologically, basal-plate development within the spinal-cord and neural-crest development, migration and phenotypic expression are the main processes involved in ANS development (Black 1978, Smith 1986, Hamill and LaGamma 1988). Interruption of mechanisms governing neuronal maturation within the first two or three weeks of life will produce lifelong developmental deficits in autonomic mechanisms (Hamill and LaGamma 1988). Postnatal human development is normally gauged by physiological observations. Certainly control over such autonomic functions as blood flow, bowel transit and bladder emptying depends upon maturation of peripheral neural structures as well as central autonomic control mechanisms. Peripherally, the differentiation of neuroblasts into enteric ganglion cells and mature plexuses is quite delayed; in fact only about a third of the neuroblasts are differentiated at birth, and development continues throughout the first five years of life (Kissel *et al.* 1981, Giacobini 1986). However, a recent report of the examination of the myenteric plexus using the silver impregnation technique indicted no clear differences between human neonatal and adult gastrointestinal (GI) tracts (Kumar and Phillips 1989). On the other hand, the development of autonomic ganglia and the innervation of pelvic structures involved in micturition is delayed. Eventually, usually by two or three years of age, voluntary control over these autonomic functions ensues. Thus autonomic control occurs in the setting of continued ANS development.

The normal development of the GI tract and its innervation has been studied and reviewed by a number of investigators (Gabella 1979, Cochard and LeDouarin 1982, Gershon *et al.* 1983, Le Douarin 1986*a*,*b*, Heaton *et al.* 1988).

Testing of autonomic functions

Details of autonomic failure and the many tests used to classify autonomic disease in adult patients have been recently reviewed (Eckberg 1980, Bergstrom *et al.* 1986, Kaijser 1986, Bannister 1988, Mustonen *et al.* 1989, Taylor and Mitchell 1990). We recommend a text recently summarising autonomic failure in the adult (Bannister 1988).

Heart-rate and blood-pressure responses to physiological perturbations (*e.g.* cough, respiration, the Valsalva manoeuvre and postural changes) have been used to assess ANS function under healthy conditions, with certain diseases and with aging (Eckberg 1980). However, only limited information about autonomic control of heart rate can be obtained by traditional statistical measures based solely on changes in mean heart rate and variance (Lipton *et al.* 1961*a*,*b*; Bannister 1988).

Monitoring of cardiovascular function

Heart rate and, to a lesser extent, blood pressure are used to evaluate development of autonomic reflex function in neonates (Lipton *et al.* 1961*a*,*b*, 1965). Effector responses in the fetus and neonates have been studied with the aid of sympathomimetic and parasympathomimetic drugs and antagonists or by means of stimuli capable of inducing reflex changes in autonomic outflow, including catecholamine levels (Lipton *et al.* 1965; Hirschman and Katkin 1974; Gootman 1983, 1986*a*,*b*, 1991; Gootman *et al.* 1987).

Heart-rate and blood-pressure responses to a variety of different stimuli have been evaluated in preterm infants and neonates of varying ages. However, when using heart rate as the criterion for changes in autonomic activity, it is essential to know the prestimulus (resting) level, state of the infant and level of arousal, since these factors all interplay with the prestimulus heart rate. The prestimulus heart rate must include the variability in 'resting' heart rate. The response to the stimulus should at least include latency to onset of response, magnitude of response and duration of response. Change in heart rate is the primary response monitored to a variety of stimuli used to elicit changes in autonomic outflow. Such changes in autonomic activity, as indexed by changes in heart rate and to a lesser extent blood pressure, have been used by psychologists to evaluate alerting and orienting responses (Lacey 1956, Prechtl 1974) and psychophysiological activity in early human life (Hirschman and Katkin 1974, Hall *et al.* 1982).

Resting values of heart rate and blood pressure in neonates

Some resting values of heart rate and blood pressure reported in the literature for both preterm and term infants are summarised in Table 10.I. Kellerova and Andrasyova (1990*b*) sequentially studied blood pressure and heart rates in 150 infants. They examined and quantitated the significant increases in pressure and decreases in heart rate (Table 10.I).* It has been suggested that there can be a problem with blood-pressure determination, which in the neonate is now more commonly determined by Doppler techniques. This method has been reported to be less accurate than direct measurements with an indwelling arterial line (Sinaiko and Wells 1990). However, Kellerova and her colleagues have validated the use of the Doppler technique using umbilical artery recordings of arterial pressure.

It has been reported that 150 term neonates, one to five days of age, had resting values of 57 ± 8/33±mmHg with heart rates of 121 ± 9 beats per minute (bpm) at 24 hours postpartum. Systolic pressure increased by 22 per cent by the fourth postnatal day while diastolic pressure increased by 19 per cent. At the same time heart rate declined by 6 per cent. The state of the neonate was important, especially by the fourth postnatal day. During sleep at the fourth postnatal day blood pressure was significantly reduced (10 to 15 per cent). Crying elicited an increase in blood pressure of 22/12mmHg, and sucking an increase of 18/14mmHg. Changes in body position were also a factor: prone 14/9mmHg and upright

*We recommend the articles by Sinaiko and Wells (1990) and Whincup *et al.* (1989) for the changes in blood pressure and heart rate occurring in the developing child from one to 18 years.

TABLE 10.I

Resting blood pressure and heart rates in term fetuses, preterm and term infants up to nine weeks of age

Age	*Blood pressure systole/diastole (mmHg)*	*Heart rate (bpm)*	*References*
Fetal (near term)		110–160	Cohen and Yeh (1986)
		140–160	Mantel *et al.* (1990*b*)
		129–169	Renou *et al.* (1969)
		120–160	Sigurd *et al.* (1985)
PCA			
25 wks PCA (3 days postnatal)		135 ± 2	Lindqvist *et al.* (1983)
26–35 wks		133 ± 5	Lindqvist (1990)
31 wks			
31–32 wks	52.7 ± 1.45/27.5 ± 9.7	140 ± 10	Kellerova (1985)
31–34 wks (8–15 days postnatal)		130 ± 8	Lindqvist *et al.* (1983)
31–35 wks (1–17 days postnatal)		126 ± 4	Lindqvist *et al.* (1983)
33–34 wks	65.7 ± 10.1/37.4 ± 11.1	132 ± 13	Kellerova (1985)
33.8 ± 2.7 wks		135 ± 21.6	Äärimaa *et al.* (1988)
35–36 wks	65.8 ± 8.9/39.1 ± 7.1	132 ± 11	Kellerova (1985)
37 wks (1 day postnatal)		115 ± 0	Lindqvist *et al.* (1983)
37–41 wks	74.7 ± 12.0/45.2 ± 11.0	120 ± 8	Kellerova (1985)
37–40 wks		123 ± 5	Lindqvist (1990)
38.9 ± 1.1 wks		122.3 ± 13	Äärimaa *et al.* (1988)
Postnatal			
1–12hrs (750g)	44/24 mean 33		Versmold *et al.* (1981)
1–12hrs (1000g)	49/26 mean 34.1		Versmold *et al.* (1981)
2–3hrs (<1000g)	35.1 ± 7.4/21.5 ± 4.5		Moscoso *et al.* (1983)
(1000–1250g)	35.3 ± 2.8/20.9 ± 2.6		Moscoso *et al.* (1983)
11–12hrs (<1000g)	40.5 ± 4.9/24.7 ± 4.7		Moscoso *et al.* (1983)
(1000–1250g)	42.7 ± 5.2/26.8 ± 3.7		Moscoso *et al.* (1983)
1–16hrs	72 ± 4.3/44 ± 2.7	132 ± 6.7	Cagnoni *et al.* (1987)
1–77hrs	64 ± 10/39 ± 8		Moss *et al.* (1963)
2–14hrs	(mean) 61 ± 6.3	118 ± 14.7	Oh *et al.* (1966)
1 day	56.7 ± 8.4/32.6 ± 6.6	121 ± 9.4	Kellerova and Andrasyova (1990)
2 days	63.6 ± 9.6/36,2 ± 6.8	118.87 ± 11.26	Kellerova and Andrasyova (1990)
3 days	68.2 ± 9.4/37.8 ± 7.4	117.53 ± 12.32	Kellerova and Andrasyova (1990)
4 days	69.1 ± 10.0/38.7 ± 6.4	114.69 ± 11.01	Kellerova and Andrasyova (1990)
4 days awake	77 ± 10		de Swiet *et al.* (1980)
asleep	71 ± 8		de Swiet *et al.* (1980)
1–5 days	57 ± 8.0/33 ± 7.0	121 ± 9	Kellerova and Andrasyova (1990)
1–5 days		122 ± 6	Lindqvist *et al.* (1983)
2 days	64 ± 10/36 ± 7	119 ± 11	Kellerova *et al.* (1990)
2–3 days		130–141	Schachter *et al.* (1971)
2–8 wks		122 ± 6 151 ± 2.8	Lewis *et al.* (1967)
5–9 wks awake	96 ± 11		de Swiet *et al.* (1980)
asleep	89 ± 11		de Swiet *et al.* (1980)

10/7mmHg (Kellerova and Andrasyova 1990*a*). A circadian rhythm in blood pressure has also been noted by this group and verified by Cagnoni *et al.* (1987). By the second postnatal day a significant decline in blood pressure was noted in term babies (9 to 10 per cent) with a smaller decline in preterm babies (post-conceptional age 33.69 weeks; postnatal age 43.8 ± 4.4 hours) of −5 to 6 per cent (Kellerova *et al.* 1985).

CHANGES IMMEDIATELY AFTER BIRTH

Contis and Lind (1963), using umbilical artery catheters to monitor blood pressure in 40 infants, found that the highest pressure recorded during the first day was at 15 minutes after birth. The blood pressure dropped to a low point on the second day. However, the most rapid decline in pressure occurred between 30 and 60 minutes after birth. By the seventh day systolic pressure reached a value higher than that observed at 15 minutes. Heart rate also declined during the first 15 to 30 minutes after birth, averaging 30bpm. Heart rate stabilised at a lower level between one and three hours after birth, followed by a gradual rise over the next six days. These results are in accord with the marked elevations in plasma catecholamines which have been reported at birth (Lagercrantz and Bistoletti 1973, Falconer and Poyser 1986, Padbury and Martinez 1988). Elevated plasma NE has also been reported in infants and children with congestive heart failure (Ross *et al.* 1987), indicating that stress stimulates the adrenal medulla.

HEART-RATE AND BLOOD-PRESSURE VARIABILITY

Increasing attention is being focused on quantifying various aspects of heart rate associated with beat-to-beat fluctuations or short-term heart-rate variability. Use of the fast Fourier transform for spectral analysis of heart rate permits characterisation of overall heart-rate variability and reveals low- and high-frequency components, which are considered to be attributable to sympathetic and vagal influences respectively (Lipsitz *et al.* 1990). Heart-rate variability is used for identification of fetal distress (Bowes *et al.* 1980; LeFevre 1984; Cohen and Yeh 1986; Koyanagi *et al.* 1988; Zimmer *et al.* 1988; Dawes *et al.* 1990; Mantel *et al.* 1990*a*,*b*). Such variability is also being studied as a means of quantitating ANS regulation of cardiac function as well as the interactions between respiratory behaviour and cardiovascular regulation in fetuses and neonates. Fluctuations with the respiratory cycle have long been known and identified as sinus arrhythmias (Lipton *et al.* 1964). Spectral analysis is one useful technique for quantifying overall heart-rate variability (Fig. 10.2, *top*), as well as specific components of this variability putatively associated with respiration, ANS innervation of the heart, and other physiological influences (Akselrod *et al.* 1981, Finley *et al.* 1987, Lipsitz *et al.* 1990). Examination of the spectrum permits evaluation of the amount of variation in the data for each frequency. The spectrum of one signal, such as heart rate, can be examined against the power of another signal such as the respiratory cycle. The two signals can be compared by examination of the cross spectrum and thus the

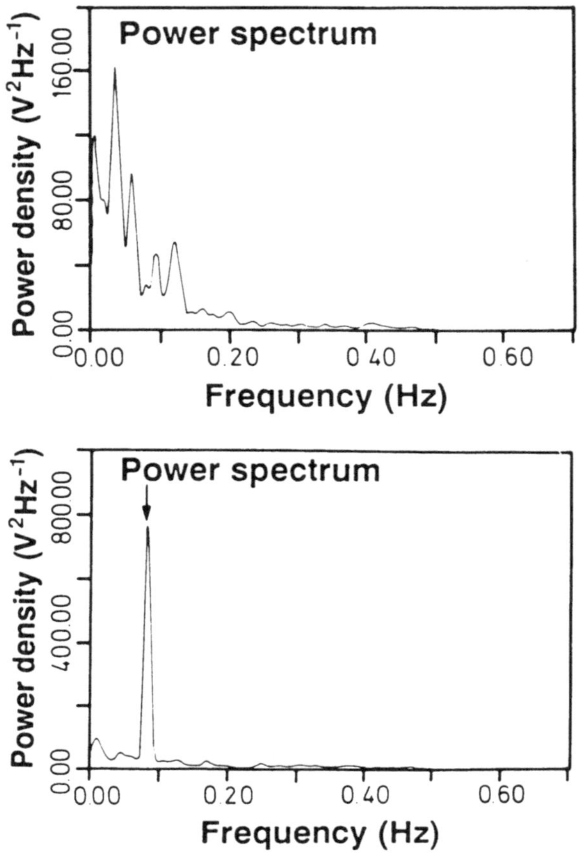

Fig. 10.2. Power spectra of heart rate during spontaneous activity (*top*) and during thermal stimulation of the foot at 0.083Hz (*bottom*) from an 11-day-old preterm infant (31 weeks PCA). (After Lindqvist 1990.)

magnitude of similar frequency components and/or their variability can be revealed (Äärimaa *et al.* 1988, Baldzer *et al.* 1989). Porges (1985) developed a technique to measure the amplitude of respiratory sinus arrhythmia or the variability in heart-rate patterns associated specifically with spontaneous breathing. Since many investigators view the variability of heart-rate pattern as a reflection principally of vagal drive to the heart, the amplitude of respiratory sinus arrhythmia has been accepted as an index of vagally mediated heart-rate patterns (Porter *et al.* 1988). However, direct recordings of sympathetic activity, at least in neonatal animals (Gootman *et al.* 1984, 1988; Sica *et al.* 1990), suggest that respiratory modulation of sympathetic activity also occurs, and therefore might be playing a role in the variability of heart rate.

Beat-to-beat variability in R-R interval has been reported to be greatest during the first two postnatal weeks and at three and four months of age (Haddad *et al.*

1980, Gootman *et al.* 1987). During the first two weeks of life the beat-to-beat variability is greater in REM sleep than in quiet sleep (Haddad *et al.* 1980).

Use of spectral analysis techniques identified fluctuations in aortic pressure related to both the respiratory cycle and the cardiac (heart-rate) cycle in preterm infants (Bignall *et al.* 1987). Such fluctuations in aortic pressure reflect the changes in autonomic activity reported to occur in neonatal animals with both the respiratory and cardiac cycles (Gootman *et al.* 1984, 1987; Sica *et al.* 1990). Slower oscillations (circadian variation) in aortic pressure have also been reported in both fullterm (two to 26 hours old) and preterm (gestational age 33 to 36 weeks) infants (Kellerova *et al.* 1985). The drop in pressure was greatest at night with a magnitude change of the order of 9 to 10 per cent in term and 5 to 6 per cent in preterm infants. This difference in amplitude of oscillation was significant.

Heart-rate variability is shown to be greatest in healthy term infants and least in sick infants (note the fixed high heart rates of infants with respiratory distress syndrome). Thus examination of heart rate and heart-rate variability can be used to identify infants at risk for subsequent developmental problems, as well as the degree of distress of a sick infant, without any intervention other than recording heart rate and carrying out analyses of heart-rate variability (Waldman *et al.* 1979, Fox 1983).

Heart-rate responses

Changes in heart rate, and less frequently blood pressure, are the primary measure of autonomic reactions. An infant's response to various stimuli must be considered in the light of the 'law of initial value' (Lacey 1956). A low resting heart rate frequently leads to a greater than average response if the stimulus elicits an increase in heart rate. On the other hand, a decrease in heart rate would be smaller with the same resting heart rate (Lipton *et al.* 1960, 1961*a*,*b*; Vranekovic *et al.* 1974). This is one reason why different laboratories can report different responses. Physiological state (*e.g.* sleep, postprandial) also changes the resting heart rate as well as blood pressure. Thus state can affect the response pattern both by the 'law of initial value' and by level of arousal/attention of the infant to the stimulus.

Autonomic reflexes

The following reflexes have been examined by different investigators examining autonomic responses in neonates and infants to pharmacologic interventions, auditory stimulation, laryngeal stimuli, feeding, postural changes, crying, airstream stimulation, visual stimuli (including oculocardiac reflex), thermal stimulation, tactile stimulation and movement. The possible use of the galvanic skin response to different stimuli will be discussed.

PHARMACOLOGICAL INTERVENTIONS

Examination of the baroreceptor reflex in young infants and newborn animals has recently been reviewed (Gootman 1991). Use of Symth *et al.*'s (1969) technique to evaluate the properties of the baroreceptor reflex has involved calculating the change in heart rate (R-R interval) plotted against experimentally induced increases and decreases in arterial pressure. Arterial pressure is usually registered via an indwelling arterial line, *i.e.* radial artery catheter (Murat *et al.* 1988, 1989). Phenylephrine and nitroglycerin are used to increase and decrease pressure respectively. Dosage is adjusted to obtain changes in baseline arterial pressure of the order of 20 to 30 per cent. The slope of the graph between change in pressure and heart period is used as the estimate of baroreflex sensitivity. An intertrial period of five to 10 minutes is required to allow the blood pressure and heart rate to return to pretest values. The infants should be maintained in a consistent state and position to allow for comparisons. Murat *et al.* (1988) reported a mean pressor slope of 8.44 ± 2.05 and a mean depressor slope 2.54 ± 0.37 in 10 newborn infants. A later study showed greater variability in these values (Murat *et al.* 1989).

AUDITORY STIMULATION

In two- or three-day-old infants a 112dB 0.3ms rectangular click was used as a stimulus against a level of 55dB random noise. The interstimulus interval varied between 99 and 118s, and 110 stimuli were given in a 2½ hour session. These sessions occurred after feeding and 80 per cent of the time the neonates were asleep to normalise state (Schachter *et al.* 1971). These investigators noted that the neonates exhibited three patterns of heart-rate response to the click stimulus: (i) deceleration alone, (ii) acceleration alone, and (iii) a biphasic response consisting of initial deceleration and a subsequent acceleration. It appeared from these data of Schachter *et al.* (1971) that prestimulus resting heart rate was an important factor in the direction of response to the click stimulus.

Term infants less than three days old respond to an auditory stimulus with increases in heart rate averaging about 19bpm followed by rebound deceleration below baseline. Preterm infants with faster resting heart rate responded with smaller increases (Vranekovic *et al.* 1974). Lagercrantz *et al.* (1990) reported that preterm infants responded biphasically to an auditory stimulus. Of the 21 infants in the latter study, three did not respond to noise, three presented solely with bradycardia and three with tachycardia. Vranekovic *et al.* (1974) also reported that infants quicker to reach peak magnitude of heart-rate responses were less likely to present with large decelerations (below resting baseline). Furthermore, term females showed significantly greater accelerations than did either term or preterm males.

Fetal heart-rate responses to vibratory acoustic stimulation were reported to be an immediate increase of 8bpm which lasted for 10 minutes (Gagnon *et al.* 1988). The external vibratory acoustic stimulus was a 5s stimulus of white noise between 10HZ and 10kHZ with a maximum sound pressure level of 110dB, with maximum vibration occurring at 450HZ.

LARYNGEAL REFLEX

Laryngeal stimulation can be carried out by injecting small amounts (0.2 to 0.5ml) of test liquid such as saline at a fixed temperature (25°c) through a gavage tube inserted into the epipharynx through a nostril. The resulting change in respiration (apnoea) and heart-rate responses should be monitored for about 30s. The test should be repeated about three times (Lagercrantz *et al.* 1990).

The laryngeal stimulation is usually used to evaluate respiratory reflexes in neonates. Stimulation of laryngeal reflexes elicited apnoea, bradycardia, increase in blood pressure, peripheral vasoconstriction and blood flow redistribution (Gootman 1986*a*, 1991). The reflex has been implicated in conjunction with the diving reflex as a possible cause of sudden infant death syndrome (SIDS) (Gootman 1983, 1986*a*; Gootman *et al.* 1987). With examination of the laryngeal reflex in human preterm infants, the respiratory component (apnoea) was present; however Perkett and Vaughan (1982) reported the absence of a cardiac response, implying immaturity of the autonomic component of this reflex. On the other hand, Lagercrantz *et al.* (1990) reported bradycardia in all infants tested, although there was considerable variability in magnitude of bradycardia and duration of apnoea.

In term infants bradycardia and apnoea are particularly pronounced (Gootman, 1986*a*, 1991; Gootman *et al.* 1987). In preterm infants there was no significant change in heart rate with laryngeal stimulation (Perkett and Vaughan 1982, Wennergren *et al.* 1989). If the infants were hypoxic, however, the laryngeal reflex elicited a marked bradycardia. In fact, there was a significant correlation between duration of apnoea and degree of decreased heart rate to laryngeal stimulation.

FEEDING (SUCKING) RESPONSES

Feeding of babies by sucking elicited a significant increase in blood pressure and heart rate independent of age (Kellerova 1980). These increases were affected by mode of feeding (breast *vs* bottle). Breast-feeding increased systolic pressure by 12 per cent, diastolic by 13 per cent and heart rate by 14 per cent. Greater changes in cardiovascular function occurred with bottle-feeding (systolic pressure increased 23 per cent, diastolic pressure 26 per cent and heart rate 20 per cent) even though the baby was kept in the same posture. Shifting the baby to a semivertical position for bottle-feeding resulted in a three times greater increase in systolic (32 per cent) and diastolic (38 per cent) pressure with no difference in heart rate (Fig. 10.3).

On the other hand, Winter *et al.* (1966), studying a total of 135 healthy infants ranging in age from six hours to eight days, reported a significant cardiac deceleration in 50 of these infants. The feeding was carried out with the infants in a supine unrestrained position and they were bottle fed a 5 per cent glucose solution. Their criterion of significant change was a change in the average R-R interval of at least 0.1s. These authors eliminated from their data analysis any response which was <0.1s and classified these infants as no significant response. The cut-off of 100ms was chosen as the threshold for significant response because that timing would eliminate sinus arrhythmias as a complication.

Sucking has an additional effect at least partly mediated via an autonomic reflex pathway. Uvnas-Moberg *et al.* (1987) found that non-nutritive sucking on a

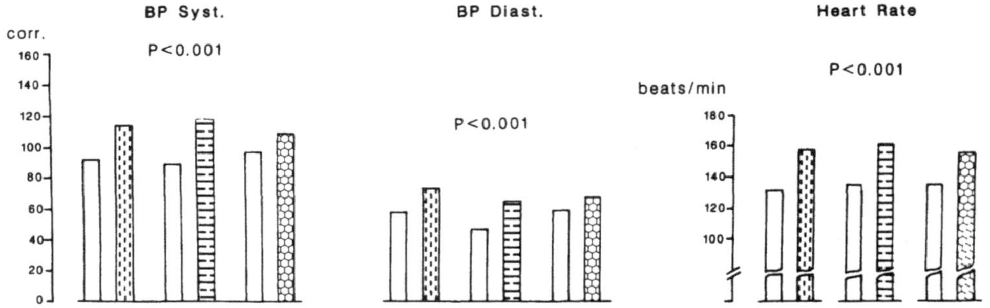

Fig. 10.3. Effects of feeding on arterial pressure and heart rate in 150 infants (mean age 10 weeks). *Open bars:* control values before feeding. *First set of bars:* bottle-feeding in supine position; *second set of bars:* bottle-feeding in semivertical position; *third set of bars:* breast-feeding. (After Kellerova 1981.)

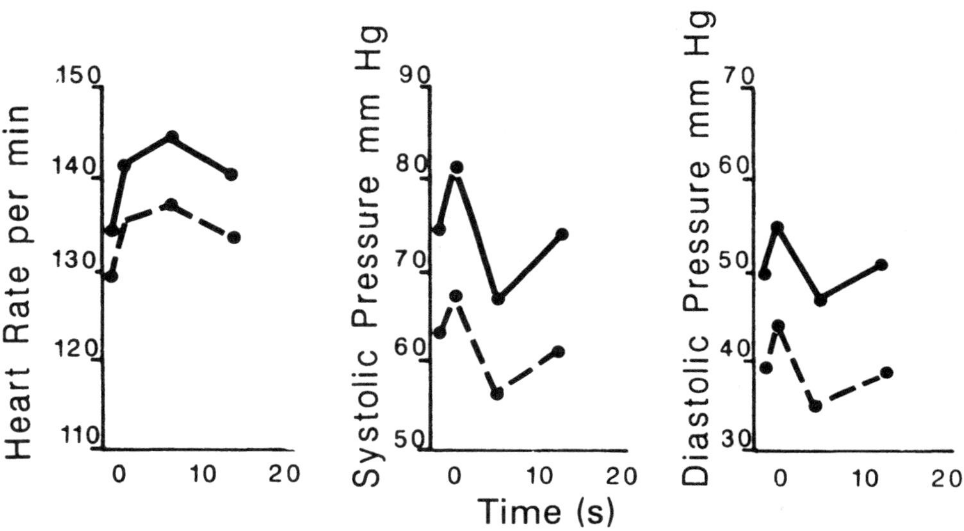

Fig. 10.4. Effects of a 70° head-up tilt on heart rate and blood pressure in 27 term (solid line) and 23 preterm (broken line) infants. (After Moss *et al.* 1963.)

pacifier activates sensory endings in the oral mucosa which result in release of vagally controlled GI hormones, gastrin and cholecystokinin. Insulin levels also rose significantly and somatostatin tended to fall. These results may contribute to the beneficial effects on maturation and growth caused by sensory stimulation.

POSTURAL CHANGES (TILT)

Contradictory reports concerning the effects of changing body position of the newborn have been obtained. In preterm infants a 45° tilt elicited no change in heart rate or blood pressure; however, there was an increase in peripheral resistance (Lagercrantz *et al.* 1990) as measured by volume changes in limbs (Whitney 1953). Waldman *et al.* (1979) reported an increase in peripheral vascular resistance, a 6 per cent fall in mean arterial pressure and no significant change in heart rate. Peripheral flow in the latter study was measured by venous occlusion plethysmography. When the same measurements were obtained in infants with respiratory distress (Waldman *et al.* 1979), the changes in vascular resistance and pressures were opposite to those in normal children. Kellerova (1985) obtained positive results in a head-up tilt of +45°. This laboratory reported a significant 14.6 per cent increase in systolic and a 25 per cent increase in diastolic pressure.

A 35 to 40° head-up tilt reduced right atrial and aortic mean pressure; in addition, the tilt reduced renal blood flow in newborn infants less than five days of age (Oh *et al.* 1966). Initially a slight increase in heart rate occurred during the first minute after the positional change, followed by a 2 to 6bpm decrease during the remainder of the observation period. Recovery from the head-up tilt to the recumbent position resulted initially in a slight increase in heart rate, followed by a similarly small decline in heart rate after the second minute (Oh *et al.* 1966).

Changing positions in 150 neonates (one to five days old) was reported to alter blood pressure: change to the prone position increased blood pressure by 14/9mmHg and to the ortho position by 10/7mmHg (Kellerova and Andrasyova 1990*a*).

A 70° head-up tilt was carried out with subjects secured to a circumcision board with the upper extremities restrained in flexion and the lower extremities in extension. The board was tilted over the edge of a table with the umbilical artery catheter tip located at the estimated level of the right atrium. Care was taken to fix the fulcrum at this level. Tilting was attained within 1s (Moss *et al.* 1963). These investigators studied 50 infants (27 term and 23 preterm) between one and 77 hours after birth, at time of study, and reported that heart rate increased in all infants. A small immediate increase in blood pressure was commonly observed but thought due to a reflection of the impact of the aortic column of blood upon the catheter. The initial increase was followed by a sharp drop in both systolic and diastolic pressure with a subsequent rapid return to the pretilt level. The investigators reported that the above pattern was observed in both term and preterm infants (Fig. 10.4).

In another study (Picton-Warlow and Mayer 1970), a 70 to 80° head-up tilt was carried out serially in 20 infants, aged between four hours and 12 days. Examinations were made on sleeping infants, half an hour postprandial, placed in a moulded foam-rubber pad on a hinged tabletop. The infants were supported by a sling under the axillae, leaving the thorax and abdomen unimpeded. Recordings in this study were made for three- or four-minute periods in each position and the tests repeated three to five times. Results were not included if a baby awoke or moved upon tilting. Heart rate was continuously recorded by cardiotachmeters. Systolic pressure was measured indirectly using a cuff and microphone and forearm blood flow by venous occlusion plethysmography. These investigators reported that on tilting to head-up position a small rise in pulse pressure occurred and was maintained until there was a rapid return to control level on resuming the supine position. Systolic pressure fell 3 to 8mmHg soon after tilting and remained at the lower level for the duration of observation period. Forearm blood flow always decreased. Respiratory rate slowed with tilting; the greater the decline in respiratory rate, the less marked was the cardiac acceleration. On the other hand, Young and Holland (1958) reported no change in systolic pressure with head-up tilt until infants were about four days old, although increases in heart rate were usually obtained.

The effect of stage of sleep on response to tilt was evaluated in 19 newborn infants (aged one to seven days) and 11 preterm infants (aged two to 19 days) by Finley *et al.* (1984). There was no significant difference in decrease in R-R interval for head-up tilt or increase in R-R interval for downward tilt between active (REM) and quiet sleep. Finley *et al.* (1984) reported that respiratory-rate changes were an important source of variability in the heart-rate responses to tilting, and were the likely source of previous inconsistencies. Tilt does not result in a change in aortic pressure in the normal adult, so the change in infants' blood pressure may reflect an immaturity of vasomotor regulation (Gootman 1983, 1991).

Upright tilt has been used in young children to elicit symptoms in patients with unexplained syncope; these patients presented with bradycardia and hypotension upon tilting (Pongiglione *et al.* 1990).

CRYING

Crying elicited an increase in blood pressure of 22/12mmHg (Kellerova and Andrasyova 1990*a*) in babies one to four days old, while Moss *et al.* (1963) reported that pressure rose from an average resting pressure of 64/39mmHg to 81/57mmHg in preterm infants and from 72/47 to 94/72mmHg in term infants. Young and Holland (1958) reported that there was no change in systolic pressure in infants one to three days of age; often rises of 20mmHg were observed after three days of age. However, crying regularly caused an increase in pulse rate of about 40bpm.

Thus there are different results concerning changes in blood pressure with crying in the first few days of age. In infants recovering from respiratory distress syndrome, prolonged crying led to significant decreases in inspiratory oesophageal pressure and a greater positive expiratory pressure (Dinwiddie *et al.* 1979). The mean age of infants at the time of the study was 66 hours old; pressures were recorded via indwelling umbilical artery catheters. Vigorous crying lasted 1½ minutes; crying was elicited by stimulating the infant's heel. These investigators reported a significant increase in heart rate of 19bpm and a progressive decline in systolic and diastolic blood pressure, following an initial increase in both pressures at the beginning of the strain.

AIRSTREAM STIMULATION

Abdominal airstream stimulation. Lipton *et al.* (1961*a*,*b*, 1966) examined responses to abdominal airstream stimulation from birth to five months of age. This method of stimulation involves a plastic cone taped above the umbilicus permitting an airstream stimulus of 1200g of pressure from a tank of compressed air or N_2 to be applied for 5s (Lipton *et al.* 1961*a*,*b*). They classify this type of stimulus as tactile (pressure) and, to a limited extent, as auditory. These investigators found that the heart-rate change to stimulation varied with the prestimulus control heart rate. No change or a decrease in rate was often associated with high prestimulus levels. These authors noted that the response pattern had changed significantly by 2½ months of age; there was a faster response, an attenuated initial rise in rate and generally a rebound below prestimulus levels.

Trigeminal airstream stimulation is another method used to elicit changes in autonomic activity in infants (one to three days, and four, eight, 12 and 16 weeks of age) as reflected by heart-rate responses (Allen *et al.* 1979). After placing a length of flexible plastic tubing (internal diameter 4.0mm) into the nostrils, short 2s streams of air (flow rate 15 l/min.) warmed to 24°. These investigators used five stimuli with 30s epochs, *i.e.* interstimulus intervals of 28s. The usual response was an acceleration of heart rate. This response was reported to depend on prestimulus heart rate and to a lesser degree on post-conceptional age (PCA). A small number of infants (<0.1 per cent) presented with a sudden bradycardia. In these cases a diving response may have been elicited (Gootman 1991).

Ramet *et al.* (1990) modified the methodology of Allen *et al.* (1979) by delivering the airstream stimulation through two parallel short plastic tubes inside both nostrils. The common proximal end of the tubing was connected to a pneumotachograph that ensured precise recording of onset and offset of airstream stimulation. Ramet *et al.* (1990) studied 33 preterm and term infants (PCA 31.5 to 50 weeks) (gestational age, GA, ranged from 26.5 to 40.5 weeks); postnatal age at time of study was five to 76 days. These investigators performed their testing during REM sleep and at least two hours postprandial. The stimulus was applied for 10 seconds. The R-R interval and duration of the total respiratory cycle changes during the stimulus were compared to the preceding 60s mean R-R interval and duration of respiratory cycle in each infant. Preterm infants responded to airstream stimulation with deceleration of heart rate and prolongation of the total respiratory cycle. The term infants' responses were limited; some responded with slight acceleration, as previously reported by Allen *et al.* (1979). The cardiac and respiratory responses significantly declined with postnatal age.

VISUAL SYSTEM STIMULATION

Studies of visual stimuli, using 12 trials of a 30s flashing light pattern with interstimulus intervals of 30s, suggest a consistent pattern of response, *i.e.* bradycardia. The magnitude of the bradycardia was greater the longer the infant fixed on the visual stimulus (Lewis *et al.* 1966, 1967; Hirschman and Katkin 1974).

The *oculocardiac reflex*, elicited by pressure on the eyeball, can be demonstrated in preterm and term newborn and older infants (Lipton *et al.* 1965). It has been further reported that the reflex is more easily elicited in younger children (less than five years of age). Of 73 preterm newborn infants, bradycardia could be elicited in 90 per cent of the healthy babies. However, when the same reflex was examined in infants with respiratory distress syndrome, only 59 per cent responded. Furthermore, the magnitudes of the heart-rate response were significantly reduced (Javorka *et al.* 1983). Sapire and Casta (1985) have successfully used this reflex in their diagnosis of increased vagal tone as the underlying cause of syncopal attacks in infants as young as two weeks of age as well as in older children.

A recent study used a standardised ocular compression test (Ramet *et al.* 1988) in which a water-filled pressure sensor with an 18mm external diameter was placed on a sleeping infant's eyelid just before testing. The pressor sensor was connected to a pressure transducer and the applied pressure recorded on a polygraph along with other variables. Mean and SD of the manually applied pressure, monitored via the water-filled sensors, was 103 ± 9mmHg. A 10s square wave stimulus was employed with identical pressure applied to both eyes. To standardise the state of infants, all were asleep on their backs and testing was carried out an hour postprandial. Ramet *et al.* (1988) reported that the reflex bradycardia was related to PCA; considerable blunting of the response was reported with maturation.

Adrenergic response of the iris of the neonate. The response of the dilator pupillae muscle to direct and indirectly acting sympathetic amines can be studied using a photograph technique (Lind *et al.* 1971). Photographs of the infants' eyes are obtained using a 35mm camera with the focal length of the camera fixed, giving constant magnification when the eye is in focus. The film is then projected to obtain a final magnification level of approximately ×15. The change in pupil diameter 30 minutes after instillation is then expressed as percentage of the original diameter of the pupil studied in each infant. One drop (0.2ml) of the drug under investigation was instilled into the conjunctival sac (phenylephrine, 5.0 per cent, hydroxyamphetamine hydrobromide, 1.0 per cent, tyramine hydrochloride, 2.0 per cent, adrenaline bitartrate, 1.0 per cent). Lind *et al.* (1971) reported a significant mydriasis to phenylephrine in all infants with wide variation between subjects. While there was no correlation with GA, a significant correlation was found between percentage of mydriasis and birthweight in infants studied within one to three days of birth. Adrenaline produced no mydriasis in six infants including the youngest. This technique has been used to identify patients with familial dysautonomia.

THERMAL STIMULATION

Cold. One cold face test (CFT), frequently used to test parasympathetic regulation of heart rate, is to take an ice cube placed within a thin plastic bag and apply to the baby's forehead for 20 seconds at least three to five times with interstimulus intervals of at least one minute (Lagercrantz *et al.* 1990). In these studies on 21 preterm infants (25 to 37 weeks PCA) one to 11 days after birth, bradycardia occurred only in the presence of apnoea. Seven infants did not respond at all or were aroused. The trigeminal CFT (*i.e.* cold applied to cheek) was examined in 73 preterm newborn infants. It was found that bradycardia could be elicited in 90 per

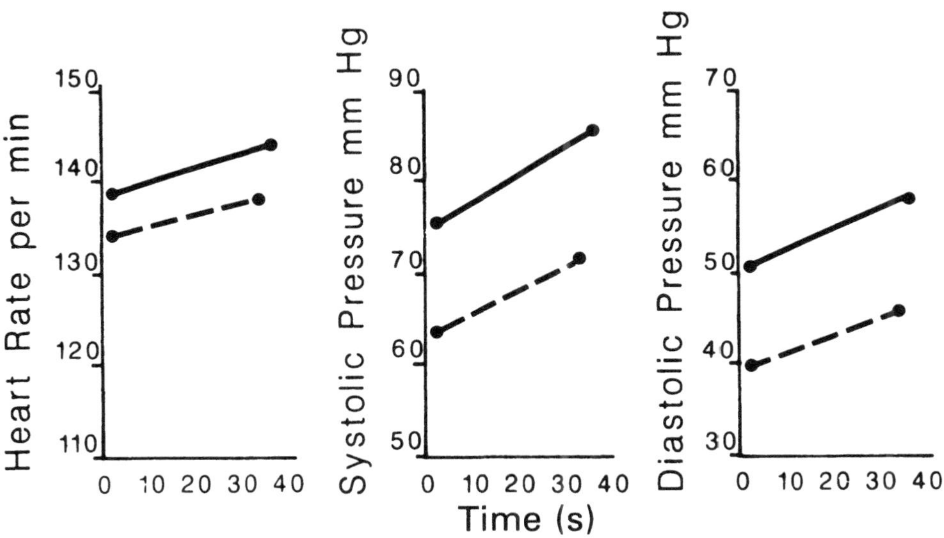

Fig. 10.5. Effects of cold pressor test on blood pressure and heart rate in 29 term (solid line) and 17 preterm (broken line) infants. (After Moss *et al.* 1963.)

cent of the healthy preterm babies. However, when the same reflex was examined in infants with respiratory distress syndrome, only 59 per cent responded (Javorka *et al.* 1983). Furthermore, the magnitudes of the heart-rate response were significantly reduced.

More elaborate cold water stimulation was used to terminate supraventricular tachycardia in a 14-day-old infant. The infant's face was placed into a basin of ice water at 5°c for five seconds with nostrils manually occluded to prevent aspiration (Hamilton *et al.* 1979). This method was successful in terminating the tachycardia where carotid massage and unilateral eyeball pressure were not.

The cold pressor test used by Moss *et al.* (1963) on 113 newborn infants (age at study range from one to 77 hours) involved immersing a foot to the level of the ankle in 4 to 5°c ice cold water for a period of one minute. These investigators directly measured arterial pressure through a catheter placed in one of the umbilical arteries. Since the initial response of all infants involved discomfort as reflected by crying, one to three pretest immersions at one-minute intervals were made until all signs of discomfort had disappeared. Moss *et al.* (1963) reported an increase in heart rate and both systolic and diastolic pressure in 80 per cent of term and 88 per cent of preterm infants (Fig. 10.5).

Heat. Another thermal test involves wrapping the infant in blankets with a lower extremity exposed to externally applied warmth (Lindqvist *et al.* 1983, Lindqvist 1990). Small preterm infants can be studied in incubators. The foot up to the ankle is placed into the jet stream of an air blower. Heart rate was monitored for one control period and for four seven-minute stimulation periods. The warm air was blown at different frequencies (0.083, 0.100, 0.042 and 0.025Hz). The warm and cool periods of the thermal stimulation were of equal duration. In these infants the heart rate was measured and heart-rate variability determined. Using power spectral analysis, Lindqvist (1990) noted a distinct and dominant peak in the heart-rate variability of the thermally stimulated power spectra corresponding to the frequency of the stimulus frequency (Fig. 10.2).

TACTILE STIMULATION

Tactile stimulation was used to examine the importance of level of arousal on the heart-rate response (Lewis *et al.* 1967). Such stimulation consisted of a calibrated series of 20 nylon filaments which were applied to the corner of the infant's mouth and run back towards the upper angle of the ear. The stimuli were presented in a monotonically increasing order and lasted approximately one second, with inter-trial intervals of 15 to 25 seconds.

Miscellaneous causes of changes in heart rate

A variety of different normal physiologic functions result in alterations in autonomic outflow such that changes in heart rate can be noticed. *Bowel evacuation* has been identified with both intermittent respiratory pauses and bradycardia. Lipton *et al.* (1964) recorded a 50 per cent decrease in heart rate in a five-month-old infant. They reported a characteristic drop in heart rate with *diaphragmatic spasms* (hiccup). A degree of bradycardia was also reported to occur with a *yawn* (large deep inspiratory effort). Lipton *et al.* (1965) also reported that *nasogastric intubation* in preterm infants would often evoke a marked bradycardia.

BODY MOVEMENTS

Motor restraint by the age-old technique of swaddling was used by Lipton *et al.* (1965) to standardise the position and behavioural state of infants in their various studies. They documented that swaddling reduced heart rate as well as body movement, and often promptly quieted the infant. A more recent study correlating body movements and heart rate employed the static charge-sensitive bed method of recordings (Erkinjuntti and Kero 1990). These investigators reported a heart-rate acceleration response to body movement with a deceleration at the end of the movements in healthy newborns. On the other hand, brain-damaged infants showed abnormal heart-rate acceleration/deceleration response patterns to body movement during sleep (Erkinjuntti and Kero 1990). They had weak deceleration responses at the end of minor movements and significantly greater increases in heart rate in response to major body movements compared with normal infants.

Electrodermal response system

A frequently used test of autonomic function in the adult involves evaluation of the changes in skin electrical resistance (galvanic skin response) to various stimuli (*e.g.* the Valsalva manoeuvre, psychic stimuli) which is considered to reflect changes in sympathetic activity innervating sweat glands, myoepithelial cells and cutaneous vessels (Bannister 1988, Ionescu-Tirgoviste and Pruna 1990). Such tests in infants have been relatively infrequent, presumably because of the complication of body movement causing false positive responses. The limited number of studies were reviewed by Hirschman and Katkin (1974). Their conclusion was that, even with the complicating factor of body movement, the neonate in the first three days of life was capable of showing a discrete electrodermal response to visual, auditory and tactile stimuli. These studies should be repeated perhaps with the equipment of the type developed by Ionescu-Tirgoviste and Pruna (1990) which is more sensitive and permits accurate individualisation of the evoked response as well as monitoring resting oscillations of the cutaneous bioelectrical activity.

Estimation of over-all autonomic reflex activity

Recently Lagercrantz *et al.* (1990) developed an arbitrary method for estimating over-all autonomic reflex responses for a given child. This score is based on calculations of multiple responses recorded in the various tests. It also requires an assumption that the direction of change in variable to a particular test is due to a change in either sympathetic (and given a + sign) or parasympathetic (– sign) discharge. Peripheral vascular resistance (PVR) (obtained from peripheral blood-flow using occlusion plethysmography) and change PVR (dPVR) during tilting and tachycardia response to noise were taken as variables of sympathetic activity and given + signs; decrease of heart rate during CFT, laryngeal reflex stimulation (LR) and bradycardia noise response (BNR) were taken as variables of parasympathetic function and given – signs. Individual responses were divided by the median response from a group of infants. The score was calculated according to the following formula:

PVR/median PVR + dPVR during tilting/median dPVR + TNR/median TNR
– (minus) CFT/median CFT – LR/median LR – BNR/median BNR.

This score represents an attempt to consolidate data from different tests and a variety of measured responses. The idea is an excellent effort to integrate the various factors. However, to arbitrarily assign a pattern of response to one or another subdivision of the ANS may lead to rigid interpretation of responses. Since usually changes in both divisions of the ANS contribute to a pattern of response, this type of consolidation would tend to fix response patterns as due solely to one subdivision or the other.

Diseases involving the ANS in neonates and infants

Two ANS developmental disorders which illustrate ontogenetic aberrations of neural crest cells are familial dysautonomia and Hirschsprung's disease.

Familial dysautonomia (Riley–Day syndrome)

Familial dysautonomia was described in 1949 by Riley and his colleagues (Riley 1957, Axelrod *et al.* 1974). Evidence to date suggests that the disease has autosomal recessive inheritance since more than 90 per cent of patients have been Jews of Ashkenazi extraction and the disease tends to occur in siblings rather than successive generations. While the majority of patients are Jewish, it has been reported to occur in other races, including a possible case in a Japanese child. However, the fact that the disease is essentially confined to Ashkenazi Jews suggests that it is due to an altered single mutant allele at one gene locus (Hamill and LaGamma 1988).

The patients are usually children and are liable to frequent infections. The disturbances of the ANS are manifested by lability of the blood pressure with both paroxysmal hypertension and orthostatic hypotension. Other evidence of sympathetic failure may include blotching of the skin, abnormal temperature regulation, excessive sweating, reduction or absence of tear production, and alterations of gastrointestinal function, *e.g.* diarrhoea or constipation, abnormal oesophageal motility, vomiting and aspiration pneumonia. Other types of neurological involvement, such as insensitivity to pain, have also been reported to occur in dysautonomia. There are abnormalities of catecholamine metabolism, including reduced plasma dopamine-beta-hydroxylase activity and norepinephrine sensitivity (Weinshilboum and Axelrod 1971, Freedman *et al.* 1972). A defect in the formation, storage or release of ACh has been postulated. There is no specific treatment for the disease and most children die from infection, although some patients survive into early adult life (Axelrod *et al.* 1987).

FAMILIAL DYSAUTONOMIA IN NEONATES

To date no specific pattern of neonatal signs of familial dysautonomia has been identified (Axelrod *et al.* 1987). The only documented sign of autonomic dysfunction reported for the neonatal period was the occurrence of hypothermia. Signs of autonomic dysfunctions such as excessive sweating, and skin mottling and absence of tears appear after one month of age (Axelrod *et al.* 1987). However, Kaplan *et al.* (1985) suggested using a histamine test performed with 1:10,000 histamine solution. Because the histamine test was unequivocally positive (weal present without a flare response), a diagnosis of familial dysautonomia was made in their patients who were noted to be extremely lethargic, refused to feed, cried weakly, sucked poorly and were extremely hypotonic. This type of investigation needs to be extended, given the importance of early diagnosis of these children.

Autonomic diseases affecting the gastrointestinal system

There are a variety of congenital diseases implicating the neural supply to the GI tract. The symptoms include poor suck, achalasia and megacolon. Diagnosis is based upon biopsy or autopsy. Treatment includes waiting because the symptoms may subside satisfactorily in several weeks when due to pharyngo-oesophageal inco-ordination (Ferguson 1971), or removal of the affected portion of gut when due to Hirschsprung's disease (Ehrenpreis 1971). If severe and extensive enough, the infant will die.

HIRSCHSPRUNG'S DISEASE

Hirschsprung's disease is a congenital disorder characterised by the absence of ganglion cells in the enteric nervous system (*i.e.* Auerbach's and Meissner's plexi), usually within the distal colon. It is thought to be caused by the interruption of caudal migration of neuroblasts. During early intrauterine life, neuroblasts enter the cranial part of the alimentary tube and migrate aborally forming the plexuses. Classic symptoms include failure to pass meconium during first 24 hours, vomiting, diarrhoea, obstipation, abdominal distention and poor feeding (Burrington and Wayne 1976). However, frequently the disease is not diagnosed early in the neonatal period so that complications such as perforation of the bowel and septicaemia occur. Recently prenatal sonography has been successfully employed to diagnose Hirschsprung's disease (Vermesh *et al.* 1986). More commonly, the results of biopsy can determine the necessity and degree of resection of the bowel. The affected areas are usually devoid of ganglion cells although large external nerve bundles may be present.

FAMILIAL ACHALASIA

Achalasia has been reported in children and may be more common than generally suspected (Ferguson 1971, Monnig 1990). A familial occurrence has been reported, suggesting that it may be transmitted as an autosomal recessive trait. The symptoms include swallowing difficulties (especially with solid food), spitting up after eating and/or at night; respiratory symptoms include cough, wheeze and pneumonia (Ferguson 1971). Treatment has frequently involved surgery: specifically, a transthoracic modified Heller procedure (oesophagogastromyotomy) (Monnig 1990).

Sudden infant death syndrome

This catch-all syndrome for sudden death of infants with no known cause reaches peak incidence between three and six months of age. A controversy as to the mode of death in SIDS continues to this day. While originally thought to be respiratory arrest, other investigators have implicated a cardiac component including imbalance of sympathetic innervation of the heart (Gootman 1983, 1991; Gootman *et al.* 1987; Schwartz *et al.* 1988; Willinger 1989). A variety of factors probably play a role in the etiology of SIDS. Given the documented interactions between respiratory regulation and autonomic outflow, it is possible that a failure within the brainstem regulatory systems results in failure of ongoing regulation of respiration and cardiac control.

Long QT syndrome

Syncope and sudden death due to ventricular fibrillation are manifestations of the condition known as long QT syndrome or Romano-Ward syndrome (Schwartz *et al.* 1975, Schwartz 1981, Vincent 1986, Gootman *et al.* 1987, Wilton and Hantler 1987). The literature to date suggests that the underlying cause of this syndrome is an imbalance of the sympathetic innervation of the heart, such that left cardiac sympathetic activity dominates. Whether the dominance is due to left side overactivity or right cardiac sympathetic underactivity is not known. However, lower than normal resting heart rate and ventricular arrhythmias suggest decreased function of sympathetic innervation on the right. This could result from an imbalance of innervation or from diminished activity due to abnormalities in brainstem regulation of sympathetic outflow.

Reflex sympathetic dystrophy in children

Reflex sympathetic dystrophy syndrome has long been considered to be rare in children, but a number of recent reports have suggested that it may be under-reported in this age group (Dietz *et al.* 1990). In the majority of cases there was dysesthesia, vasomotor instability and swelling of the affected area. Vasomotor instability must be present for the diagnosis of reflex sympathetic dystrophy to be made. Vasomotor instability most commonly presented as discoloration, temperature differences between adjacent skin regions and an erythematous line 15 to 30s after stroking the affected area with a blunt object and comparing response with the unaffected limb. In children the sympathetic dystrophy tended to affect the legs in at least 80 per cent of reported cases. The pathophysiology of reflex sympathetic dystrophy and causalgia involves both peripheral and central mechanisms that remain incompletely understood.

Summary

Variability in pulse interval (heart rate) occurs substantially with respiration, sleep stage and age. Such findings indicate developmental changes in heart-rate regulation and are a reflection of the postnatal maturation of ANS regulation of cardiovascular function (Katona *et al.* 1980; Gootman 1983, 1991; Hathorn 1987; Äärimaa *et al.* 1988; Äärimaa and Välimäki 1988; Baldzer *et al.* 1989). Thus autonomic responses to certain stimuli may be present in term infants (*e.g.* tilt), diminished in preterm infants (*e.g.* laryngeal stimulation), or delayed and develop postnatally (Gootman 1991). Some reflex responses apparently diminish with postnatal maturation (*e.g.* tilt). Finally, testing of autonomic function in the neonate and both term and preterm infant is more difficult than in the older child or adult due to the inability of the infant to co-operate during the testing. Therefore choice of test employed, stability of state and repetition of the stimulus are essential for confirmation of findings.

The authors would like to acknowledge the library research of Ms Karen Ambrowitz and Mr Clement Medford. This chapter was supported by National Institutes of Health Grants from the National Heart, Lung and Blood Institute (HL-20864) and from the National Institute of Child Health and Human Development (HD-28931).

REFERENCES

Äärimaa, T., Oja, R., Antila, K., Välimäki, I. (1988) 'Interaction of heart rate and respiration in newborn babies.' *Pediatric Research*, **24**, 745–750.

—— Välimäki, I.A.T. (1988) 'Spectral analysis of impedance respirogram in newborn infants.' *Biology of the Neonate*, **54**, 188–194.

Akselrod, S., Gordon, D., Ubel, F.A., Shannon, D.C., Barger, A.C., Cohen, R.J. (1981) 'Power spectrum analysis of heart rate fluctuation: a quantitative probe of beat-to-beat cardiovascular control.' *Science*, **213**, 220–222.

Allen, L.G., Howard, G., Smith, J.B., McCubbin, J.A., Weaver, R.L. (1979) 'Infant heart rate response to trigeminal airstream stimulation: determination of normal and deviant values.' *Pediatric Research*, **13**, 184–187.

Axelrod, F.B., Nachtigal, R., Dancis, J. (1974) 'Familial dysautonomia: diagnosis, pathogenesis and management.' *Advances in Pediatrics*, **21**, 75–96.

—— Porges, R.F., Sein, M.E. (1987) 'Neonatal recognition of familial dysautonomia.' *Journal of Pediatrics*, **110**, 946–948.

Baldzer, K., Dykes, F.D., Jones, S.A., Brogan, M., Carrigan, T.A., Giddens, D.P.P. (1989) 'Heart rate variability analysis in full-term infants: spectral indices for study of neonatal cardiorespiratory control.' *Pediatric Research*, **26**, 188–195.

Bannister, R. (1988) *Autonomic Failure. A Textbook of Clinical Disorders of the Autonomic Nervous System, 2nd Edn.* New York: Oxford University Press.

Bergstrom, B., Lilja, B., Rosberg, K., Sundkvist, G. (1986) 'Autonomic nerve function tests. Reference values in healthy subjects.' *Clinical Physiology*, **6**, 523–528.

Bignall, S., Rivers, R.P.A., Lissauer, T.J. (1987) 'Spectral analysis of aortic blood pressure and cerebral blood flow velocity in premature infants.' *Journal of Physiology*, **390**, 213P.

Black, I.B. (1978) 'Regulation of autonomic development.' *Annual Review of Neuroscience*, **1**, 183–214.

Bornstein, J.C., Costa, M., Furness, J.B. (1988) 'Intrinsic and extrinsic inhibitory synaptic inputs to submucous neurones of the guinea-pig small intestine.' *Journal of Physiology*, **398**, 371–390.

Bowes, W.A., Gabbe, S.G., Bowes, C. (1980) 'Fetal heart rate monitoring in premature infants weighing 1,500 grams or less.' *American Journal of Obstetrics and Gynecology*, **137**, 791–796.

Burrington, J.D., Wayne, E.R. (1976) 'Modified Duhamel procedure for treatment of total aganglionic colon in childhood.' *Journal of Pediatric Surgery*, **11**, 391–398.

Cagnoni, M., Tarquini, B., Halberg, F., Marz, W., Cornelissen, G., Mainardi, G., Panero, C., Shinoda, M., Scarpelli, P., Roman, S., Bingham, C., Hellbrugge, T. (1987) 'Circadian variability of blood pressure and heart rate in newborns and cardiovascular chronorisk.' *In* Pauly, J.E., Scheving, L.E. (Eds) *Advances in Chronobiology, Part B.* New York: Alan R. Liss. pp. 145–151.

Chiba, T. (1978) 'Monoamine fluorescence and electron microscopic studies on small intensity fluorescent (granule-containing) cells in human sympathetic ganglia.' *Journal of Comparative Neurology*, **179**, 153–168.

Cochard, P., Le Douarin, N.M. (1982) 'Development of the intrinsic innervation of the gut.' *Scandinavian Journal of Gastroenterology*, **17** (Suppl. 71), 1–14.

Cohen, W.R., Yeh, S.-Y. (1986) 'The abnormal fetal heart rate baseline.' *Clinical Obstetrics and Gynecology*, **29**, 73–82.

Contis, G., Lind, J. (1963) 'Study of systolic blood pressure, heart rate, body temperature of normal newborn infants through the first week of life.' *Acta Paediatrica Scandinavica*, Suppl., **146**, 41–47.

Dawes, G.S., Moulden, M., Redman, C.W.G. (1990) 'Criteria for the design of fetal heart rate analysis sytems.' *International Journal of Biomedical Computing*, **25**, 287–294.

DeGroat, W.C., Booth, A.M. (1980) 'Inhibition and facilitation in parasympathetic ganglia of the urinary bladder.' *Federation Proceedings*, **39**, 2990–2996.

—— —— (1984) 'Autonomic systems to the urinary bladder and sexual organs.' *In* Dyck, P.J., Thomas, P.K., Lambert, E.H., Bunge, R. (Eds) *Peripheral Neuropathies.* Philadelphia: W.B. Saunders. pp. 285–299.

de Swiet, M., Fayers, P., Shinebourne, E.A. (1980) 'Systolic blood pressure in a population of infants in the first year of life: the Brompton study.' *Pediatrics*, **65**, 1028–1035.

Dietz, F.R., Mathews, K.D., Montgomery, W.J. (1990) 'Reflex sympathetic dystrophy in children.' *Clinical Orthopaedics and Related Research*, **258**, 225–231.

Dinwiddie, R., Pitcher-Wilmott, R., Schwartz, J.G., Shaffer, T.H., Fox, W.W. (1979) 'Cardiopulmonary changes in the crying neonate.' *Pediatric Research*, **13**, 900–903.
Eckberg, D.L. (1980) 'Parasympathetic cardiovascular control in human disease: a critical review of methods and results.' *American Journal of Physiology*, **239**, H581–H593.
Ehrenpreis, T. (1971) 'Hirschsprung's disease.' *Digestive Diseases*, **16**, 1032–1052.
Eränkö, L., Päivärinta, H., Soinila, S., Häppölä, O. (1986) 'Transmitters and modulators in superior cervical ganglion of the rat.' *Medical Biology*, **64**, 75–83.
Eränkö, O. (1976) *SIF Cells. Structure and Function of the Small Intensely Fluorescent Cells.* DHEW Publication No. NIH 76–942. Washington: US Government Printing Office.
Erkinjuntti, M., Kero, P. (1990) 'Pathological heart rate responses associated with body movements in neurologically damaged infants during sleep.' *Acta Paediatrica Scandinavica*, **79**, 558–562.
Falconer, A.D., Poyser, L.M. (1986) 'Fetal sympatho-adrenal mediated metabolic responses to parturition.' *British Journal of Obstetrics and Gynaecology*, **93**, 747–753.
Ferguson, C.F. (1971) 'Esophageal dysfunction and other swallowing difficulties in early life.' *Annals of Otology, Rhinology and Laryngology*, **80**, 541–548.
Finley, J.P., Hamilton, R., MacKenzie, M.G. (1984) 'Heart rate response to tilting in newborns in quiet and active sleep.' *Biology of the Neonate*, **45**, 1–10.
—— Nugent, S.T., Hellenbrand, W. (1987) 'Heart rate variability in children. Spectral analysis of developmental changes between 5 and 24 years.' *Canadian Journal of Physiology and Pharmacology*, **65**, 2048–2052.
Fox, N.A. (1983) 'Maturation of autonomic control in preterm infants.' *Developmental Psychobiology*, **16**, 495–504.
Freedman, L.S., Ohuchi, T., Goldstein, M., Axelrod, F., Fish, I., Dancis, J. (1972) 'Changes in human serum dopamine-β-hydroxylase activity with age.' *Nature*, **236**, 310–311.
Freire-Maia, L., Azevedo, A.D. (1990) 'The autonomic nervous system is not a purely efferent system.' *Medical Hypothesis*, **32**, 91–99.
Gabella, G. (1979) 'Innervation of the gastrointestinal tract.' *International Review of Cytology*, **59**, 129–193.
Gagnon, R., Hunse, C., Carmichael, L., Fellows, F., Patrick, J. (1988) 'Fetal heart rate and fetal activity patterns after vibratory acoustic stimulation at thirty to thirty-two weeks gestational age.' *American Journal of Obstetrics and Gynecology*, **158**, 75–79.
Gershon, M.D., Payette, R.F., Rothman, T. F. (1983) 'Development of the enteric nervous system.' *Federation Proceedings*, **42**, 1620–1625.
Giacobini, E. (1986) 'Development of peripheral parasympathetic neurons and synapses.' *In* Gootman, P.M. (Ed.) *Developmental Neurobiology of the Autonomic Nervous System.* New Jersey: Humana Press. pp. 29–67.
Gootman, P.M. (1983) 'Postnatal development of central nervous regulation of cardiovascular function.' *In* Gootman, N., Gootman, P.M. (Eds) *Perinatal Cardiovascular Function.* New York: Marcel Dekker. pp. 265–328.
—— (1986*a*) *Developmental Neurobiology of the Autonomic Nervous System.* New Jersey: Humana Press.
—— (1986*b*) 'Development of central autonomic regulation of cardiovascular function.' *In* Gootman, P.M. (Ed.) *Developmental Neurobiology of the Autonomic Nervous System.* New Jersey: Humana Press. pp. 279–325.
—— (1986*c*) 'Cardiovascular regulation in developing swine.' *In* Tumbleson, M.E. (Ed.) *Swine in Biomedical Research.* New York: Plenum. pp. 1161–1178.
—— (1991) 'Developmental aspects of reflex control of the circulation.' *In* Gilmore, J.P., Zucker, I.H. (Eds) *Reflex Control of the Circulation.* Boca Raton, FL: CRC Press. pp. 965–1027.
—— Cohen, H.L., DiRusso, S.M., Rudell, A.P., Eberle, L.P. (1984) 'Characteristics of spontaneous efferent splanchnic discharge in neonatal swine.' *In* Usdin, E., Dahlstrom, A., Engel, J., Carlsson, A. (Eds) *Catecholamines. Part A: Basic and Peripheral Mechanisms.* New York: Alan R. Liss. pp. 369–374.
—— —— Gootman, N. (1987) 'Autonomic nervous system regulation of heart rate in the perinatal period.' *In* Lieberman, J., Plonsety, R., Rudy, Y. (Eds) *Pediatric and Fundamental Electrocardiography.* The Hague: Martinus Nijhoff. pp. 137–159.
—— Sica, A.L., Steele, A.M., Cohen, H.L., Griswold, P.G., Gandhi, M.R., Eberle, L.P., Hundley,

B.W. (1988) 'Spontaneous efferent preganglionic sympathetic (SYMP) activity in neonatal swine.' *In* Dahlstrom, A., Belmaker, R.H., Sandler, M. (Eds) *Progress in Catecholamine Research, Part A: Basic Aspects and Peripheral Mechanisms.* New York: Alan R. Liss. pp. 449–453.

Greengard, P., Kebabian, J.W. (1974) 'Role of cyclic AMP in synaptic transmission in the mammalian peripheral nervous system.' *Federation Proceedings*, **33**, 1059–1067.

Haddad, G.G., Epstein, R.A., Epstein, M.A.F., Leistner, H.L., Mellins, R.B. (1980) 'The R-R interval and R-R variability in normal infants during sleep.' *Pediatric Research*, **14**, 809–811.

Hall, P.S., Thomas, S.A., Friedmann, E., Lynch, J.J. (1982) 'Measurement of neonatal blood pressure: a new method.' *Psychophysiology*, **19**, 231–236.

Hamill, R.W., LaGamma, E. (1988) 'Autonomic nervous system development.' *In* Bannister, R. (Ed.) *Autonomic Failure. A Textbook of Clinical Disorders of the Autonomic Nervous System. 2nd Edn.* New York: Oxford University Press. pp. 23–43.

Hamilton, J., Moodie, D., Levy, J. (1979) 'The use of the diving reflex to terminate supraventricular tachycardia in a 2-week-old infant.' *American Heart Journal*, **97**, 371–374.

Hathorn, M.K.S. (1987) 'Respiratory sinus arrythmias in new-born infants.' *Journal of Physiology*, **385**, 1–12.

Heaton, N.D., Garrett, J.R., Howard, E.R. (1988) 'The enteric nervous system: structure and pathology.' *In* Bannister, R. (Ed.) *Autonomic Failure. A Textbook of Clinical Disorders of the Autonomic Nervous System. 2nd Edn.* New York: Oxford University Press. pp. 238–263.

Hirschman, R., Katkin, E.S. (1974) 'Psychophysiological functioning, arousal, attention and learning during the first year of life.' *Advances in Child Development and Behaviour*, **9**, 115–150.

Ionescu-Tirgoviste, C., Pruna, S. (1990) 'Quantitative noninvasive electrophysiological evaluation of the activity of the cutaneous division of the sympathetic nervous system.' *Archives Internationales de Physiologie et de Biochimie*, **98**, 111–119.

Javorka, K., Zavarska, L., Tomori, Z. (1983) 'Some cardiorespiratory reflexes in newborns.' *Bulletin of European Physiopathyology Research*, **19**, 42P.

Kaijser, L. (1986) 'Autonomic nerve function tests—need for standardization?' *Clinical Physiology*, **6**, 475–479.

Kanerva, L., Hervonen, A. (1976) 'SIF cells, short adrenergic neurons and vacuolated nerve cells of the paracervical (Frankenhouser) ganglion.' *In* Eranko, O. (Ed.) *SIF Cells. Structure and Function of the Small Intensely Fluorescent Cells.* DHEW Publication No. NIH 76-942. Washington: US Government Printing Office.

Kaplan, M., Schiffman, R., Shapira, Y. (1985) 'Diagnosis of familial dysautonomia in the neonatal period.' *Acta Paediatrica Scandinavica*, **74**, 131–132.

Katona, P.G., Frasz, A., Egbert, J. (1980) 'Maturation of cardiac control in full-term and preterm infants during sleep.' *Early Human Development*, **4**, 145–159.

Kellerova, E. (1981) 'Physiological responses of blood pressure and heart rate in neonate and infants.' *In* Kovach, A.G.B., Sandor, P., Kollai, M. (Eds) *Advances in Physiological Science, Vol. 9. Cardiovascular Physiology, Neural Control Mechanisms.* Budapest: Pergamon. pp. 367–375.

—— (1985) 'Physiological aspects of blood pressure development in early life of term and premature infants.' *Ergebnisse der Experimental Medizin*, **46**, 314–319.

—— Javorka, K., Zavarska, L. (1985) 'Circadian variation of blood pressure in term and premature neonates.' *Physiologia Bohemoslovaca*, **34**, 263.

—— Andrasyova, D. (1990*a*) 'Physiological factors influencing the blood pressure in neonates.' *Journal of Hypertension*, Suppl. 3, S129.

—— —— (1990*b*) 'Normal blood pressure values and physiologic factors of their variability in neonates.' *Bratislavske Lekarske Listy*, **91**, 241–246.

Kissel, P., Andre, J.M., Jacquier, A. (1981) *The Neuroscristopathies.* Chicago, IL: Year Book Medical.

Kogner, P., Bjork, O., Theodorsson, E. (1990) 'Neuropeptide Y as a marker in pediatric neuroblastoma.' *Pediatric Pathology*, **10**, 207–216.

Koyanagi, T., Nakahara, H., Hori, E., Hara, K., Nakano, H. (1988) 'A mathematical model for analyzing beat-to-beat difference in the human fetal heart rate during gestation and labor.' *International Journal of Biomedical Computing*, **22**, 29–37.

Kumar, D., Phillips, S.F. (1989) Human myenteric plexus: confirmation of unfamiliar structures in adults and neonates.' *Gastroenterology*, **96**, 1021–1028.

Lacey, J.I. (1956) 'The evaluation of autonomic responses: towards a general solution.' *Annals of the*

New York Academy of Sciences, **67**, 123–164.

Lagercrantz, H., Bistoletti, P. (1973) 'Catecholamine release in the newborn infant at birth.' *Pediatric Research*, **11**, 889–893.

—— Edwards, D., Henderson Smart, D., Hertzberg, T., Jeffery, H. (1990) 'Autonomic reflexes in preterm infants.' *Acta Paediatrica Scandinavica*, **79**, 721–728.

Langley, J.N. (1921) *The Autonomic Nervous System, Part 1.* Cambridge: A.W. Heffer.

Le Douarin, N.M. (1986*a*) 'Cell line segregation during peripheral nervous system ontogeny.' *Science*, **231**, 1515–1522.

—— (1986*b*) 'Ontogeny of the peripheral nervous system from the neural crest and the placodes. A developmental model studied on the basis of the quail-chick chimaera system.' *Harvey Lectures Series*, **80**, 137–186.

LeFevre, M.L. (1984) 'Fetal heart rate pattern and postparacervical fetal bradycardia.' *Obstetrics and Gynecology*, **64**, 343–346.

Lewis, M., Kagan, J., Campbell, H., Kalafat, J. (1966) 'The cardiac response as a correlate of attention in infants.' *Child Development*, **37**, 63–71.

—— Bartels, B., Goldberg, S. (1967) 'State as a determinant of infants' heart rate response to stimulation.' *Science*, **155**, 486–488.

Lind, N.E., Shinebourne, E., Turner, P., Cottom, D. (1971) 'Adrenergic neurone and receptor activity in the iris of the neonate.' *Pediatrics*, **47**, 105–112.

Lindqvist, A. (1990) 'Noninvasive methods to study autonomic nervous control of circulation.' *Acta Physiologica Scandinavica*, **138** (Suppl. 588), 9–107.

—— Oja, R., Hellman, O., Välimäki, I. (1983) 'Impact of thermal vasomotor control on the heart rate variability of newborn infants.' *Early Human Development*, **8**, 37–47.

Lipsitz, L.A., Mietus, J., Moodt, G.B., Goldberger, A.L. (1990) 'Spectral characteristics of heart rate variability before and during postural tilt. Relations to aging and risk of syncope.' *Circulation*, **81**, 1803–1810.

Lipton, E.L., Steinschneider, A., Richmond, J.B. (1960) 'Autonomic function in the neonate: II. Physiologic effects of motor restraint.' *Psychosomatic Medicine*, **22**, 57–67.

—— —— —— (1961*a*) 'Autonomic function in the neonate: III. Methodological considerations.' *Psychosomatic Medicine*, **23**, 461–471.

—— —— —— (1961*b*) 'Autonomic function in the neonate: IV. Individual differences in cardiac reactivity.' *Psychosomatic Medicine*, **23**, 472–484.

—— —— —— (1964) 'Autonomic function in the neonate: VIII. Cardio-pulmonary observations.' *Pediatrics*, **33**, 212–215.

—— —— —— (1965) 'The autonomic nervous system in early life.' *New England Journal of Medicine*, **273**, 147–153.

—— —— —— (1966) 'Autonomic function in the neonate: VII. Maturational changes in cardiac control.' *Child Development*, **37**, 1–16.

Mantel, R., van Geijn, H.P., Caron, F.J.M., Swartjes, J.M., van Woerden, E.E., Jongsma, H.W. (1990*a*) 'Computer analysis of antepartum fetal heart rate: 1. Baseline determination.' *International Journal of Biomedical Computing*, **25**, 261–272.

—— —— —— —— —— —— (1990*b*) 'Computer analysis of antepartum fetal heart rate: 2. Detection of accelerations and decelerations.' *International Journal of Biomedical Computing*, **25**, 273–286.

Monnig, P.J. (1990) 'Familial achalasia in children.' *Annals of Thoracic Surgery*, **49**, 1019–1022.

Moscoso, P., Goldberg, R.N., Jamieson, J., Bancalari, E. (1983) 'Spontaneous elevation in arterial blood pressure during the first hours of life in very low-birth-weight infant.' *Journal of Pediatrics*, **103**, 114–117.

Moss, A.J., Duffie, E.R. Jr, Emmanouilides, G. (1963) 'Blood pressure and vasomotor reflexes in the newborn infant.' *Pediatrics*, **32**, 175–179.

Murat, I., Levron, J.C., Berg, A., Saint-Maurice, C. (1988) 'Effects of fentanyl on baroreceptor reflex control of heart rate in newborn infants.' *Anesthesiology*, **68**, 717–722.

—— Lapeyre, G., Saint-Maurice, C. (1989) 'Isoflurane attenuates baroreflex control of heart rate in human neonates.' *Anesthesiology*, **70**, 395–400.

Mustonen, J., Länsimies, E., Uusitupa, M., Talwar, S., Hyödynmaa, S., Kärkkäinen, A. (1989) 'Testing of autonomic cardiovascular regulation—methodological considerations.' *Clinical Physiology*, **9**, 249–257.

Oh, W., Arcilla, R.A., Oh, M.A., Lind, J. (1966) 'Renal and cardiovascular effects of body tilting in the newborn infant.' *Biology of the Neonate*, **10**, 76–92.
Padbury, J.F., Martinez, A.M. (1988) 'Sympathoadrenal system activity at birth: integration of postnatal adaptation.' *Seminars in Perinatology*, **12**, 163–172.
Perkett, E.A., Vaughan, R.L. (1982) 'Evidence for a laryngeal chemoreflex in some human preterm infants.' *Acta Paediatrica Scandinavica*, **71**, 969–972.
Picton-Warlow, C.G., Mayer, F.E. (1970) 'Cardiovascular responses to postural changes in the neonate.' *Archives of Disease in Childhood*, **45**, 354–359.
Pongiglione, G., Fish, F.A., Strasburger, J.F., Benson, D.W. Jr (1990) 'Heart rate and blood pressure response to upright tilt in young patients with unexplained syncope.' *Journal of the American College of Cardiology*, **16**, 165–170.
Porges, S.W. (1985) *Method and Apparatus for Evaluating Rhythmic Oscillations in Aperiodic Physiological Response Systems.* Patent no. 4,510,944.
Porter, F.L., Porges, S.W., Marshall, R.E. (1988) 'Newborn pain cries and vagal tone: parallel changes in response to circumcision.' *Child Development*, **59**, 495–505.
Potter, E.K. (1988) 'Neuropeptide as an autonomic neurotransmitter.' *Pharmacology and Therapeutics*, **37**, 251–273.
Prechtl, H.F.R. (1974) 'The behavioural states of the newborn (a review).' *Brain Research*, **76**, 185–212.
Prechtl, J.C., Powley, T.L. (1990) 'B-afferents: a fundamental division of the nervous system mediating homeostasis?' *Behavioural and Brain Sciences*, **13**, 289–331.
Ramet, J., Praud, J.P., D'Allest, A.M., Carofilis, A., Dehan, M., Guilleminault, C., Gaultier, Cl. (1988) 'Effect of maturation on heart rate response to ocular compression test during rapid eye movement sleep in human infants.' *Pediatric Research*, **24**, 477–480.
—— —— —— Dehan, M., Gaultier, Cl. (1990) 'Trigeminal airstream stimulation. Maturation-related cardiac and respiratory responses during REM sleep in human infants.' *Chest*, **98**, 92–96.
Renou, P., Newman, W., Wood, C. (1969) 'Autonomic control of fetal heart rate.' *American Journal of Obstetrics and Gynecology*, **105**, 949–953.
Riley, C.M. (1957) 'Familial dysautonomia.' *Advances in Pediatrics*, **9**, 157–190.
Ross, R.D., Daniels, S.R., Schwartz, D.C., Hannon, D.W., Shukla, R., Kaplan, S. (1987) 'Plasma norepinephrine levels in infants and children with congestive heart failure.' *American Journal of Cardiology*, **59**, 911–914.
Sapire, D.W., Casta, A. (1985) 'Vagotonia in infants, children, adolescents and young adults.' *International Journal of Cardiology*, **9**, 211–224.
Schachter, J., Williams, T.A., Khachaturian, Z., Tobin, M., Kruger, R., Kerr, J. (1971) 'Heart rate responses to auditory clicks in neonates.' *Psychophysiology*, **8**, 163–179.
Schwartz, P.J. (1981) 'The sudden infant death syndrome.' *In* Scarpelli, E.M., Cosmi, E.V. (Eds) *Reviews in Perinatal Medicine, Vol. 4.* New York: Raven Press. pp. 475–524.
—— Periti, M., Malliani, A. (1975) 'The long Q-T syndrome.' *American Heart Journal*, **89**, 378–390.
—— Southall, D.P., Valdes-Dapena, M. (Eds) (1988) 'The sudden infant death syndrome.' *Annals of the New York Academy of Sciences*, **533**, 1–474.
Sica, A.L., Siddiqi, Z.A., Gandhi, M.R., Condemi, G. (1990) 'Evidence for central patterning of sympathetic discharge in kittens.' *Brain Research*, **530**, 349–352.
Sigurd, J., Löfgren, O., Joelsson, I. (1985) 'Cardiotocographic distortion of fetal heart rate variability. Theoretical considerations and examplification by computerized simulation.' *Acta Obstetrica et Gynecologica Scandinavica*, **64**, 255–258.
Sinaiko, A.R., Wells, T.G. (1990) 'Childhood hypertension.' *In* Laragh, J.H., Brener, B.M. (Eds) *Hypertension, Pathophysiology, Diagnosis and Management.* New York: Raven Press. pp. 1853–1868.
Smith, J. (1986) 'Ontogeny of the autonomic nervous system. Cell line divergence and differentiation.' *In* Gootman, P.M. (Ed.) *Developmental Neurobiology of the Autonomic Nervous System.* Clifton, NJ: Humana Press. pp. 1–28.
Smyth, H.S., Sleight, P., Pickering, G.W. (1969) 'Reflex regulation of arterial pressure during sleep in man. A quantitative method of assessing baroreflex sensitivity.' *Circulation Research*, **24**, 109–121.
Surprenant, A. (1986) 'Muscarinic receptors in the submucous plexus and their roles in mucosal ion transport.' *Trends in Pharmacological Sciences* (Suppl. II), 23–27.
Taylor, A.A., Mitchell, J.R. (1990) 'Laboratory evaluation of autonomic nervous system function. *In*

Laragh, J.H., Brener, B.M. (Eds) *Hypertension, Pathophysiology, Diagnosis and Management.* New York: Raven Press. pp. 1461–1478.

Tsuto, T., Obata-Tsuto, H.L., Iwai, N., Takahashi, T., Ibata, Y. (1989) 'Fine structure of neurons synthesizing vasoactive intestinal peptide in the human colon from patients with Hirschsprung's disease.' *Histochemistry*, **93**, 1–8.

Uvnas-Moberg, K., Widstrom, A.M., Marchini, G., Winberg, J. (1987) 'Release of GI hormones in mother and infant by sensory stimulation.' *Acta Paediatrica Scandinavica*, **76**, 851—860.

Vermesh, M., Mayden, K.L., Confino, E., Giglia, R.V., Gleicher, N. (1986) 'Prenatal sonographic diagnosis of Hirschsprung's disease.' *Journal of Ultrasound in Medicine*, **5**, 37–39.

Versmold, H.T., Kitterman, J.A., Phibbs, R.H., Gregory, G.A., Tooley, W.H. (1981) 'Aortic blood pressure during the first 12 hours of life in infants with birth weight 610–4,220 grams.' *Pediatrics*, **67**, 607–613.

Vincent, G.M. (1986) 'The heart rate of Romano-Ward syndrome patients.' *American Heart Journal*, **112**, 61–64.

Vranekovic, G., Hock, E., Isaac, P., Cordero, L. (1974) 'Heart rate variability and cardiac response to an auditory stimulus.' *Biology of the Neonate*, **24**, 66–73.

Waldman, S., Krauss, A.N., Auld, P.A.M. (1979) 'Baroreceptors in preterm infants: their relationship to maturity and disease.' *Developmental Medicine and Child Neurology*, **21**, 714–722.

Weinshilboum, R.M., Axelrod, J. (1971) 'Reduced plasma dopamine-β-hydroxylase activity in familial dysautonomia.' *New England Journal of Medicine*, **285**, 938–942.

Wennergren, G., Hertzberg, T., Milerad, J., Bjure, J., Lagercrantz, H. (1989) 'Hypoxia reinforces laryngeal reflex bradycardia in infants.' *Acta Paediatrica Scandinavica*, **78**, 11–17.

Whincup, P.H., Cook, D.G., Shaper, A.G. (1989) 'Early influences on blood pressure: a study of children aged 5–7 years.' *British Medical Journal*, **299**, 587–591.

Whitney, R.J. (1953) 'The measurement of volume changes in human limbs.' *Journal of Physiology*, **121**, 1–27.

Willinger, M. (1989) 'SIDS. A challenge.' *Journal of NIH Research*, **1**, 73–80.

Wilton, N.C.T., Hantler, C.B. (1987) 'Congenital Long QT syndrome: changes in QT interval during anesthesia with thiopental, vecuronium, fentanyl, and isoflurane.' *Anesthesia and Analgesia*, **66**, 357–360.

Winter, S.T., Samueloff, M., Cohen, N.J., Porges, A., Gross, E. (1966) 'Neonatal cardiac deceleration on suckle feeding.' *American Journal of Diseases of Children*, **112**, 11–20.

Young, I.M., Holland, W.W. (1958) 'Some physiological responses to neonatal arterial blood pressure and pulse rate.' *British Medical Bulletin*, **2**, 276–278.

Zimmer, E.Z., Divon, M.Y., Vadasz, A. (1988) 'Fetal heart rate beat-to-beat variability in uncomplicated labor.' *Gynecological and Obstetrical Investigations*, **25**, 80–82.

11
THE ASSESSMENT OF BRAIN DEATH IN THE NEWBORN INFANT

Andrew R. Wilkinson

Brain death is a relatively new concept, and several aspects are still not clearly defined or understood. Physicians may unintentionally contribute to the confusion by using the term 'brain death' as an abbreviated phrase for a very complex physiological state. This may lead nurses, technical staff and relatives to use the term in different ways. Understandably the brain is viewed with special reverence, but separating the death of this organ from all others in the body has clarified only some of the issues. Brain death describes the absence of all function in the central nervous system (CNS), cerebri and brainstem, which is followed inevitably by cardiovascular death.

Before the development of intensive care, death was defined as the irreversible cessation of circulatory and respiratory functions. But this is indicative of death only when these functions persist long enough for the brain to die. In most developed countries the recent introduction of technology to maintain cardiopulmonary functions has sometimes resulted in a state where irreversible cessation of the functions of the brain can occur while the heart continues to beat. This is death too. Misunderstandings and anxieties surround the state of brain death and the means whereby it can be diagnosed. This is partly because of the problems of prolonged existence of a patient in a vegetative state. However, criteria for brain death apply only to those who die despite vigorous support (Black 1978). Neuronal function is not fully developed in the newborn infant, making clinical assessment and the interpretation of neurophysiological measurements difficult. This leads to problems in defining valid and reliable criteria for recognising brain death in the newborn infant.

The philosophical problems surrounding any definition of the onset of functional activity in the human CNS, and the criteria of 'brain life', are the symmetrical counterpart of the difficulties in defining criteria for 'brain death' (Lockwood 1988). The criteria that have been proposed for adults and evaluated in some prospective studies are not thought to be valid in young children, hence the recommendations that there should be a combination of clinical and laboratory criteria for brain death. This view is highly controversial and some maintain that a clinical examination should suffice. The role of neurophysiological investigations is therefore undecided and not advanced by the view that a test, or battery of tests, is currently more reliable and valid than a carefully conducted clinical examination, with or without tests.

Beecher (1968) proposed criteria for the determination of brain death in adults. Further experience since then has caused many other committees of official bodies on both sides of the Atlantic to put forward modified criteria. Few of the proposals have been tested prospectively, though some have been incorporated into law. All the most recent pronouncements on the determination of brain death have emphasised the lack of information about the newborn infant, and the uncertainties about using criteria applicable to older children and adults.

The primary requirement in determining brain death is to be certain about the cause of coma. This can pose serious problems, particularly in the first few days after birth. One must exclude reversible causes of coma such as the effects of hypothermia and hypotension, infection and sedative drugs (*e.g.* phenobarbitone and morphine derivatives). If pancuronium has been given, the effect must be reversed by neostigmine or edrophonium given with atropine.

Until recently little attention was paid to the systematic determination of brain death in newborn babies, infants or children, because decisions concerning intensive care centred on when to discontinue artificial ventilation or whether to withhold further medical interventions. Developments in organ transplantation have emphasised the need to resolve the medical uncertainty relating to brain death in this age group. Experience is limited by the infrequent occurrence of a baby in a condition where brain death is considered. The need to consider this diagnosis has led to the publication of three new sets of guidelines for the determination of brain death in children (Cronc 1987; Special Task Force 1987; Ashwal and Schneider 1987*a*, *b*).

There are no fundamental reasons why the standards used in children should not be applicable to the newborn infant. Since the brainstem differentiates early in gestation, sensitive tests of function ought to be equally convincing. However, the available tests have not been fully evaluated and some conflicting statements have been made.

Precise recognition of the cause of coma in a newborn baby is complicated by a number of perinatal factors, each of which could be contributory. The importance of events occurring prior to delivery may be difficult to judge because the measurements of fetal well-being are too imprecise. The major changes that occur in the baby's circulation, particularly in relation to abnormalities in cerebral bloodflow (CBF) may lead to irreversible neonatal injury. So it is unclear which clinical and neurophysiological tests to use, when to use them and how often to repeat them.

Although a diagnosis of brain death is primarily a clinical one, the particular problems in the newborn infant justify the acquisition of as much information as possible from neurophysiological tests. Further research is essential.

Ashwal and Schneider (1989) made the most comprehensive report of systematic assessments of brain death in preterm and term infants. They reviewed retrospectively the clinical course of 18 preterm and term infants under one month of age in whom brain death was diagnosed. These data were collected during 14 years at Loma Linda University, California, which was the first major centre for neonatal heart transplantation. Further details were given in the review by Ashwal (1989), highlighting the inadvisability of relying solely on clinical or neurophysiological tests to determine brain death. They must be used together.

Clinical criteria

The most important factor in the history is to determine the cause of coma and to establish that it is irreversible. Deep unconsciousness and apnoea must coexist, necessitating artificial ventilation. The pupils should be fixed and dilated without response to light and the eyes should not move by oculocephalic (doll's eyes) or caloric (oculovestibular) testing. There should be absent corneal and bulbar reflexes, and no cough reflex on suctioning the trachea. The latter reflex is present from 35 weeks post-conceptional age. The cause of irreversible coma may be determined if there is a well documented perinatal history, though in most infants the cerebral insult occurs before birth over a period of time that is difficult to document. Only in the rare cases of an intrapartum catastrophe such as a ruptured uterus, or a postnatal intracerebral haemorrhage from a vascular malformation, can the timing and the severity of the insult be more precise.

These difficulties have been recognised in individual commentaries that emphasise the need to delay decisions and await further developments (Freeman and Rogers 1980, Robinson 1981, Coulter 1987). Anxieties are sometimes expressed that by delaying a decision the patient may enter a persistent vegetative state which may last for months or years. These concerns are misplaced in the context of a diagnosis of brain death. Patients who survive in a persistent vegetative state usually breathe spontaneously and have alternating periods of apparent wakefulness and sleep. Even the most heroic efforts cannot maintain patients who are brain-dead: they inevitably die, usually in less than 72 hours. The guidelines all incorporate a period of observation, in an attempt to expose the uncertainties in the history, to diagnose the cause of coma and to confirm the clinical examination, while at the same time recording the consistency of additional neurophysiological measurements. It must be stressed that the time limit for an 'appropriate period of observation' (Cronc 1987) is arbitrary and not based on prospectively collected data. The Special Task Force (1987) concluded that a diagnosis could not be made under the age of seven days, and proposed that between one week and two months of age the clinical examination and an electroencephalogram (EEG) should be repeated after 48 hours. This was reduced to 24 hours after the age of two months. No explanation or justification for this change in threshold was presented. Ashwal (1989) gave details of five preterm infants in whom a clinical diagnosis of brain death was suspected by day five after birth and supported by diagnostic studies obtained during the next two to five days. Further details of these neurophysiological measurements are given below. Details of a term infant diagnosed in the first week after birth, and five more between one week and one month, are given in the same publication. The experience at Loma Linda University is unique, but unfortunately the rarity of the diagnosis and the difference in clinical presentation have resulted in an approach which has not been uniform over the years. Comparisons are made harder by the retrospective aspect of analysis and the introduction of new but not necessarily better neurophysiological measurements.

Neurophysiological measurements

Electroencephalogram

The role of neurophysiological tests to determine brain death in the newborn infant is a subject of considerable disagreement. Although the first criteria proposed for brain death in adults included a requirement of an isoelectric EEG subsequent experience has shown this to be unreliable in the newborn infant. Pezzani *et al.* (1986) reported on 17 infants with absent electrocortical activity in the neonatal period. Two babies survived; one was normal and the other had epilepsy. Ashwal *et al.* (1977) reported a term infant with clinical criteria of brain death and an isoelectric EEG. A repeat study 24 hours later showed electrocortical activity, and the baby survived. The American Electroencephalographic Society (1986) established a standardised technique for the performance of EEG studies at higher amplification to document electrocerebral silence. However, the small size of the neonatal skull makes it difficult to comply with the recommended electrode spacing, and other electrical apparatus in the intensive care nursery can introduce artificial signals to the recording. In Ashwal's (1989) series, nine of the 18 patients had electrocerebral silence on their initial EEG. One term baby had a serum level of phenobarbitone of 30μg/mL on day 1 at the time of the first recording, but when this was repeated six days later, when phenobarbitone was not detected in the serum, there was return of some electrical activity. Nevertheless the patient died of cardiac arrest. Of nine patients with initial EEG activity five developed electrocortical silence, three continued to have activity and one died before the study was repeated.

Interpretation of the EEG must take into account normal developmental changes, from the discontinuous pattern seen in the preterm infant to the continuous record with the sleep state related changes in voltage, characteristic of the term infant (Eyre *et al.* 1988). The extent to which the pattern of the EEG can be altered either permanently or temporarily by a severe perinatal insult is not known. If the effect is reversible it becomes extremely difficult to predict the outcome from a single isoelectric recording of the EEG. Case reports have described infants who have survived after electric cortical silence was documented (Green and Lauber 1972). On the other hand low-voltage EEG activity can occur in babies who are by all other criteria brain-dead (Ashwal and Schneider 1979). This is well established in older children (Drake *et al.* 1986) and adults (Pallis 1983). The EEG alone is not able to confirm or refute brain death. In a patient with all the clinical criteria of brain death, an isoelectric EEG is supportive evidence provided other extrinsic factors have been excluded. As already mentioned, the most recent report for the detection of brain death in children (Special Task Force 1987) recommends that, for infants over seven days and less than two months, two examinations and EEGS should be carried out 48 hours apart. It should be emphasised that these recommendations are not based on any study and so far have not been validated prospectively.

Cerebral blood flow

The absence of CBF is well established as a corroborative test in the assessment of adults when brain death is suspected. Cerebral angiography has been replaced by radionuclide bolus angiography (Ashwal *et al.* 1977). In this technique the cerebral circulation is assessed by isotopic scanning of the skull after a bolus injection of 1 millicurie of 99mTC (pertechnetate). The method is applicable at the bedside (Holzman *et al.* 1983) but has not been validated in the newborn infant.

Over the last decade there has been intensive research into the quantitative measurement of CBF in newborn babies. Using the 133 xenon technique, Greisen (1986) reported flow rates as low as 4.3ml/min/100g in a baby who survived with normal neurological function. In studies using positron emission tomography, values ranged from 7 to 11ml/min/100g (Altman *et al.* 1988). Ashwal *et al.* (1989) determined CBF by stable xenon-enhanced computed tomography. During the inhalation of 35 per cent non-radioactive xenon, saturation in blood can be followed by repeated CT scanning. In normal infants values of 15ml/min/100g were obtained, while in 10 brain-dead infants and children aged between one month and 11 years, CBF was 1.3 ± 6ml/min/100g. Few studies have compared different techniques. There was poor correlation in the only study to combine radionuclide studies with EEG recordings (Ashwal 1989). Some babies who were clinically brain-dead showed EEG activity, despite the absence of radionuclide uptake, and conversely the EEG was isoelectric when radionuclide uptake was present. In four patients both investigations were negative and in two both were positive. Neurophysiological tests such as EEG or radionuclide scanning reconfirmed clinically determined brain death in only 50 to 65 per cent of patients, but electrocerebral silence confirmed brain death if the patient remained clinically brain dead for a further 24 hours and in this situation a repeat EEG is not necessary. It is proposed that the persistence of radionuclide uptake indicating some CBF may occur because the open fontanelles and sutures of the newborn skull allow it to expand under the influence of increasing intracranial pressure. This may not exceed mean arterial pressure (Altman *et al.* 1986) and therefore some intracerebral blood flow is preserved.

Doppler ultrasonography has been used to study the changes in bloodflow velocity pattern in the anterior cerebral and the common carotid arteries. A characteristic pattern of deterioration in the flow velocity waveform has been reported in newborn infants with clinical criteria for brain death (McMenamin and Volpe 1983). The demonstration of either flow reversal in the extracranial arteries or absence of pulsatile flow in the larger intracranial arteries was interpreted to indicate a progressive increase in cerebral vascular resistance and a decrease in cerebral perfusion. Unfortunately this non-invasive technique has not been correlated with radio-isotopic brain scanning. The other disadvantage with the Doppler technique is that it only detects cessation of cortical bloodflow and gives no information about brainstem bloodflow or function. Of concern are the reports of some babies in whom flow has apparently resumed after two to three days (Ashwal 1989). It thus appears that at the present time techniques are not reliable enough or validated to distinguish between the low CBF rate of 4 to 12ml/min/100g that can occur in the newborn infant and zero flow.

Evoked potentials

The extremely low microvoltage electrical response of the brain to a standardised repeated stimulus can be computer summated and averaged. The final wave pattern represents the normal passage of activity in neuronal pathways. Three types have been described, but their use in the assessment of brain death has not been validated in the newborn baby, older infants or children.

Brainstem auditory evoked potentials are produced by a click at the ear and abnormal records revealing only the first wave (from the auditory nerve), or no response at all, have been found in patients who were brain-dead (Setzer *et al.* 1983). Clearly abnormalities of the auditory nerve must be excluded. Dear and Godfrey (1985) reported two babies after severe perinatal asphyxia who had absent auditory evoked brainstem potentials, but who showed a gradual return of the responses on repeat studies. One was developmentally normal at 18 months. Unfortunately neither baby had confirmatory measurements of brain death at the time of the first study.

Visual evoked potentials record the response of the occipital cortex to repetitive flashing light stimuli. Absence of a response may occur as a result of damage to the optic pathway anywhere from retina to cortex and so may not be useful in corroborating brain death.

Somatosensory evoked potentials. The response to electrical stimulation of a peripheral nerve is recorded at the parietal cortex. This technique enables the assessment of pathways which in infants are otherwise difficult to examine. Despite various reports the recording technique is not yet standardised, and failure to record a response in 10 to 20 per cent of well infants restricts the interpretation that can be made in sick infants and those in whom brain death is suspected. With improvements in technology and future research into the relationship between abnormal responses, brain damage and subsequent disability, it may be possible to evaluate this test (in conjunction with others) in brain-dead newborn babies.

Measurements of cerebral metabolites and oxygenation

Two new methods have recently begun to be evaluated in the noninvasive investigation of brain injury in the newborn infant, but neither has reached the stage where the results would contribute to a determination of brain death.

Magnetic resonance spectroscopy (MRS) measures the concentration of phosphorus metabolites in the brain: the energy-rich adenosine triphosphate (ATP), phosphocreatine and inorganic phosphate as well as intracellular pH. The spectra produced from the brain when studied at different times after an asphyxial insult have been characterised (Azzopardi *et al.* 1989). In 28 infants with PCr/Pi ratio less than 95 per cent confidence intervals for normal infants, there was 93 per cent positive predictive value for death or survival with serious multiple impairment. In 12 infants with low ATP/total P ratio, 11 died. As yet we have no information on MRS studies in brain-dead patients, but the technique of spatial localisation may give more information, particularly if studies are repeated (Moorcraft *et al.* 1991). While this method has the disadvantage of requiring the baby to be transported from the intensive care unit to the magnet, there is the potential to document the progressive disruption of cerebral oxidative metabolism. In future it may be possible to measure the concentrations of other metabolites, as well as the neurotransmitters.

Near infrared spectroscopy records changes in the concentration in the brain of oxyhaemoglobin and oxidised cytochrome aa3. Near infrared light penetrates tissues to a distance of about 8cm, so transmission studies can be carried out in the newborn brain. The absorption characteristics reveal changes that occur over time. This technique has the great advantage of being applicable at the cotside. Cerebral blood volume, vascular response to changes in carbon dioxide tension and CBF can be estimated by this method (Wyatt *et al.* 1989).

The criteria for brain death in the newborn urgently need clarification as the success of neonatal transplantation improves: though the prospects of organ donation should not play any part in the diagnosis. Freeman and Ferry's criticism of the guidelines (1988) centres on an interpretation that the criteria may be cited in medico-legal issues or used by residents-in-training who might be pressurised by transplantation teams to vary the guidelines. They demand better scientific data while maintaining that the diagnosis of brain death remains a clinical one. This approach has the merits of enabling the consultant responsible to co-ordinate the difficult decisions that must be made. On the other hand the scientific information by which the decisions might in the future be improved will not be available unless we continue to investigate the wide range of neurophysiological measurements that can be applied. While uncertainties persist, it is acceptable to wait for the clinical condition to evolve. However the aim should be to minimise these uncertainties by establishing the proper diagnosis and providing the appropriate support for parents and siblings.

Summary

Brain death only occurs in about 1 per cent of neonatal deaths (Ashwal 1989). Despite a succession of published guidelines for the determination of brain death in adults and children, the experience of applying the criteria in the neonatal period is limited. There are numerous difficulties both in clinical examination and in neurophysiological measurements. No single test is reliable. Correlation between tests has not been systematically studied, but when reported is poor. Tests with a negative result, such as radionuclide brain imaging and EEG, support a clinical diagnosis and could shorten the interval between examinations. In order to improve the determination of brain death, particularly in the first week after birth, we must combine experience from different centres. We need to correlate a prospective systematic evaluation of the clinical criteria of brain death with the results of a number of neurophysiological measurements. Attention needs to be applied to the possible significance and subtle changes in some neuroendocrine functions such as the excretion of growth hormone in response to releasing factor. The almost complete lack of neuropathological studies in infants after brain death must be rectified if a definitive correlation between the clinical neurophysiological and histological signs of brain death is to be made.

When determining brain death, the impact on parents, siblings and other relatives is enormous. This is particularly the case in the newborn infant when a cause of coma may still be in doubt. Family counselling by senior medical and nursing staff and by social workers with special responsibilities should be provided. Training in this difficult area of acute medicine is available and should be acquired by all who make a career in perinatal medicine.

REFERENCES

Ashwal, S. (1989) 'Brain death in the newborn.' *Clinics in Perinatology*, **16**, 501–518.

—— Smith, A.J.K., Torres, F., Loken, M., Chou, S.N. (1977) 'Radionuclide bolus angiography: a technique for verification of brain death in infants and children.' *Journal of Pediatrics*, **91**, 722–728.

—— Schneider, S. (1979) 'Failure of electroencephalography to diagnose brain death in comatose children .' *Annals of Neurology*, **6**, 512–517.

—— —— (1987*a*) 'Brain death in children. Part I.' *Pediatric Neurology*, **3**, 5–11.

—— —— (1987*b*) 'Brain death in children. Part II.' *Pediatric Neurology*, **3**, 69–77.

—— —— (1989) 'Brain death in the newborn.' *Pediatrics*, **84**, 429–437.

—— —— Thompson, J. (1989) 'Xenon computed tomography cerebral flow in the determination of brain death in children.' *Annals of Neurology*, **25**, 539–546.

Altman, D.I., Powers, W.J., Perlman, J.M., Herscovitch, P., Volpe, S.L., Volpe, J.J. (1988) 'Cerebral blood flow requirement for brain viability in newborn infants is lower than in adults.' *Annals of Neurology*, **24**, 218–226.

American Electroencephalographic Society (1986) 'Minimum technical standards for EEG recording in suspected cerebral death.' *Journal of Clinical Neurophysiology*, **3**, 144–149.

Azzopardi, D., Wyatt, J.S., Hamilton, P.A., Cady, D.T., Hope, P.L., Reynolds, E.O.R. (1989) 'Phosphorus metabolites and intracellular pH in the brains of normal and small for gestational age infants investigated by magnetic resonance spectroscopy.' *Pediatric Research*, **25**, 440–444.

Beecher, H.K. (1968) 'A definition of reversible coma. Report of the Ad Hoc Committee of the Harvard Medical School to examine the definition of brain death.' *Journal of the American Medical Association*, **205**, 337–340.

Black, P. McL. (1978) 'Brain death.' *New England Journal of Medicine*, **299**, 338–344, 393–401.

Coulter, D.I. (1987) 'Neurologic uncertainty in newborn intensive care.' *New England Journal of Medicine*, **316**, 840–844.

Cronc, R.K. (1987) 'Determination of brain death.' *Journal of Pediatrics*, **110**, 15–19.

Dear, P.R.F., Godfrey, D.J. (1985) 'Neonatal auditory brainstem responses cannot reliably diagnose brainstem death.' *Archives of Disease in Childhood*, **60**, 17–19.

Drake, B., Ashwal, S., Schneider, S. (1986) 'Determination of cerebral death in the pediatric intensive care unit.' *Pediatrics*, **78**, 107–112.

Eyre, J.A., Nanei, S., Wilkinson, A.R. (1988) 'Quantification of changes in normal neonatal EEGs with gestation from continuous five-day recordings.' *Developmental Medicine and Child Neurology*, **30**, 599–607.

Freeman, J.M., Rogers, M.C. (1980) 'On death, dying, and decisions.' *Pediatrics*, **66**, 637–638.

—— Ferry, P.C. (1988) 'New brain death guidelines in children: further confusion.' *Pediatrics*, **81**, 301–303.

Green, J.B., Lauber, A. (1972) 'Return of EEG activity after electrocerebral silence: two case reports.' *Journal of Neurology, Neurosurgery and Psychiatry*, **35**, 103–107.

Greisen, G. (1986) 'Cerebral blood flow in preterm infants during the first week of life.' *Acta Paediatricia Scandinavica*, **75**, 43–51.

Holzman, B.H., Curless, R.G., Sfakianakis, G.N., Ajmone-Marsan, C., Montes, J.E. (1983) 'Radionuclide cerebral perfusion scintigraphy in determination of brain death in children.' *Neurology*, **33**, 1027–1031.

Lockwood, M. (1988) 'When does life begin?' *In* Lockwood, M. (Ed.) *Moral Dilemmas in Modern Medicine.* Oxford: Oxford University Press. pp. 9–31.

McMenamin, J.B., Volpe, J.J. (1983) 'Doppler ultrasonography in the determination of neonatal brain death.' *Annals of Neurology*, **14**, 302–307.

Moorcraft, J., Bolas, M.F., Ives, N.K., Sutton, P., Blackledge, M.J., Rajagopalan, B., Hope, P.L., Radda, G.K. (1991) 'Spatially localized magnetic resonance spectroscopy of the brains of normal and asphyxiated newborns.' *Pediatrics*, **87**, 273–282.

Pallis, C. (1982) 'ABC of brainstem death. Reappraising death.' *British Medical Journal*, **285**, 1409–1412. 'From brain death to brainstem death.' ibid, 1487–1490. 'Diagnosis of brainstem death—I.' ibid, 1558–1560. 'Diagnosis of brainstem death—II.' ibid, 1641–1644.

—— (1983) 'ABC of brainstem death. Prognostic significance of a dead brainstem.' *British Medical Journal*, **286**, 123–124. 'The position in the USA and elsewhere.' ibid, 209–210. 'The arguments about the EEG.' ibid, 284–287.

Pezzani, C., Radvanyi-Bouvet, M.F., Relier, J.P., Monod, N. (1986) 'Neonatal electroencephalography during the first twenty-four hours of life in full-term newborn infants.' *Neuropediatrics*, **17**, 11–18.

Robinson, R.O. (1981) 'Brain death in children.' *Archives of Disease in Childhood*, **56**, 657–658.

Setzer, N.A., McPherson, R.W., Johnson, R.M., Gioia, F.G. (1983) 'Evoked potential determinations in children with brain death.' *Anesthesiology*, **59**, A130.

Special Task Force (1987) 'Guidelines for the determination of brain death in children.' *Pediatrics*, **80**, 298–300.

Wyatt, J.S., Edwards, A.D., Azzopardi, D., Reynolds, E.O.R. (1989) 'Magnetic resonance and near infrared spectroscopy for investigation of perinatal hypoxic-ischaemic brain injury.' *Archives of Disease in Childhood*, **64**, 953–963.

INDEX

www.ingramcontent.com/pod-product-compliance
Lightning Source LLC
LaVergne TN
LVHW011802200926
848484LV00003B/757